Foreword

In 1996 homeopathy celebrated its 200th anniversary. It originated with the seminal publication *Essay on New Curative Principle*, written by Dr. Samuel Hahnemann in 1796. The use of medicines on the basis of similarity was not new, and can be traced much earlier in the history of medicine, but Hahnemann was the first to systematize it and to introduce the very high dilutions or homeopathic potencies, which are the source of most of the controversy which surrounds homeopathy.

Over the last two centuries, the fortunes of homeopathy have fluctuated widely: for most of the 19th century, despite the sometimes vehement opposition of the medical establishment, it enjoyed a period of rapid growth, spreading widely and increasing in popularity throughout Europe and North America. This was followed by an equally dramatic decline in the 20th century, so that it had almost disappeared in the USA and been reduced to a shadow of its former self in Europe by the 1970s. Yet, in what must be one of the least anticipated recent developments in medicine, it has staged a strong, worldwide resurgence in the 1980s and 90s.

How are we to account for this roller-coaster evolution? Some of it can be explained by cultural and political factors, for instance, its decline in the USA was certainly hastened by the 1910 Flexner Report on medical education which resulted in the closure of most of the homeopathic medical colleges. While its recent renewal has been associated with growing disillusionment with conventional drug treatment and its adverse effects, the growth of a 'counter-culture' in the West, and the promotion of acupuncture in the Chinese Cultural Revolution in the 1960s and 70s.

But these cultural and political factors are not the motor driving the evolution of homeopathy. The roots of these fluctuations lie in its relationship with the evolving concepts of science, a relationship which has not always been comfortable, but which has had a profound influence on the perception of homeopathy by scientists, doctors, and the general public. The origins of the tangled relationship between homeopathy and science are to be found with the Italian aristocrat-scientist Count Amodeo Avogadro who, in 1811, enunciated the principle now known by his name, which enables the number of particles in a given mass of a substance to be calculated. The correctness and significance of Avogadro's Law was not generally appreciated until the mid-19th century. But when its implications for homeopathy were understood, the effect was profound, since it implies that none of the starting substance is present in the high "ultra-molecular" dilutions used in homeopathy.

This realization triggered a split in the homeopathic movement in the latter half of the 19th century, between the so-called "highs," led by the American homeopath James T. Kent, who used very high dilutions on a theoretical basis influenced by Swedenborgian metaphysical concepts, and the "lows," associated with the British homeopath Richard Hughes, who attempted to reconcile homeopathy with contemporary pathophysiological concepts.

But apparent scientific improbability is a two-edged sword, and, at the beginning of the 21st century, it is cutting the other way. Earlier, scientific preconceptions appeared to make homeopathy impossible. But we now have scientific methods sufficiently sensitive to demonstrate the actions of the very high dilutions used in homeopathy, providing empirical evidence of the reality of some of the claims made for homeopathy. At the same time theoretical concepts deriving from the leading edge of science are starting to provide a theoretical underpinning to the growing body of experimental evidence. The problem of "ultramolecular" dilutions are no longer the fundamental barrier to an understanding of homeopathy that were for earlier scientific conceptions. Homeopathy is now stimulating theoretical innovation, instead of theory inhibiting the acceptance of homeopathy.

Paolo Bellavite and Andreas Signorini provide an authoritative, up-to-date and comprehensive survey of the exciting empirical and theoretical developments in homeopathy. In addition to a thorough account of the empirical evidence, they give the best account I have read of the theoretical implications for homeopathy of the new sciences of chaos, complexity and information. I warmly recommend their book to all who are interested in understanding homeopathy, a therapy whose scientific time has finally arrived.

Dr. Peter Fisher
Director of Research
Royal London Homeopathic
Hospital, England

Preface to the Second Edition

This book is a compendium of the experience and ideas of its authors, a University Professor of General Pathology (P.B.) and a medical doctor using homeopathy as his main therapeutic method (A.S.), together with an updated review of the evidence emerging from the international literature in this field. The original core of the book was a research project, drafted in 1990 as a grant application to the Italian National Research Council. Drafting the project forced us to do a major rethink of the entire domain in order to pinpoint the most promising lines of experimental research. The sheer body of data collected, the vast array of problems encountered, and the interest they aroused in our minds prompted us to write this book.

The book first came out in Italian in 1993 and as the American edition in 1995 (Homeopathy: A Frontier in Medical Science), but the problems dealt with here not only have remained unsolved over the past years, but have increased in interest and relevance from both the scientific and the health and welfare standpoints. This is also the reason that we decided to adopt a new title focused more precisely on positioning this text in homeopathic and scientific literature.

As the term "nanotechnology" refers to the study and use of hyper-miniaturized technologies that can carry more and more bodies of information in smaller and smaller chips, likewise the term "nanopharmacology" may be appropriate to the newly defined field of homeopathic pharmacology. Here the term is not used to designate a precise dose/dilution (literally, the prefix "nano" would indicate one billionth of a unit) but simply the extremely low doses or even the high dilutions/dynamizations of medicines that are utilized in homeopathy. To understand the nature and the rationale of homeopathic nanopharmacology, it is important to know how the medicines are made (i.e. the role of drug potentiation) and how they could affect the behaviour of the system where such vectors of information act (i.e. the rules of complex biological networks that justify the specific hypersensitivity of the sick person to a specific medicine). Here we present a number of paths to understanding from a scientific standpoint how these extremely diluted medicines may act and, as a consequence, how the field of homeopathy could become a legitimate part of united medicine.

The book thus continues to grow and improve, but the original core of scientific ideas and proposals has maintained its soundness and validity. The information reported in the first version has been updated and amplified, with the addition of over two hundred new references. Several chapters have been supplemented and enlarged with additional evidence coming to light in the mean time in our and other laboratories worldwide.

Besides updating the references with particular regard to clinical research, which in recent years has given controversial results, we have added as an appendix two chapters that include a full rethinking of our view on homeopathic theory. By picking up qualifying points from the main text and revising them in light of subsequent published findings, we come to a more convincing re-evaluation of the two fundamental achievements of Hahnemann, i.e. the "simile" as a founding principle, and the homeopathic concept of drug "potency". We present the basic research supporting the *"similia similibus curantur"* as a major principle in biology and pathology (appendix n. 1), then we suggest that the apparent homeopathic paradoxes can be understood only by using a logic based on dynamic systems theory (appendix n. 2). The old "vital force" is replaced with biodynamics and bioenergetics: many things are explained, but homeopathy still holds in part its mystery.

We were pleased with the enthusiastic response to this publication, which has been acknowledged as the first serious attempt to bridge the gap between two apparently conflicting medical approaches. In the introduction to the first edition, we expressly invited critical and even contradictory contributions to the theories that are expounded here. We have yet to receive any serious negative comments, but, needless to say, we remain open to criticism and indeed welcome it. In science, it is only by observing new phenomena and by eliminating errors in the antecedent theories that a more accurate picture of reality can be depicted.

During our work, we have benefited from the ideas and reference material provided by a large number of colleagues, among whom we would like to mention Jacques Benveniste, Sandro Bettini, Ivo Bianchi, Francesco Borghini, Adriana Carluccio, Maurizio Castellini, Anita Conforti, Elisabeth Davenas, Emilio Del Giudice, Emilio Dido, P. Christian Endler, Michael Kofler, Klaus Linde, Riccardo Ortolani, Pietro Piovesan, Bernard Poitevin, Fritz A. Popp, Giuliano Preparata, Giuliana Rapacioli, Beverly Rubik, Cyril W. Smith, Paolo Sommaruga, Massimo Sperini, Rosy Tommasoli, Roeland van Wiik, Hildebert Wagner, Harald Walach, and Otto Weingartner. Particular thanks are due to Dana Ullman for his enthusiastic support and advice, to Sarah Serafimidis for editorial assistance with the second edition of the book, to Mario Zatti for his help and encouragement and to Anthony Steele for his painstaking English translation.

We dedicate our efforts to the memory of our friend and colleague, Giovanni Scolaro.

—The Authors

"Test everything;
hold fast what is good"
—(St. Paul, I Thess., 5, 21)

1 Introduction

Homeopathy is a distinctly singular phenomenon in the history of medicine. It came into being as a result of the ideas and experiments of C.F.S. Hahnemann, and was initially developed over the decades spanning the late eighteenth and early nineteenth centuries. It met with mixed fortunes, and spread to varying extents to the other continents, but what is most astonishing is that even today, some 200 years later and despite the enormous advances in the field of the instruments available to biomedical research, there is no consensus of opinion either as to its efficacy or as to its mechanism of action. On the other hand, in view of the increasing practical applications of homeopathy, which in Europe alone is now used by some 30 million people and has recently been accorded a form of recognition even at the level of the European Parliament (i.e. Resolution A4-0075, 1997), there can be no denying the fact that studies on its efficacy, a working definition of its fields of application, and some degree of rationalization of its theoretical basis are not only scientifically desirable, but also necessary in view of the public-health, social-welfare, and economic implications involved. These fundamental issues are addressed in this book on the basis of a critical and rational approach.

The basic hypothesis presented here is that *the progress of biomedical research, on the one hand, and the evolution of homeopathy, on the other, are leading to an increasing degree of convergence of the two systems*, which are usually regarded as alternatives. An open-minded scientific approach to homeopathy can thus be a source of major surprises and of fascinating fields of investigation for both the medical practitioner and the biological researcher. This study aims at comparing certain aspects of basic research and homeopathy, according to a methodology firmly rooted in the practices of general pathology. The ideas and experience reported here are thus an attempt to construct a common ground or, at any rate, a dialogue between medical systems with very different histories and conceptual bases.

A widely held view among doctors is that there is no convincing proof of the efficacy of homeopathy, which is regarded essentially as a commercial ploy exploiting the placebo effect. This view is based on the existence both of the placebo effect and, unfortunately, of various forms of commercial abuse and exploitation. Another common way of viewing homeopathy tends to class it alongside other alternative practices such as touch therapy, herbalism, and oriental medicine.

As we see it, such attitudes fail to grasp all the complexity and realty of the phenomenon, particularly owing to the fact that they are often expressed without a thorough review of the literature available on the topic. The fact is that the published literature in the sector proves by no means easy to retrieve in our libraries, the subject is not taught in faculties of medicine (with only a few exceptions) and, what is more, such limited and often inaccurate information as manages to filter through, mainly via the pharmaceutical companies, tends to pass largely unnoticed amidst the plethora of data, news, and messages in which doctors and researchers in the biological field today are literally submerged.

The main reason for this paucity of information on homeopathy among the public at large lies, however, in the almost total lack of communication between medical systems viewed on both sides as alternatives. This lack of communication has both historical and socio-economic roots, and is influenced by terminological and lexical difficulties, as well as by epistemological problems (relating to the process of acquiring scientific knowledge) which will be extensively illustrated here below. Homeopathic experience and literature have often been relegated to a self-contained, self-sufficient world which at the same time proves difficult to judge according to the categories of modern medicine.

This situation today is slowly but steadily changing. In February 1991, the British Medical Journal published a paper entitled Clinical Trials in Homeopathy, produced by researchers from the Department of Epidemiology of Limburg University (Netherlands), and reviewing 107 publications on controlled trials in homeopathy [Kleijnen et al., 1991]. Despite the fact that most of the trials were of poor quality, the authors of the review article (not themselves homeopaths) claim to have been amazed at the bulk of positive evidence found in these trials, and suggest there is an urgent need for a major effort to glean further evidence by means of well designed trials in strict double-blind conditions. It is therefore not true that there are no serious controlled trials on homeopathic medicine, though it must be admitted that such trials are too few to allow any very firm conclusions to be drawn [similar conclusions in Linde *et al.*, 1997; 1998].

One of the aims of this work is precisely to present an overview of the literature on clinical and basic research relevant to an understanding of homeopathy. The search for such literature proved fairly painstaking and time-consuming, and the result therefore probably cannot claim to be complete or exhaustive, though it certainly represents a valid sample of studies conducted in the past and of those currently in progress. We often had to ask the researchers concerned directly for reference material or to consult the volumes of the congress proceedings of homeopathic associations or of the International Study Group on Very Low Dose and High Dilution Effects (GIRI). The overview emerging is that of an expanding sector, where, however, the groups involved in serious research are still few and far between in relation to the size, scale, and importance of the issues to be tackled. The current state of the art in homeopathy thus strongly prompts the conducting of further studies and trials to establish whether significant effects of homeopathic remedies can be unequivocally demonstrated, while, at the same time, *there is a need for a theory or, at any rate, for viable hypotheses, to provide reasonable explanations* for the effects observed. What clearly emerges from the above-cited review by Kleijnen and coworkers (and also from joint discussions on the topic) is that *the subject of the efficacy of homeopathy can hardly be tackled without providing some plausible explanation as to its mechanism of action*: "The amount of positive evidence even among the best studies came as a surprise to us. Based on this evidence we would readily accept that homeopathy can be efficacious, if only the mechanism of action were more plausible" [Kleijnen *et al.*, 1991, p. 321]. The attempt to construct a plausible model of the mechanism(s) of homeopathic action is the main aim of the present work.

The scientific validity of a therapeutic method does not depend so much on its success rate as on the fact that the clinical result should be consistent with a pathophysiological, biochemical, and pharmacological theory or rationale. It is only through patient, unrestricted, and methodical research conducted on several planes—clinical, laboratory, epidemiological, and physicochemical—that we shall be able to shed light on the many issues which so far remain unsolved.

In future, the study of the scientific basis of homeopathic medicine will have substantial repercussions on the world of homeopathy itself, which is divided into various distinct schools often in conflict with one another. In all probability, this fragmentation and the impossibility of settling doctrinal disputes is almost certainly due to the total lack of a scientific theory. This not only has an adverse effect on results but also seriously compromises any possible future development in this sector of medicine matching up to the quality standards required today, and capable of coping with the new diseases emerging. Our intention here is not so much to discuss the pros and cons of the arguments put forward in these disputes, which mainly have to do with clinical methodology, as to review from a modern standpoint the basic principles such as the *law of similars* and the *principle of dilution/potentiation* which are accepted by all schools of homeopathy.

The various chapters of this book examine different aspects of the problem, seeking to expound the data and theories already figuring in the published literature, sift them critically and, where possible, propose areas of common ground and working hypotheses. Our study begins with a summary of the main concepts underlying homeopathy, examining the basic principles and history from the origins to the present day (Chapter 2). Since it is not the aim of this study to provide a practical manual for learning about homeopathy, we have confined our account to essentials.

Chapter 3 addresses the empirical and clinical evidence suggesting that homeopathy is really effective and that this efficacy is not simply definable as a placebo effect. Though such evidence to date is clearly poor and only very preliminary in both qualitative and quantitative terms, particularly if judged using the touchstones of conventional medicine, the explanation based solely on the placebo effect is steadily losing ground, while at the same time there is a growing demand for some kind of theory, model or explanation in modern pathophysiological terms.

Like any scientific theory, hypotheses regarding the mechanism of action of homeopathy can only be based on experimentation or on other currently accepted theories. A substantial body of experimental evidence (Chapter 4) has been obtained in *in vitro* cells or in animal models according to the accepted methodologies codified by conventional science and by western biomedical reasoning. Experimental studies of this type, therefore, cannot be contested as being non-scientific (which would be a contradiction in terms), and the results can be read, discussed and interpreted according to the paradigms used for any other subject of investigation. Admittedly, many studies published to date may fail to prove convincing because of their poor quality, but, in any case, they are part and parcel of the overall frame of methodological and conceptual reference of modern science. The debate regarding the quality of trials is not confined merely to homeopathic medicine.

In an attempt to construct a new explanatory model of the action of homeopathic drugs, the notion of the biological *complexity* of the regulation of homeostatic systems has been introduced. Complexity in biology and in medicine is illustrated in Chapter 5, which deals at great length with the most recent developments in knowledge in the fields of inflammation and cancer. Though the treatment of this subject, rich in biochemical and biological detail, may not seem to have any direct bearing on homeopathy, it will be seen that it is precisely from our current scientific knowledge that any possibility of a reasoned appraisal of the potentiality and the limits of homeopathy (as, indeed, of any other therapeutic method) is beginning to emerge.

On the strength of the experimental studies available and with the aid of these new conceptual instruments, explanatory hypotheses will be synthetically elaborated for the law of similars, the cornerstone of homeopathy

(Chapter 6), and for the principle of dilution (Chapter 7). The new conceptual approaches which will be introduced here represent an open frontier in the future of medicine and rest both upon physical and mathematical theories and upon recent advances in immunological and pharmacological theories. We are entering here into the sphere of models of complexity, chaos, fractals, quantum physics, coherence phenomena, electromagnetic phenomena, and the relationships between homeopathy and acupuncture. These new standpoints for viewing homeopathy will make for a greater understanding of the phenomenon in rational terms.

As regards the *"law of similars,"* which is unquestionably the cornerstone of homeopathy, we present a model based on analysis of the functioning of homeostatic biological systems and cellular receptors. The subject is developed analytically and consequentially in a series of stages starting from the functioning of homeostatic systems and ending up with analysis of the pharmacologically active ingredients of homeopathic solutions. In a nutshell, it is claimed that homeopathic remedies activate the homeostasis control systems via receptors other than those for endogenous mediators, but which achieve the same effect as the endogenous mediators themselves, i.e. they cause resumption of production of regulatory signals and thus activate a negative feedback mechanism in relation to the spontaneous progression of the disease process. Homeopathic drugs are thus thought to act as substitutes for an endogenous regulatory signal which, for various reasons, may be inadequate or ineffective because the system is no longer sensitive to it, being "blocked" by the disease itself.

As regards the possible clinical effects and, according to a number of groups of investigators, also the possible biological effects of highly diluted solutions, this clearly goes beyond the bounds of classic pharmacology. Here there is less scope for certainty and more for hypotheses which, however plausible they may be, still require clear, objective substantiation. The scientific research data so far available can only partly explain what homeopathy claims to achieve. The essential items in our treatment of this topic are the following:

a) The physical properties of water are still in many respects unknown.

b) It is by no means absurd to think that information can be stored in water in the form of vibrational frequencies of molecular dipoles (*"superradiance"*) or in the form of *"hollow hydration shells"* (or *"clathrates"*).

c) There is evidence that the treatment of pure water with electromagnetic waves endows it with new physicochemical properties which may be conserved for many days.

d) Highly sensitive subjects can present allergic manifestations to contact with water treated with electromagnetic frequencies.

e) According to Voll's electroacupuncture, a highly diluted homeopathic drug may restore the electrical conductivity of the skin over the acupuncture points if such conductivity has been deranged as a result of disease.

f) There is evidence that many types of cellular receptors and enzymes are activated or inhibited in various experimental systems by the application of low-frequency electromagnetic fields.

g) There is some preliminary evidence demonstrating a homeopathic effect not only of solutions but also of closed ampoules containing solutions and placed in contact with the system to be regulated (human or animal).

In the text these concepts are expounded systematically, though in hypothetical form. Science, however, should not be afraid to draw up hypotheses, even daring ones, if they lend themselves to experimental verification or invalidation.

This study is targeted mainly at doctors, whether homeopaths or otherwise. Homeopathic doctors will find stimuli in the book for a more thorough investigation into the biological basis of the therapeutic system they adopt. The technological spirit of our age demands explanations. In this day and age, when homeopathy still often comes under attack as being "nonscientific," the data and theories reported here may constitute an updated instrument for documentation and discussion. The authors also hope that the line they have taken in investigating the basis of homeopathy will lead to an increasing measure of confidence in the possibility, even in this field with its many mysterious aspects, of using a rational approach and a scientific method capable of contributing towards keeping this clinico-therapeutic method as far away as possible from unscrupulous forms of exploitation which have nothing to do with the practice of medicine.

Nonhomeopathic doctors may find the book useful as a first approach to the problematical issue of homeopathy, viewed not as an alternative but according to a perspective which, at least in many respects, is consistent with the tenets of modern biomedicine, in which they (like the authors of this work) have been trained and which they regularly abide by in their day-to-day practice. Homeopathy is a practice which came into being and gained widespread notoriety "too early" in the history of medicine, at a time when it was impossible to provide any kind of explanation for it. Since, however, it is a form of empirical medicine, it cannot fail to contain elements which are essentially relevant to the realities of human health and disease. It is thus a macroscopic set of "preliminary observations," where strong elements of interpretative and methodological confusion have built up and stratified alongside an undeniable measure of clinical far-sightedness and therapeutic accuracy. To reject everything *en bloc*, as many are tempted to do, means throwing out the observations along with the interpretations, an operation which may be the line of least resistance, but which is not scientific because unexplained observations have always been the main hive of ideas for research. For these reasons, homeopathy and the critical reappraisal and integration of the various therapeutic systems in general will prove increasingly necessary in medicine in the near future, contributing towards overcoming the difficulties involved in solving complex problems from blinkered, reductive viewpoints.

The ideas and experience reported here thus constitute an attempt to produce a résumé of medical systems usually regarded as alternatives, or at least some form of dialogue between these systems. Such a project promises to be extremely difficult, in view of the vast body of knowledge built up, on the one hand, by homeopathy and, on the other, by modern biomedicine. If to this we add the fact that such knowledge is continually evolving, the task seems well nigh impossible. From this standpoint there is a risk that the contents of the book may discontent the various "specialists." Both homeopaths and scientists expert in their specific fields may find shortcomings and perhaps even inaccuracies at various points of the treatise. The authors, who welcome criticism and correction, trust that any discordance over specific points will not be to the detriment of the main message of this work, which we modestly believe may make a contribution to the current debate on this subject. Though any form of complete synthesis is objectively impossible, there is nothing to prevent us from directing study, research, and reasoning in this direction.

2 Basic Principles and Brief History of Homeopathy

Homeopathic medicine is a clinico-pharmaceutical system which uses microdoses of substances derived from plants, minerals or animals for the purposes of stimulating the natural healing response [Coulter, 1976; Dujany, 1978; Vithoulkas, 1980; Reckeweg, 1981; Charette, 1982; Julian and Haffen, 1982; Meuris, 1982; Del Giudice and Del Giudice, 1984; Lodispoto, 1984; Bianchi, 1987; Gibson and Gibson, 1987; Brigo and Masciello, 1988; Tetau, 1989; Ullman, 1991a; Bianchi, 1990; Granata, 1990; Mossinger, 1992; Jonas and Jacobs, 1996; Ullman, 1996; Candegabe and Carrara, 1997; Swayne, 1998; Vickers, 1999]. This system claims to cure diseases using drugs (usually called "remedies") which are prepared according to particular procedures of dilution and dynamization and chosen according to a complex methodology based essentially on the so-called "law of similars."

2.1

The Law of Similars

The "law" or "principle" of similars (or similarity) constitutes the main acquisition of homeopathy and the basis for its understanding, though today, as we shall see, it is no longer regarded as a universal "law" valid in all cases. According to this principle, which already figured in certain medical and philosophical systems of antiquity (Hippocrates, St. Augustine, Paracelsus), but which was rediscovered mainly by the German physician Samuel Hahnemann (1755-1853), a disease can be cured by administering the patient a substance which, in healthy human subjects, causes symptoms similar to those of the disease (hence the dictum *"similia similibus curentur"* [Hahnemann, 1796]). In practice, this means that:

a) Every biologically active substance (drug or remedy) produces *characteristic symptoms* in healthy bodies which are *susceptible* to being in some way perturbed by that substance.

b) Every sick body expresses a series of *characteristic symptoms* which are typical of the pathological alteration of that *particular* subject.

c) The healing of a sick body, characterized by the progressive disappearance of all symptoms, may be obtained by targeted administration of the drug which produces a similar symptom picture in healthy bodies.

For example, the homeopath, starting from the observation that bee venom causes a characteristic wheal with pain and erythema mitigated by the application of cold compresses, administers bee extract in a homeopathic presentation (diluted and dynamized) to cure patients presenting urticaria with wheals and pain similar to those of bee stings, albeit of different etiology.

In its early formulations, which are still present in a number of schools, the remedy is prescribed not only on the basis of the diagnosis, this being of secondary importance, but also by seeking with the utmost care the correspondence between the symptomatological picture of the disease and the symptom picture caused by a given substance in healthy subjects. If the match is substantial or perfect (the remedy is a "*simillimum*" or "most similar medicine"), the administration even of only a minimum dose of the remedy triggers a reaction in the patient which leads, often after an initial aggravation of the disease, to healing. The healing, then, would appear not to be a direct suppressive effect of the substance administered ("law of opposites"), but the result of the subject's reaction, due, according to classic homeopathy, to the action of the so-called "*vital force*," or life force [Hahnemann, 1994].

For the purposes of identifying the remedies most suited to the individual circumstances, the homeopathic pharmacopoeia has been gradually built up right from the early days of homeopathy on the strength of tests of a "toxicological" type, performed by administering small doses of a whole variety of substances to healthy volunteers and painstakingly recording the symptomatological results as soon as a reaction is observed. These experiments, called *drug provings*, have been collected in the so-called *materia medicas* (encyclopedias of drug effects), which have been and are being continually updated and contain data on hundreds of different mineral, vegetable, and animal substances. The materia medicas have been and continue to be checked, modified, and updated also on the basis of the experience gained with patients. In fact, for a particular remedy to be introduced and used in the homeopathic pharmacopoeia, it is not enough for it to be capable of causing symptoms in a healthy subject; it must show proven ability to cure patients presenting the symptoms detected during the provings.

Another aspect which should be stressed, inasmuch as it is a recurrent feature of the literature, is the fact that, in this patient, thorough analysis of the symptoms (called *repertorization*), a great deal of importance is attributed to the more unusual symptoms, which may reveal a particular type of individual reactivity, as well as to those in the psychological sphere, which are regarded as no less important than the somatic symptoms. Correct repertorization, in fact, requires an analytical and at the same time a holistic all-embracing approach to the sick person. According to homeopathic methodology, it is only in this way that the correct choice of drug indicated for each patient can be made.

The concept of the choice of drug on the basis of the law of similars can be illustrated here with an example [Gibson and Gibson, 1987]. Three patients with influenza are treated with three different remedies: the first patient presents chills, is anxious and restless, and wants to be covered up and drink fresh water; his eyes and nose are producing an irritating mucous runny discharge causing reddening of the nose and upper lip; he also presents gastrointestinal symptoms (vomiting and diarrhea). The remedy indicated for this patient is *Arsenicum album* (arsenic). The second patient with influenza in the same epidemic feels tired and lethargic, experiences chills, and complains of occipital headache; he wants something to warm his back, wants to stay stock-still in bed, and not make any kind of physical effort. In this case the remedy indicated is *Gelsemium* (yellow jasmine). The third person has influenza with a feverish temperature and the most striking symptom is achiness throughout the entire body, as if all his bones were broken. The remedy indicated in his case is *Eupatorium perfoliatum* (boneset). All three patients have contracted the same influenza virus, but their individual reactions to the disease are different and thus their treatment has to be differentiated.

To the homeopathic practitioner, a symptom like fever says very little, in that it is a very nonspecific reaction of the inflammatory process, but he will take great care to analyze the types of fever and the concomitant symptoms as a guide to establishing the right remedy: fever with heat sensations, reddening of the skin, perspiration, a very high pulse rate, a throbbing headache, mydriasis, and photophobia indicates that the patient needs *Belladonna* (deadly nightshade). Fever of sudden onset after a cold, with anxiety even to the point of fearing death, reddening of the skin (without perspiration), and a strong, hard pulse, but also with miosis, intense thirst, and an aversion to blankets, indicates *Aconitum* (monkshood) as the remedy of choice. It is thus particular details and subtle differences which guide the doctor in his choice.

2.2

Homeopathic drugs (or "remedies")

Not only the clinical methodology, but also the preparation of the substances used in homeopathy is quite unique. As is known, they are produced by means of a process of serial dilution and succussion aimed at endowing the solutions with a greater therapeutic effect (*dynamization*).

There are precise historical reasons for the use of highly diluted substances: many substances which right from the outset were tested and introduced into the homeopathic pharmacopoeia were of empirical origin, derived from biologically highly potent or toxic compounds, *such as certain mineral elements, organic and inorganic chemical poisons, and animal or plant poisons.* The symptoms they caused were deduced from accidental intoxication, but obviously they could not be used as such in human experimentation. It was thus that their effects were tested in healthy subjects (provings) and in patients (curative homeopathy) at low and very low doses, administered repeatedly until symptoms appeared (or disappeared, as the case may be).

In the course of these initial trials, Hahnemann himself claimed to have observed the following phenomena:

a) If a patient needed a remedy, i.e. if there was a match within the framework of the law of similars, he or she tended to be very sensitive to the remedy itself. Thus, the doses necessary and sufficient to obtain a positive reaction, were much lower than those needed to cause symptoms in healthy subjects or to cure a sick person who did not present a perfect symptom match.

b) On the strength of this observation, he began to dilute the remedies in order to find curative doses that did not produce unwanted side effects. Experience led him to note an increase in the curative potency on reducing the dose, i.e. on increasing the dilutions.

c) The early dilution procedures also included the process of succussion or trituration of the raw materials (according to whether they were liquid or solid) for a wholly practical reason, consisting in the homogeneousness of the diluted product; only later was it observed that this procedure was necessary to increase the effect of the dilutions. For this reason the progressively increasing dilutions were also called *potencies* and the dilution and succussion process was called *potentization* or *dynamization*.

In practice, the raw materials are extracted by solubilization in alcohol containing various percentages of water, or, if insoluble, they are initially pulverized and triturated with lactose and then diluted in a water-alcohol solution. The initial solutions, containing the maximum concentrations of active ingredients, are called *mother tinctures* (MT). Successive dilutions are then operated, followed by vigorous shaking.

The preparation techniques for the various types of remedies used today are codified in detail in the various pharmacopoeias, the most important of which are the French and German ones, though there is a tendency to find a consensus, at least at the level of the European Union.

The most commonly used dilutions/potencies are: 1:9 (labelled "D," "DH," "X, "or "x"), when 1 part of the most concentrated solution is diluted in 9 parts of solvent; or 1:99 (labelled "C," "CH," or "c"), when 1 part of the most concentrated solution is diluted with 99 parts of solvent. There are also dilutions labelled "LM," based on 1:50,000 serial dilutions, and even *Korsakovian* dilutions (labelled "K"), based on dilutions produced by emptying the recipient containing the most concentrated solution, leaving a few droplets in the bottom, and filling it with solvent (obviously, this latter method is harder to standardize, despite being simple to perform). Lastly, mechanized continuous-flow procedures are also used today.

It is well known that often—though not as a rule—extremely high dilutions are used, with the result that theoretically there is no longer so much as a single molecule of the original substance remaining. This constitutes one of the cornerstones of homeopathy, and at the same time is perhaps the main problem which research is called upon to confirm and possibly explain.

Another very important point has to do with the so-called *dynamization*. In the procedure for the preparation of homeopathic drugs, the rule is that, after each dilution, the resulting solution be subjected to vigorous shaking. Classic standard practice prescribes 100 downward shakes, but other succussion procedures have been developed, including automated techniques.

Lastly, there are also preparations in granule or globule form, consisting in small spheres of sucrose or lactose impregnated with the Hahnemann dilution, from which they take their name. For example, *Arnica montana* (mountain daisy) 9c granules are granules which have been impregnated with the 9c dilution of *Arnica montana*.

Further details on the preparation techniques for homeopathic remedies can be found in other reviews [Vithoulkas, 1980; Del Giudice and Del Giudice, 1984; Brigo and Masciello, 1988; Winston, 1989; Majerus, 1991].

2.3 Hahnemann's Organon

The history of homeopathy [Lodispoto, 1984; Gibson and Gibson, 1987; Haehl, 1989; Majerus, 1991; Ullman, 1991a; Ullman 1991b] begins with the ideas and discoveries of its founder C.F.S. Hahnemann. It was he who first coined the term homeopathy from the Greek *homoios* ("similar") and *pathos* ("suffering"), referring to the law of similars which is its basis. Hahnemann's first real insight into the law of similars came in 1789, when he was translating a book by W. Cullen, one of the most eminent physicians of the era. At a certain point, Cullen attributed the efficacy of Peruvian bark (cinchona) in the treatment of malaria to its bitter and astringent properties. Hahnemann, who was also an expert chemist and keen experimenter, was not happy with this explanation, since he was well aware that there were many other more bitter and astringent substances than Peruvian bark, which, however, were devoid of efficacy in antimalarial treatment. He therefore began to experiment on himself by taking repeated doses of Peruvian bark extract until he reached a stage where he started to manifest fever, chills, and other symptoms similar to those of malaria.

Hahnemann thought that the reason for the efficacy of Peruvian bark in patients suffering from malaria had in some way to be related to the fact that this substance caused symptoms similar to those of the disease it was used to treat. He then tested other drugs in use at the time on himself as well as on friends and relatives, and, using his vast knowledge of botany, chemistry and toxicology, he studied the effects of many plants and medicinal substances. Over the next 20 years, on the basis of patient and meticulous provings, he laid the foundations for the *materia medica*. As early as 1796 he published an article [Hahnemann, 1796] in which he indicated the existence of three types of approach to the treatment of disease: the first (which he defined as the most "sublime") consisted in removal of the cause, if known; the second type consisted in treatment by means of opposites, in other words treatment which he defined as "palliative," such as, for instance, the use of laxatives for constipation; the third type was treatment by means of similars, which he regarded as the only valid approach, apart from prevention. He also suggested the importance of diet, physical exercise, and hygiene, factors which at that time were practically ignored by medical science.

In addition to his activity as a medical practitioner and experimenter, Hahnemann wrote many articles and books, in which he laid the foundations for the entire edifice of homeopathy [cf. review by Aulas and Chefdeville, 1984]. The first complete text on homeopathy was published under the title *Organon of Rational Medical Science* in 1810. Nine years later, in 1819, a second edition of the work was published, entitled *Organon of the Art of Healing*, which was then followed by other editions, up to the sixth, published posthumously in 1921. It obviously encompasses Hahnemann's complete thinking, as well as all the wealth of experience of the author and his followers, who applied and publicized homeopathy in the early decades of the nineteenth century. In view of the historical importance and also the intrinsic cultural interest of the *Organon*, it may be worth devoting more than merely passing attention to the text and quoting some of its more significant statements. The quotations cited here are from the *Organon of Medicine* edited by Joseph Reves, from the 5th and 6th editions [Hahnemann, 1994].

The *Organon* was written as a series of 291 paragraphs and starts with this basic claim: "*The physician's highest and only mission is to restore the sick to health, to cure, as it is termed.*" Then, in a footnote to the first paragraph, we read: "It is not, however, to construct so-called systems, by interweaving empty speculations and hypotheses concerning the internal essential nature of the vital processes and the mode in which diseases originate in the invisible interior of the organism, (whereon so many physicians have hitherto ambitiously wasted their talents and their time)... in order to astonish the ignorant—whilst sick humanity sighs in vain for aid." These sentences effectively convey the main objective of a physician who was always actively engaged in medical practice, as well as revealing his combative and fairly undiplomatic character, which made no small contribution towards getting him ostracized by most of the medical establishment of his day and age.

The claim as to the primacy of practical interests over the construction of theories and hypotheses regarding *"the internal essential nature of the vital processes and the mode in which diseases originate in the invisible interior of the organism"* can be explained on the grounds of the scientific backwardness of the era (early nineteenth century), in which really very little was known about such processes. On the other hand, such a claim might appear thoroughly unscientific: for a scientist, giving up any attempt to understand the mechanisms underlying vital processes is unacceptable. In actual fact, the most likely interpretation of this first paragraph is that Hahnemann was not disputing the study of the natural laws governing the functioning of vital processes, since all the rest of the work bears witness to a substantial rational and investigatory effort, this being the only approach allowing an effective form of therapy based on real awareness. The author, evidently, wished to stress that the *"internal essential nature"* of vital processes is unknowable, and in this sense his claim could hardly be more modern, in the light of recent discoveries regarding biological complexity and chaotic systems, as we shall see in detail below (Chapters 5 and 6). It is likely that the author also intended to criticize those in medicine who limited themselves to devising hypotheses and theories which, though appearing complicated and astonishingly impressive, actually proved utterly useless when it came to solving the patients' practical problems.

In the third paragraph, Hahnemann states: "If the physician clearly perceives what is to be cured in diseases, that is to say, in every individual case of disease (*knowledge of disease, indication*), if he clearly perceives what is curative in medicines, that is to say, in each individual medicine (*knowledge of medicinal powers*), and if he knows how to adapt, according to clearly defined principles, what is curative in medicines to what he has discovered to be undoubtedly morbid in the patient, so that the recovery must ensue—to adapt it, as well in respect to the suitability of the medicine most appropriate according to its mode of action to the case before him (*choice of the remedy, the medicine indicated*), as also in respect to the exact mode of preparation and quantity of it required (*proper dose*), and the proper period for repeating the dose;—if, finally, he knows the obstacles to recovery in each case and is aware how to remove them, so that the restoration may be permanent: *then he understands how to treat judiciously and rationally, and he is a true practitioner of the healing art.*" In the fourth paragraph we read: "He is likewise a preserver of health if he knows the things that derange health and cause disease, and how to remove them from persons in health." These quotations could hardly fail to be endorsed by any medical practitioner operating today, but, in the pre-scientific medical context obtaining at the time, they undoubtedly represented a novel and original approach. The whole basis of Hahnemann's clinical reasoning—and thus of homeopathy—is avowedly rational and logical.

The reasoning of the *Organon* proceeds in the following paragraphs with the statement that the fundamental factor in man's state of health is the *"vital force"* and that any disturbance of this "dynamic inner principle" is responsible for onset of disease, just as, conversely, the *"restitutio ad integrum* of the vital force necessarily presupposes the return to health of the entire organism"* (Paragraph 12). The author was certainly perfectly aware of the existence of pathogens and was fully familiar with the work of his contemporaries, including Sydenham, Jenner, and others (paragraph 38), but strongly emphasized factors related to the medium, host, and subject.

Paragraphs 29-31 clearly define what Hahnemann meant by disease, i.e. *"every disease (not entirely surgical) consists only in a special, morbid, dynamic alteration of our vital energy"* (paragraph 29), whereas the pathogens are only trigger factors: "The inimical forces, partly psychical, partly physical, to which our terrestrial existence is exposed, which are termed morbific noxious agents, do not possess the power of morbidly deranging the health of man unconditionally; but we are made ill by them only *when our organism is sufficiently disposed* and susceptible to the attack of the morbific cause that may be present, and to be altered in its health, deranged and made to undergo abnormal sensations and functions—hence they *do not produce disease in every one nor at all times*" (Paragraph 31). Also in the presence of this key passage of the original theory of homeopathy we are amazed at how concepts which have only recently been espoused by the modern sciences of pathology and immunology could be so clearly perceived and expressed over 150 years ago.

The concept of *vital force* (paragraphs 9-17) has aroused a great deal of discussion. The author undoubtedly ascribed an "intangible" essence to what he understood as vital force (paragraph 10) and, being a man of strong religious beliefs, he also called it the *"spirit-like dynamis"* (Paragraph 16). We should not, however, mistake his statements for an arbitrary attempt to resort to metaphysics. In his day and age, talking about a vital force as something mysterious was simply a way of acknowledging the body's ability to defend and heal itself, without being in a position to provide any explanation of it in physiological or immunological terms. The author himself, in a footnote to paragraph 31, says: "When I call disease a derangement of man's state of health, I am far from wishing thereby to give a hyperphysical explanation of the internal nature of diseases generally, or of any case of disease in particular..." The criticism of Hahnemann's notion of life force is therefore anachronistic and ill-conceived: life force is no more than a metaphor to indicate *a dynamic self-regulatory capability which all living creatures are undeniably endowed with* in order to give them a better chance of survival. That this capability is simply the fruit of evolution or, as Hahnemann puts it, a gift of God (note to paragraph 17), is a problem akin to that of the origin of the universe, which, because of its philosophical implications, goes beyond the bounds of scientific investigation.

Be that as it may, while maintaining a clear distinction between metaphysical and scientific issues, there can be no doubt that, right from the outset, homeopathy has always represented a form of medicine which is very open to the spiritual dimensions of human existence. As Hahnemann himself affirms: "In the healthy condition of man, the spiritual *Vital Force* (autocracy), the dynamis that animates the material body (organism), rules with unbounded sway, and retains all the parts of the organism in admirable, harmonious, vital operation, as regards both sensations and functions, so that our indwelling, reason-gifted mind can freely employ this living, healthy instrument for the higher purpose of our existence" (Paragraph 9).

In the following paragraphs (32-70) the author expounds the experiences and reflections that led him to formulate the law of similars, defined as "*the great, the sole therapeutic law of nature: cure by symptom similarity!*" (Paragraph 50). These experiences are based on careful observation of the courses of natural diseases and the interactions between similar or different diseases, on the effect of smallpox vaccines, on experiments with remedies tested in healthy and sick persons, and on noting the deficiencies of the allopathic approach (paragraphs 54-61, an uncompromising indictment of therapies based on Galen's law of the "*contraria contrariis*" and of other widespread practices at the time such as purging and bloodletting, or the administration of alcoholic beverages and opium).

The explanation of the efficacy of cures using "similars" is given in paragraphs 63-68 and is based essentially on the concept of activation of the reactive response of the vital force: "Every agent that acts upon the vitality, every medicine, deranges more or less the Vital Force, and causes a certain alteration in the health of the individual for a longer or a shorter period. This is termed *primary action*. Although a product of the medicinal and vital powers conjointly, it is principally due to the former power. To its action our Vital Force endeavours to oppose its own energy. This resistant action is a property, is indeed an automatic action of our life-preserving power, which goes by the name of *secondary action or counteraction*" (Paragraph 63).

Many examples are adduced, including: "Excessive vivacity follows the use of strong coffee (primary action), but sluggishness and drowsiness remain for a long time afterwards (reaction, secondary action), if this be not always again removed for a short time by imbibing fresh supplies of coffee (palliative). After the profound stupefied sleep caused by opium (primary action), the following night will be all the more sleepless (reaction, secondary action). After the constipation produced by opium (primary action), diarrhea ensues (secondary action); and after purgation with medicines that irritate the bowels, constipation of several days' duration ensues (secondary action). And in like manner it always happens, after the primary action of a medicine that produces in large doses a great change in the health of a healthy person, that its exact opposite, when, as has been observed, there is actually such a thing, is produced in the secondary action by our Vital Force" (Paragraph 65).

As a result of this principle, by experimentation in healthy human subjects we can know the primary and secondary effects of a large number of remedies, which is precisely what Hahnemann did. "There is, therefore, no other possible way in which the peculiar effects of medicines on the health of individuals can be accurately ascertained—there is no sure, no more natural way of accomplishing this object, than to administer the several medicines experimentally, in moderate doses, to *healthy* persons, in order to ascertain what changes, symptoms and signs of their influence each medicine individually produces on the health of the body and of the mind; that is to say, what disease elements they are able and tend to produce, since, as has been demonstrated, all the curative power of medicines lies in this power they possess of changing the state of man's health, and is revealed by observation of the latter. Not one single physician, as far as I know, during the previous two thousand five hundred years, thought of this so natural, so absolutely necessary and only genuine mode of testing medicines for their pure and peculiar effects in deranging the health of man, in order to learn what morbid state each medicine is capable of curing, except the great and immortal Albrecht von Haller. (...) I was the first that opened up this path, which I have pursued with a perseverance that could only arise and be kept up by a perfect conviction of the great truth, fraught with such blessings to humanity, that it is only by the homeopathic employment of medicines that the certain cure of human maladies is possible" (Paragraphs 108,109).

The author of the *Organon* shows his flair as a keen experimenter and his unquestioned moral stature in this other passage: "As certainly as every species of plant differs in its external form, mode of life and growth, in its taste and smell from every other species and genus of plant, as certainly as every mineral and salt differs from all others, in its external as well as its internal physical and chemical properties (which alone should have sufficed to prevent any confounding of one with another), so certainly do they all differ and diverge among themselves in their pathogenetic—consequently also in their therapeutic—effects. If this be pure truth, as it undoubtedly is, then no physician who would not be regarded as devoid of reason, and who would not act contrary to the dictates of his conscience, the sole arbiter of real worth, can employ in the treatment of diseases any medicinal substance but one with whose real significance he is thoroughly and perfectly conversant, *i.e.*, whose positive action on the health of healthy individuals he has so accurately tested. (...) In all former ages—posterity will scarcely believe it—physicians have hitherto contented themselves with blindly prescribing for diseases medicines whose value was unknown, and which had *never been tested* relative to their highly important, very various, pure dynamic action on the health of man; and, moreover, they mingled several of these unknown medicines that differed so vastly among each other in one formula, and left it to chance to determine what effect should thereby be produced on the patient. This is just as if a madman should force his way into the workshop of an artisan, seize upon *handfuls of very different tools, with the uses of all of which he is quite unacquainted*, in order, as he imagines, to work at the objects of art he sees around him. I need hardly remark that these would be destroyed, I may say utterly ruined, by his senseless operations" (Paragraphs 119 and 168-169).

The *Organon* then goes on to describe in detail all the procedures used both in the experiments ("provings") in groups of healthy volunteers and for the use of the homeopathic method in clinical practice. These practical and applicational aspects lie outside the scope of this book, and therefore we refer the interested reader to the original work, which, in any event, would be quite difficult to summarize here.

The last part of the treatise describes the preparation of homeopathic remedies (trituration, extraction of the active ingredients, various methods of dilution and dynamization), aspects which are clearly important as regards the problem of their possible mechanism of action: "The homeopathic system of medicine develops for its special use, to a hitherto unheard degree, the inner spirit-like medicinal powers of the crude substances by means of a process peculiar to it and which has hitherto never been tried, whereby only they all become immeasurably and penetratingly effi-

[Handwritten margin notes: "Hahneman vs Isopathy"; "PREPARATION OF REMEDIES"; "DEFINITION HomEo."]

cacious and remedial, *even those that in the crude state give no evidence of the slightest medicinal power on the human body.* This remarkable change in the qualities of natural bodies develops the latent, hitherto unperceived, as if slumbering hidden, dynamic powers which influence the life principle, change the well-being of animal life. This is effected by mechanical action upon their smallest particles by means of rubbing and shaking *and through the addition of an indifferent substance, dry or fluid, are separated from each other.* This process is called *dynamizing, potentizing* (development of medicinal power) and the products are dynamizations or potencies in different degrees. (...) On this account it refers only to the increase and stronger development of their power to cause changes in the health of animals and men if these natural substances in this improved state, are brought very near to the living sensitive fibre or come in contact with it (by means of intake or olfaction)" (Paragraphs 269, 295).

DYNAMIZATION

The problem of the routes and modalities of administration is also addressed. In paragraph 272 the author ascribes the effect of the medicine to contact with the nerves of the tongue and oral cavity, and later (paragraph 284) adds that, in addition to the tongue, mouth, and stomach, also the airways (inhalation) and skin (friction) are potential administration routes for the medicines.

As regards the doses, Hahnemann asks himself "how small, in other words, must be the dose of each individual medicine, homeopathically selected for a case of disease, to effect the best cure?" (Paragraph 278); he recommends the use of the lowest possible doses, but does not establish rigid criteria, claiming, amongst other things, that to solve this problem "is, as may easily be conceived, not the work of theoretical speculation. (...) Pure experiment, careful observation of the sensitiveness of each patient, and accurate experience can alone determine this *in each individual case*" (Paragraph 278).

DOSES

More important than the dose is the correct choice of remedy, which must be the one most closely matching the patient's symptom picture and his or her particular sensitivity to the drug: "And because a medicine, provided the dose of it was sufficiently small, is all the more salutary and almost marvellously efficacious the more accurately homoeopathic its selection has been, a medicine whose selection has been accurately homoeopathic must be all the more salutary the more its dose is reduced to the degree of minuteness appropriate for a gentle remedial effect" (Paragraph 277).

An analysis of the basic content of the *Organon* is of interest not merely from the historical point of view, in the sense that it constitutes the cornerstone of the entire homeopathic edifice, but also because even today it is still the main reference text for anyone wishing to learn about homeopathy. In actual fact, despite the fact that at a very early stage (even during Hahnemann's lifetime, as he mentions in his works) various different schools of thought and different methodological orientations were to emerge in homeopathy, the authority of the founder has always remained of paramount importance. It may indeed seem most surprising that the basic principles and methodologies discovered by Hahnemann have practically never been questioned, disputes, if any, being confined to the interpretation of his teachings.

At the same time, another indicative aspect is the fact that over the following 150 years Hahnemann's homeopathic disciples never saw fit to operate any very substantial revision of his original insights and discoveries in more up-to-date terms. The reasons for this are probably related to the fact that homeopathy presented itself as an effective curative method, based on very mysterious and almost unfathomable principles, which therefore were essentially indisputable. A procedure which claims to work, but without any very substantial scientific explanation, can only be accepted or rejected according to personal experience. It is also undeniable that the fact that this therapeutic approach was developed without reference to any kind of pathophysiological explanation (Hahnemann even went so far as to claim that there was no point in searching for the "hidden causes" of disease) is the main obstacle to its acceptance. On the other hand, any attempt to provide a rational explanation of how the law of similars and microdoses works is a daunting task, even with all the knowledge and instruments available to us today, and thus, in a certain sense, the refusal on the part of the world of homeopathy to undertake serious scientific research is justifiable. As we shall see, it was only recently that homeopaths began to do something about this state of affairs.

2.4

Opposition to the development of homeopathy

The concepts and observations expounded in the *Organon* are one of the first attempts in the history of medicine to codify the principles and laws governing human health and disease in an organic manner on the basis of reasoning and experimentation. This indisputable fact has been overlooked in most treatises on the history of medicine. Homeopathy brought ideas which were apparently too advanced for the primitive state in which medicine found itself at the time and which over the years have never been understood by more than a minority of those working in the field of conventional medicine, incapable as most of them are of embracing ideas and insights far ahead of contemporary thought.

Homeopathic medicine has undergone substantial ups and downs in its historical development: the rapid early boom throughout the world in the last century was followed by a head-on clash with orthodox medicine, which stopped homeopathy in its tracks and then led to its progressive decline, particularly in Western countries, where in some cases it all but disappeared altogether. Over the past few decades, however, we have been witnessing a steady recovery of homeopathic practice, even in very technologically advanced countries such as France, Germany, and Italy.

Hahnemann himself, right from the outset, found himself faced with stern opposition from colleagues and even more so from the apothecaries, who felt that he was undermining the foundations of their profession: since he was recommending the use of small doses and was against multiple prescriptions, this new medicine was perceived as a serious threat to their profits. Moreover, he was accused of dispensing his own medicines and administering them to his patients, which was illegal at the time. He was thus arrested in Leipzig in 1820, convicted, and forced to leave the city. He then obtained special permission from Grand Duke Ferdinand to practice homeopathy in the town of Köthen, where he continued to work, write, and instruct his followers who were swiftly increasing in numbers and spreading their wings further afield. At his death (1843), homeopathy was known in all European countries (except Norway and Sweden), as well as in the United States, Mexico, Cuba, and Russia, and not long after his death it was soon to reach India and South America.

The rapid initial spread of homeopathy was probably due, on the one hand, to the fact that the orthodox medicine of his day and age was still extremely backward and lacked truly effective therapeutic remedies, and, on the other, to the distinct superiority of homeopathy in treating the various epidemics of typhoid fever, cholera, and yellow fever which raged across Europe and America in the 1800s.

For instance, in the 1854 London cholera epidemic the mortality rate was 53.2 percent for patients treated in conventional hospitals as against only 16.4 percent in those treated in the homeopathic hospital. During the yellow fever epidemic which spread throughout the southern states of America in 1878 the statistics show that the mortality rate in patients receiving homeopathic treatment was one-third of that in patients on conventional treatment [Gibson and Gibson, 1987; Ullman, 1991a].

In the nineteenth century homeopathy was immensely popular in the United States where major figures such as Hering, Kent, and Farrington were practicing. Homeopathy was taught at Boston University and at the Universities of Michigan, Minnesota, and Iowa. By the turn of the century as many as 29 homeopathic journals were being published. 1844 marked the founding of the American Institute of Homeopathy, which thus became the first American national medical society. Despite this, strong organized opposition was soon forthcoming from "orthodox" medicine, which viewed the growth of homeopathy as a major threat: homeopathy was calling into question the very philosophical basis, clinical methodology and official pharmacology of orthodox medicine. Right from the very beginning the new approach embodied a strong critical attitude towards the use of conventional medicines, which were judged to be harmful, toxic and counterproductive for the practice of homeopathy, in that they were all based on suppression of symptoms. What is more, good homeopathic practice called for a long apprenticeship and individualization of treatment, both of which demanded more time than physicians were normally prepared to give their patients.

1846 marked the foundation of the American Medical Association (AMA), one of the first objectives of which was to combat homeopathy: homeopaths could not be members of the AMA, and AMA members were not allowed even to consult a homeopath, the penalty for this being expulsion from the Association; legal recognition was denied to graduates with diplomas from universities with full professors of homeopathy on their academic boards. In 1910, a classification of American medical schools was drawn up (the Flexner Report) on the basis of criteria which assigned high ratings to schools which placed the emphasis on a physicochemical and pathological approach to the human body and strongly penalized the homeopathic approach. The homeopathic colleges obviously obtained poor ratings, and as only the graduates of schools with high ratings had their qualifications recognized, this was a mortal blow to the teaching of homeopathy. Of 22 homeopathic colleges operating in 1900, only two were still teaching homeopathy in 1923. By 1950 there was not a single school in the United States teaching homeopathy and it was estimated that there were only about a hundred practicing homeopaths, almost all over 50 years of age, throughout the US. For similar reasons, there was also a parallel decline in homeopathic practice in Europe in the early decades of the twentieth century.

We should not conclude, however, that the decline of homeopathy was due only to political and economic reasons. At least two other factors played a decisive role, namely the internal struggles within homeopathy itself and the new major scientific and pharmacological discoveries. As regards the splits in the homeopathic world, there were disputes between the various schools over dilutions (high or low potencies), over single or multiple prescriptions, and over whether prescribing should be based on total symptoms or on the main disease present. The various different schools developed their own organizations, hospitals and journals, thus making it very hard even for doctors seriously interested in learning about homeopathy to get their bearings in this field.

A severe blow to homeopathic theory was delivered by the chemical sciences and in particular by Avogadro's law, published initially as a hypothesis in 1811 and then tested experimentally by Millikan in 1909 [studies cited by Majerus, 1991]: as is well known, this law establishes that one mole of any substance contains 6.02254×10^{23} molecular or atomic units. As a result, a simple calculation demonstrated that dilutions of any substance beyond 10^{24} (24x or 12c in homeopathic terms) presented an increasingly remote chance of containing even only a single molecule or atom of the original compound. From this it was obviously but a short step to ridiculing the use of homeopathic medicines, and homeopaths were branded by their adversaries as being on a par with some kind of esoteric sect. Such opinions have continued to be voiced virtually unaltered up to the present day and can still be encountered in certain authoritative texts [Meyers *et al.*, 1981].

The decisive factor, however, permitting conventional scientific medicine to prevail over homeopathy was its own development as a science capable of identifying the causes of many diseases and as a source of effective techniques and technologies for curing them. Lister's discoveries in the antiseptic field and the development of anesthesiology greatly increased the success, indications, and popularity of surgery. While chemistry, physiology, and pathology were making giant strides in the theoretical sphere, the discovery of vitamin and hormone replacement therapies and, above all, the advent of antibiotics, analgesics, and antiinflammatory drugs enabled orthodox therapy to demonstrate its practical superiority. The possibility of interpreting pathological phenomena rationally on the basis of a scientifically validated model of the human body and the availability of chemical, physical or technological means capable of repairing defects detected with the utmost precision by increasingly sophisticated and reliable instruments was (and is) altogether too attractive and convincing a prospect to allow scope for exploring alternatives based on outdated and mysterious theories.

2.5

Variants of classic homeopathy

As we have already mentioned and as is only logical, further discoveries and applications have gradually added themselves to the initial concepts and groundrules. Among these, particularly worthy of note are *"isopathy"* and the introduction of the use of the so-called *"nosodes."*

ISOPATHY (handwritten)

2.5.1 History of isopathy

One of the earliest and most notable innovations of homeopathy, mentioned even in the later editions of the *Organon*, is isopathy. The term was probably coined by the veterinarian Wilhelm Lux somewhere around 1831–1833 [Lux, 1833]: after starting to treat his animals with the homeopathic method, he became convinced that every contagious disease bears within itself the means whereby it can be cured. He observed that the technique of dilution and dynamization of a contagious product (bacterium, virus or infected secretions, and organic material) would put such a product in a position to exert a therapeutic action on the disease resulting from the contagion. The law of similars *Similia similibus curentur* thus becomes: *Aequalia aequalibus curentur*, or the law of sameness.

LAW of SIMILARS (handwritten margin note) *LAW of SAMENESS* (handwritten margin note)

In actual fact, the principles underlying isopathy can be traced to roots dating back even further than those of homeopathy [Julian, 1983]. Attempting to treat a disease by administering the agent capable of causing it or transmitting it is one of the most general acquisitions of empirical medicine. Numerous primitive peoples defend themselves against the effects of snake venoms by repeatedly inoculating themselves with them or with materials extracted from the venom apparati of snakes. In the Far East the Chinese practiced a form of preventive smallpox vaccination both by wearing the clothes worn by a smallpox victim in the full suppuration phase of the disease and by inhaling dried smallpox pustules after storing them for one year. Pliny claimed that the saliva of a rabid dog can afford protection against rabies. Dioskurides of Anazarbo recommended that hydrophobia sufferers eat the liver of the dog that bit them. Aetius of Antioch recommended eating the meat of the viper that had just bitten you. In the seventeenth century the Irishman Robert Fludd cured the victims of consumption with dilutions of their own sputum after suitable preparation.

It was only at the beginning of the nineteenth century, however, with the birth of homeopathy, that isopathy was fully developed [for a review see Julian, 1983]. Three authors dominate the history of isopathy, and all three were homeopaths: Constantine Hering, Wilhelm Lux, and Denys Collet.

NB (handwritten margin note)

Constantine Hering was born in Saxony in 1800 and became an assistant to the surgeon Robbi, who entrusted him with the task of writing a book for him confuting homeopathy once and for all, as had already been requested by the publisher Baumgartner. After taking a closer look at Hahnemann's works, Hering was not only intrigued, but ended up by defending Hahnemann and coming out in favor of the new method. Hering contributed a great deal to homeopathy, but above all it is to him that we

PROPHYLAXIS
prevention of or protection against disease often involving
use of a biological/chemical or mechanical agent to destroy or prevent
the entry of infectious organisms

owe the *Lachesis* experimentation and the preparation of homeopathic remedies from pathological excretions and secretions, which he terms *nosodes*. Originally this term denoted any remedy extracted from pathological excretions or secretions obtained from human subjects or animals. Animal poisons were included in this definition, so much so indeed that Hering was the first to "prove" *Lachesis* (venom of the bushmaster snake, the first nosode in history, later to become a homeopathic remedy to all intents and purposes) and the rabies "poison." Convinced that every disease contains within it its own remedy and prophylaxis, he extended his studies to the scabies "virus," extracting the alleged "virus" from blisters from a subject with well developed scabies.

Hering also maintained that products of the human body and the various parts of the body in the healthy state all have a preferential action on the corresponding diseased parts, and as early as 1834 he advised the use of diluted and dynamized homologous organs ("iso-organotherapy"). Finally, he assumed that the chemical elements exerted a particular action on those organs in which they were mainly contained. His studies and papers on minerals and salts preceded the work of Schüssler on biochemical salts.

ISO-ORGANOTHERAPY

The second great isopath was the veterinarian Joseph Wilhelm Lux, born in Silesia in 1776. Lux was appointed Professor of Veterinary Science at the University of Leipzig in 1806, and his work constituted a landmark in the history of veterinary medicine. From 1820 onwards he was familiar with Hahnemann's works and applied the new method in veterinary medicine, becoming a staunch advocate of veterinary homeopathy.

In 1831 Valentin Zibrik asked him for a homeopathic remedy for distemper and anthrax. As he knew of no homeopathic remedies for these epidemics at the time, his advice was to replace the homeopathic "similar" (i.e. the drug prescribed on the basis of the symptoms) with a 30c dilution of a drop of nasal mucus from an animal with distemper and a 30c dilution of a drop of blood of an animal with anthrax, and get all the animals suffering from distemper and anthrax, respectively, to take them.

He was thus the first to create the strain called *Anthracinum*. In 1833 Lux published the results obtained in a booklet entitled *Isopathik der Contagionen* [Lux, 1833], in which he claimed that all contagious diseases bear within their pathological phenomena and products their own means of cure. It thus proved possible to dilute and dynamize not only the "known" disease agents, but also any type of human or animal secretion or excretion. Moreover, Lux also extended the principle to substances which had become iatrogenic as a result of abuse, so that a method which was originally used only in contagious diseases was also applied to noncontagious illnesses.

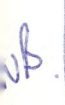
NB.

[handwritten marginalia: OPOTHERAPY / use of dessicated healthy animal tissues or their juices or the active principles extracted from them — may be administered by gastrointestinal route or injection]

Hering and Lux's ideas were supported and defended by Hahnemann's ablest disciple, Dr. Ernst Staph, and spread to France and Germany. In 1836, Weber, medical adviser to the Court of Hessen, published a study on the isotherapy of anthrax using a 30c dilution of purulent fluid from a gangrenous spleen (specific localization in animals). Joly wrote to Hahnemann from Constantinople in 1835 claiming to have achieved numerous cures for bubonic plague in leper colonies, using 30c dilutions of serous fluid from plague bubos.

Some years later, J.F. Herrmann of Thalgau (Salzburg) took up Hering's ideas and in 1848 published "*The true isopathy or the use of healthy animal organs as remedies for similar diseases in man.*" His own ideas were later to be developed by C.E. Brown-Séquard, the father of modern opotherapy.

Nevertheless, after this early period of expansion, the new method ran into continuous and increasingly severe criticism, so much so that isopathy went into decline for several years, even within the homeopathic community. Only a very few solitary practitioners went on using isopathic remedies. It was Father Denys Collet, a doctor and Dominican friar born in 1824, who eventually brought isopathy back onto the scene. In 1865 he witnessed a homeopathic healing which convinced him to devote himself to the new method. He rediscovered isopathy alone and after several decades of practice published a book entitled *Isopathie, Méthode Pasteur par Voie Interne* at the age of 74. According to Collet, there are three ways of healing, namely allopathy, homeopathy, and isopathy, all of which are useful depending on the clinical indications. In addition, he distinguishes between three types of isopathy:

[handwritten marginalia: COLLET; YES!]

a) "Pure isopathy," which uses secretion products from the patient to cure the same disease.

b) "Organic isopathy," which cures the diseased organs with dynamized derivatives from healthy organs.

c) "Serotherapeutic isopathy" or "serotherapy" (dilutions of hyperimmune serum). The book also contains 42 personal observations and the rules of isopathic pharmacopraxis, which is the starting point for a substantial renewal of the method.

In the twentieth century two works devoted entirely to nosodes have been published: the first in 1910 by H.C. Allen, entitled *The Materia Medica of the Nosodes* [Allen, 1910]. The second is by the Frenchman O.A. Julian, who first published *Materia Medica der Nosoden* in German in 1960, later to come out in two French versions, one in 1962 entitled *Biothérapiques et Nosodes* and the other in 1977 entitled *Traité de Micro-Immunothérapie Dynamisée.*

The above-mentioned book by O.A. Julian in 1960 was a great success in Germany, where it revived the study of nosodes. In particular, R. Voll accorded therapy with nosodes a central role in his diagnostic-therapeutic procedure called electroacupuncture-organometry (see Chapter 7, Section 3), and H.H. Reckeweg, the founder of homotoxicology, made extensive use of nosodes in his biotherapy (see Chapter 2, Section 6).

2.5.2 Terminology and definitions of isotherapy, nosodes, and biotherapeutic substances

As can be seen from the history of isopathy, there is a major degree of confusion over terminology. Hering was the first to talk about nosodes, by which he meant a homeopathic dilution extracted from pathological excretions or secretions derived from human subjects or from animals. On the other hand, it was probably Lux (see Chapter 2, Section 5.1.) who first coined the term "*isopathy*," referring to a therapeutic method based on the principle of sameness—*Aequalia aequalibus curentur*—whereby an infectious substance, diluted and dynamized according to homeopathic practice, is capable of healing the same contagious disease that it causes.

More recently, in France, in the December 29, 1948 issue of the *Journal Officiel*, a decree was published called *Codification of homeopathic herbal preparations*, in which the term "*nosode*" was defined as follows: "Nosodes are homeopathic preparations obtained from microbial cultures, viruses, or pathological secretions or excretions. (...) Nosodes are never sold to the public in the natural state, but only from the 3c dilution or 6x dilution upwards." They need to pass sterility tests. The 1c dilution, and obviously all subsequent dilutions, when seeded on various bacteriological media, must not produce a culture.

The definition of the term "*isopathic*" is different and does not refer directly to the term "*isopathy*." Again according to the French decree of 1948, "the term isopathic refers to those nosodes whose strain comes from the sick person himself." They are dispensed in an extempore manner starting from substances coming from the patient (blood, urine, and pathological secretions), the first liquid dilution of which must be sterilized, or they are supplied by the patient (vaccine, medicine, allergen, and other products). An isopathic substance can be distinguished from a nosode on the basis of its individual nature, being destined for use only in the person who supplied the strain, after which it is immediately destroyed.

Even more recently, in the Codex to the 1965 eighth edition of the French Pharmacopoeia, the terms "*nosode*" and "*isopathic substance*" are replaced by the terms "*biotherapeutic*" and "*isotherapeutic*" substance, respectively. Lastly, it was O.A. Julian in the late 1970s who proposed an update of terminology in line with modern medical vocabulary and suggested calling biotherapeutic and isotherapeutic substances *"Dynamized Micro-Immunotherapy."* The idea he wanted to get across was that the preferential action of these medicines is regulation of the immune system at the level of production of antibodies and/or autoantibodies. However, even the term introduced by Julian has not met with universal acceptance, amongst other things because the very concept of *dynamization* is much debated and controversial, inasmuch as no physicochemical basis for it has been defined.

In conclusion, what is meant by *isopathy* today is the use as remedies of dilute, dynamized preparations of the etiological agents responsible for the diseases themselves, based not on the principle of similarity of symptoms, but on the remedy being identical to the etiological agent. For example, the use of pollens in allergic asthma, the use of the same poisons to cure poisoning, and the use of "homeopathized" preparations of allopathic drugs to combat the toxic side effects of the drugs themselves.

What is meant by *isopathic* is the therapeutic use of pathological material, secretions, and excretions coming from the patient himself. For example, for the patient supplying it, matter taken from a boil constitutes an isopathic remedy (obviously after suitable preparation) for his or her chronic furunculosis.

What is meant by *nosodes* are those homeopathic preparations which consist of extracts of pathological materials (scabies blisters, urethral pus, initial syphiloma material), pathogen cultures (microbes, viruses), human or animal metabolic products (bile juices), or pathologically abnormal organs or tissues (tonsillitis, ulcers, osteomyelitis, etc.), suitably dispensed in sterile, dilute, and dynamized form according to homeopathic methodologies. By way of examples, *Tuberculinum* is a nosode prepared from the lesion induced by the Koch mycobacterium, *Variolinum* the nosode prepared from matter obtained from a smallpox pustule, and *Carcinosinum* the nosode from a carcinoma, and so on.

A particular form of isopathy is autohemotherapy, in which the patient's own blood is used, usually administered intramuscularly after suitable treatment (e.g. dilution-dynamization, ozonization, addition of homeopathic drug). This aspect will be dealt with in greater detail in Chapter 6, Section 4.

2.6

Homotoxicology

As a result of the development of the chemical, biochemical, and immunological sciences, which around the middle of this century began to provide a glimpse of a truly scientific interpretation of biological and pathological phenomena, various authors started to undertake a reappraisal of home-

DIATHESIS — inherited physical constitution *
predisposing to certain diseases/conditions believed
associated with Y chromosome — cos o⁷ more affected than ♀

Basic Principles and Brief History of Homeopathy **29**

opathy within the framework of strictly modern scientific criteria. The law
of similars, the active ingredients of homeopathic drugs, and the mechanisms of the effect of low and very low doses were subjected to critical
review. This attempt was (from the 1950s on) and still is being made mainly
by the German school of homotoxicology [Reckeweg, 1981; Bianchi, 1987;
Maiwald, 1988; Bianchi, 1990] whose starting point was a reconsideration
of the inflammatory process, seen essentially not as a pathological process,
but as an organic defense reaction. The concept of vital force was restored
to the sphere of biochemical, physiological, and immunological discovery.

Homotoxicology thus represents that branch of homeopathy which has
attempted and is still attempting to link homeopathy scientifically to the
chemical and therapeutic inroads made in the field of modern medical
knowledge. We should note, however, that this attempt is still incomplete
both on account of the limited effort and resources so far devoted to the
purpose and owing to the vastness of the subject which potentially embraces all sectors of biomedical science.

The word homotoxicology derives from the concept of *homotoxins*, which
basically mean any molecule, whether endogenous or exogenous, capable
of causing biological damage. The concept probably came from the theories and experiences of classic homeopathy, which talked about endogenous
toxins present in pathological "diatheses." — *

Though somewhat generic, this definition is of indicative value in medical
theory and practice. Reckeweg, in fact, defines the homotoxicological conception of disease as follows: "All those processes that we call diseases are
an expression of biologically appropriate defense mechanisms against exogenous or endogenous homotoxins (excretion, reaction, and deposition
phases) or of the attempt on the part of the body to compensate for the
homotoxic damage sustained (impregnation, degeneration, and neoplastic
phases) so as to stay alive as long as possible" [Reckeweg, 1981, p. II (Fore-
word)].

We have no intention here of analyzing the applicational aspects of
homotoxicology, which, in many respects, are just as intensely debated and
controversial as those of homeopathy in general, but prefer rather to confine our attention to the basic theoretical concepts. To illustrate the
homotoxicological type of approach, we can take a starting point, for instance, which is apparently common to both conventional medicine and
homeopathy, namely vaccination. On considering this immune system manipulation practice, what clearly emerges is the ability of the organism to
react to a disturbance of the system (in this case, the foreign antigen), producing a specific integrated response aimed at safeguarding its own structural and functional integrity. This response is excessive in relation to the

Reckeweg

HomoTox .
embraces
all sectors
of
Biomedical
Science

HomoToxin .

initial stimulus and is relatively stable (memory), so much so, indeed, that it can be used to neutralize a hypothetical second disturbance (in this case, an infection). Furthermore, it is well known that the immune response is specific to the antigen triggering it, but may also direct itself against any target that is in some way "similar" (even only a part of the molecule). In the complex network of the immune system, the antibody spectrum may be broadened for the purposes of attacking and neutralizing not only identical antigens, but also those which merely resemble the original.

These concepts, which are the subject matter of modern immunology, serve to illustrate one type of behavior of living creatures which homotoxicology exploits and studies. The real contribution of homotoxicology is the extension of this concept from the field of vaccination and immunity to the body as a whole, with all its systems responsible for preserving physiological integrity. As far as homotoxicology is concerned, the factors impairing this integrity are not merely foreign antigens, but also toxic chemicals, radiation, endogenous molecules deriving from inflammatory processes (especially if these are impeded pharmacologically in their normal evolution), excessive or unbalanced nutrition, variations in the pH of connective tissues, stress, particular psychological states, and many other factors. We define as *homotoxins* all endogenous or exogenous molecules which mediate damage to cells, tissues, and organs. The body's highly integrated response to the pathogenetic noxa involves everything which is called the "*major defense system*" and which comprises:

a) The immune system.

b) The connective tissue where the various toxic substances are "burnt" by the inflammatory reaction, or are accumulated pending their elimination.

c) The hypothalamo-pituitary-adrenal mechanism.

d) The sympathetic and parasympathetic neural reflex system.

e) The detoxifying function of the liver, such as microsomal systems and glucuronic acid conjugation.

This formulation of the *major defense system* concept dates back to the mid-60s; today, other important elements could be added (we need only mention the soluble polymolecular systems of plasma, the neuropeptides, the multiform functions of prostaglandins, the new functions of the endocrine glands and the gastrointestinal system) without this changing its essential pathophysiological significance.

In normal circumstances the activity of the defense system is characterized by normal physiological function, whereas in the case of an excess of toxic factors (or their permanence in the system) an activity level sufficient to produce symptoms is encountered in the various systems. If the defense system fails to eliminate the pathogenetic noxa, or itself introduces other pathogenetic elements, the picture changes and becomes complicated. According to the homotoxicological view, on analyzing the processes detectable in disease, we can distinguish between 6 basic phases, which are, in a certain sense, progressive:

a) The *excretion* phase, in which the body activates all the processes of excretion via the skin, bowels, kidneys, nose, lungs, etc.

b) The *inflammation* phase, with the formation of exudate, pus, fever, activation of the immune system.

c) The *deposition* phase, with processes such as steatosis, glycogenosis, atherosclerosis, amyloidosis, calculosis, in which the body tends to confine the toxic or excess substances to particular regions.

d) The *impregnation* phase, in which the toxic substances (including any endogenous toxins produced in the previous phases) spread in tissues and organs owing to initial blockade of cell and enzyme disposal systems.

e) The *degeneration* phase, in which cellular damage of cytotoxic, anoxic, dystrophic origin, prevails.

f) The *neoplastic* phase, in which genetically damaging factors, in conjunction with the presence of growth or hormonal factors, and possibly with depression of the immune system, lead to the occurrence of tumors.

One positive aspect of this model is that it provides a picture and an understanding of the evolution of the disease and, above all, it serves as a guide to the physician when it comes to making a rational choice of therapeutic action. In fact, once the possible causes of the disease have been removed, it is up to the physician to get the patient's body to work "backwards" through the various phases, using biological drugs and not enzyme inhibitors. From this standpoint, the inappropriate use of drugs which inhibit, for instance, the excretion phases (perspiration, exudates, peeling of the skin, catarrh, diarrhea, etc.) or the reaction phases (fever, acute inflammation) may even cause progression of the disease towards degenerative or neoplastic phases because the unremoved pathogenetic factors ("homotoxins") direct themselves towards other cell targets.

In its pharmacological repertory homotoxicology recuperates much of the homeopathic empirical tradition, preferring the use of low-dilution homeopathic drugs (i.e. drugs containing substantial amounts of active ingredient), though not openly opposing the classic approach, i.e. the quest for the *simillimum* and the use of high dilutions. The basic thinking, however, is the same: the aim is to stimulate the intrinsic healing and detoxifying power of the body by means of biological drugs at low doses. According to this approach, there will inevitably be areas of convergence with conventional medicine and modern pharmacology: new therapeutic agents are conceived which were not identified by homeopathic methodology, such as, for instance, the use of quinones or intermediate products of the Krebs cycle as catalysts of cell energy regeneration processes, the use of various oligoelements and vitamins, the use of natural and synthetic immunostimulants, including interferons and cytokines recently produced by genetic engineering.

It is obvious that the homotoxicological theory was bound to meet with criticism from the advocates of classic homeopathy, who maintained that the basic principles of homeopathy (similarity and potentized microdoses) are almost entirely neglected. The debate hinges basically on the fact that the aim of the homotoxicological approach is detoxification and elimination of "homotoxins," which in itself is valid, but the risk is that perhaps not *all* the levels of potential dysregulation of the body will be considered, including the predispositions and particular "terrain" of each individual.

Despite the fact that such issues are still very much a matter of debate, homotoxicology, which acts as a bridge between homeopathy and conventional medicine, does not wish to clash head on with either of them. Above all, there is a possibility that the experimental criterion whereby theories are subjected to vetting in the form of clinical and laboratory tests may constitute a firm point of reference for further progress and clarification as to the relationships between homeopathy and homotoxicology.

2.7 Homeopathy today

As we have already stated, the enormous progress of conventional medicine in this century has reinforced the opinion that allopathic treatment by means of "opposites" is the only effective form of treatment and, generally speaking, has also strengthened the view that it is only a question of time before a treatment is found for every disease. The great epidemics of infectious diseases have been defeated by a combination of improvements in living conditions, hygiene, vaccinations, and antibiotics. Our knowledge of disease due to vitamin, enzyme or hormone deficiencies has furnished new weapons in the struggle against diseases such as pernicious anaemia, dwarfism, and diabetes. If it were not for the problem of finding donors, transplants would already be routine therapy for a sizeable number of diseases. Cortisone and its derivatives are solving many problems of immune hypersensitivity. Recent developments in molecular biology give us good reason to believe that not even the genetic sphere will be able to escape our manipulative capability.

Against this backcloth, one cannot see any real scope for homeopathy, though at present its use is still spreading. This spread of homeopathy is happening in countries such as Italy, France, and Germany, and parallels the renewed interest in homeopathy in many other countries throughout the world [Gibson and Gibson, 1987; Ullman, 1991a; Ullman, 1991b]. In Great Britain, visits to homeopathic physicians are increasing at a rate of 39 percent per year, and in a survey of 28,000 members of a consumer organization as many as 80 percent reported using some form of complementary medicine at some time; in a *British Medical Journal* survey, 42 percent of the physicians interviewed referred patients to homeopaths [Wharton and Lewith, 1986].

A recent survey in the same Journal reported that in the Netherlands 47% of general pratictioners use complementary therapeutic methods, most commonly homeopathy (40%), up to 37% of British general pratictioners use homeopathy, and over a third of France's general pratictioners use complementary therapeutic methods (5% exclusively, 21% often, and 73% occasionally) [Fisher and Ward, 1994].

Of 100 recently graduated British doctors, 80 percent expressed an interest in being trained in either homeopathy, acupuncture or hypnosis [Taylor Reilly, 1983; Ullman, 1991b]. It is well known that even the British Royal Family uses homeopathy as the main form of therapy. In France, some 11,000 physicians prescribe homeopathic remedies, and according to statistics 30 percent of French people have used such medicines [Bouchaier, 1990]. The French magazine *Le Nouvel Observateur* reports that President Mitterand and six medical school deans are pressing for a greater commitment to homeopathic research. In Germany, 20 percent of doctors use homeopathic medicines at least occasionally [Ullman, 1991b]. A study conducted in a Norwegian university hospital showed that 51.1 percent of patients with atopic dermatitis and 42.5 percent of patients with psoriasis had resorted to alternative therapies (mostly homeopathy and phytotherapy) [Jensen, 1990].

Homeopathy is even more popular in Asia, most notably in India, Pakistan, and Sri Lanka. Great support for the spread of homeopathy in India came from Mahatma Gandhi, and it goes without saying that in the countries of the Third World where the health system is as primitive as it was a century ago and there are no facilities or infrastructures for the application of western-style medicine, homeopathy finds plenty of scope for development, not least because of the low production costs of the medicines. This is also confirmed by the fact that Mother Teresa took steps to introduce homeopathic care in the reception centers for poor patients and sick children in Calcutta back in 1950 and today there are four homeopathic dispensaries run by the Missionary of Charity Sisters. The same is true of other countries: in Brazil there are approximately 2,000 physicians using homeopathic medicines and many medical schools hold courses in homeopathy. In Mexico, homeopathy is very popular, with five colleges of homeopathic medicine, two of which in Mexico City. In the United States, too, we are witnessing a revival of homeopathic practice: the sales of homeopathic medicines showed a ten-fold increase from the late 1970s to the early 1980s, and by the mid '80s there were as many as approximately 1000 physicians specializing in homeopathy [Ullman, 1991a]. Sales of homeopathic medicines in the USA have been growing at an annual rate of 20-25% during the 1990s.

Throughout Europe, many young doctors are "specializing" in this sector which they regard as very promising from both the professional and occupational points of view. Schools of homeopathy are coming into being in many cities, issuing diplomas, and applying for official recognition. These considerations alone should be enough to justify a greater commitment on the part of the official scientific institutions towards monitoring and clinically verifying the efficacy of the therapeutic agents and measures adopted. A need is also felt for at least some teaching of the basics of homeopathy to the doctors trained in universities, since, at general practitioner level particularly, patients often tend to be keenly interested in homeopathy and to ask their GPs for information and advice on the subject. subject.

Homeopathic medicines have obtained an official status in the European Community (Directory n. 92/73/CEE) and the Belgian Parliament has recognized the practice of homeopathy [van Wassenhoven, 2000].

There may be any number of reasons for the revival of homeopathy, despite the lack of university teaching in the field and of support on the part of public health authorities (homeopathic drugs are not available on the NHS), but it can hardly be accounted for merely on commercial grounds. The main reason for the success of the so-called "alternative" medicines lies in the fact that they offer something which today's physician is unable to provide. This "something" can be traced, on the one hand, to the greater degree of individualization of the treatment, attention being paid to the human and psychological elements, which are becoming increasingly neglected in this era of ultra-high-tech medicine; on the other hand, it is due to the awareness that many of the challenges still facing us today in the fight against disease call for a different approach from that adopted to date. In fact, the public at large and also the medical profession itself are becoming increasingly aware that modern medicine must come up with new means and new ideas for tackling problems such as the contamination of the environment by toxic agents, the ever-growing numbers of diseases induced by the increasingly potent drugs themselves, the degenerative diseases to which errors of diet or life-style contribute, allergies, autoimmunity and immune deficiency, large numbers of neurological and psychiatric diseases, psychosomatic disorders, and tumors. Despite the undoubted progress made over the past decades in these crucial fields of medicine, despite the fact that we so often hear of new "major break-throughs" paving the way towards achieving a definitive cure for this or that disease, and despite the fact that our knowledge of the intimate mechanisms of the various diseases has increased enormously as a result of the techniques of molecular biology, it has to be admitted that, as far as general practice and the vast majority of patients suffering from the above-mentioned diseases are concerned, the actual practical benefit of such knowledge is not exactly spectacular.

Anyone who denies that conventional medicine, in its large-scale application, currently finds itself in a kind of impasse is closing a blind eye to realty, which at every turn dramatically reveals this gap between scientific knowledge and practical results, or between outstanding diagnostic capability and poor curative means. Not only general practitioners, but also the specialists in many sectors are displaying a lack of confidence in the real ability of medicine to "heal" the sick [Muller, 1992]. Sophisticated systems are available for implementing investigations, therapies, treatments, monitoring operations, follow-ups, statistical analyses, but there are many more stumbling-blocks when it comes to healing patients. In view of the high standards of medical schools, this impasse cannot be ascribed to a lack of will-power, expertise, and commitment on the part of health care providers, just as it cannot be attributed to lack of means, if we consider the budgets which western societies devote to the public health sector. There is clearly something wrong with the system itself and this some-thing is not of a quantitative type (amount of knowledge, amount of re-sources), but is qualitative, having to do with the basic approach.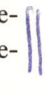

These observations do not lead to the conclusion, as people often mis-takenly claim, that the entire system has to be called into question; they merely serve to explain why an increasingly vast public is resorting to the use of the so-called alternative forms of medicine. One of the aims of this work is to show that there is no very substantial clash between scientific medicine and the empirical forms, the latter representing a kind of reser-voir of experience, insights, guesswork, and traditions, which, once they have been thoroughly vetted and rid of their spurious elements, may spear-head a process of renewal, which, though by no means easy or painless, is of interest to both medical science and medical practice.

That this is not merely a commercial phenomenon is also suggested by the fact that we are witnessing a renewed interest on the part of scientists in experimental trials in this field. Studies are beginning to appear on the biological effects of homeopathic drugs, as well as studies on the so-called "*high-dilution effect,*" or double-blind placebo-controlled clinical trials. The debate in scientific circles is becoming increasingly heated, and many researchers are setting themselves the objective of developing reliable methods for tackling the problem. For example, P. Turner, in an editorial in the journal *Human Toxicology* writes: "An explanation of the activity of homeopathic preparations might be found more readily if cellular or animal models could be developed for their investigation" [Turner, 1987, p. 267], and C.D. Berkowitz, in a commentary in the journal *Lancet* writes: "Despite these barriers to universal acceptance of homeopathy, physicians should maintain an open mind about potential benefits" [Berkowitz, 1994, p. 702]. Though the international allopathic literature still takes a very prudent stance, these are topical scientific problems which are addressed in international meetings not only of homeopathic specialists, but also of biochemists, physicists, and biologists (cf., for instance, the annual GIRI meetings, the 8th edition of which was in 1994).

Over the past few years there has been a growing demand for scientific explanation and rigorous clinical trials both from medical practitioners and from the health authorities. Unfortunately, we are faced with the considerable problem of the funding of the staff and institutions engaged in this activity. From the early 1960s research in the field of homeopathy has been boosted by the companies operating in the sector, who have started financing university institutes or setting up their own research laboratories [Majerus, 1991]. The main aims of the research are to test efficacy in double-blind controlled trials and to pinpoint the mechanism of action of the homeopathic drug at molecular, cellular and/or complex body systems level.

An important way to implement the dialogue between different medical systems is to develop a common homeopathic terminology to improve communication. Following the initiative of Dr. Gujardo-Bernal, an international group of experts suggested that a number of terms that are inaccurate, unclear, or have become outdated should be replaced by new terms. The main areas in which terminology should be updated are: concepts relating to homeopathic pharmacology, research, homeopathic medicine, the principle of similarity, homeostasis and disease imitation, miasms, experimental homeopathy, provings, and pathogenic trials [Gujardo-Bernal *et al.*, 1999].

3 *Is Homeopathy Effective?*

There still exists a great deal of skepticism in the field of conventional medicine as to the real efficacy of homeopathy, which is largely judged to be a kind of placebo treatment, or as a form of treatment which is, in any event, harmless. This skepticism is not entirely unjustified, inasmuch as it is due, on the one hand, to a lack of information about the problem, as already mentioned above in the Introduction, and, on the other, to an "epistemological" difficulty regarding the philosophical outlook and methodological approach apparently emerging from the mechanistic and reductive way of reasoning upon which medical thinking has been based for centuries (see Chapter 4, Section 5).

We have no intention here of claiming that there is not a placebo effect in homeopathy. This phenomenon is well known even with conventional treatments and is one of the main problems in research in the field of clinical pharmacology. In the particular homeopathic methodology, where the physician pays the utmost attention to the symptoms the patient complains of and to the patient's personal and family medical history, where a very profound relationship is set up between patient and doctor, and where numerous socio-cultural factors come into play (renewed interest in the health of the mind-body, concern for ecology, fear of drug toxicity, lack of confidence in the health system, and similar factors), the efficacy of therapy is obviously strongly influenced by subjective elements. There are, however, many signs that the placebo effect is not the only possible explanation for the action of homeopathic drugs. These signs are illustrated here below, according to two distinct lines of approach, one based on empirical evidence (Chapter 3, Section 1) and the other on clinical studies conducted in groups of patients (Chapter 3, Section 2).

An initial type of evidence of the efficacy of homeopathy is based on a series of data and experiences figuring in the tradition and reported in the homeopathic literature, which are not presented in the form of controlled clinical trials, but which may, all the same, be regarded as worthy of serious reflection and discussion. As emphasized elsewhere, the homeopathic tradition, though being the result essentially of an experimental approach, later came to devote little effort to conducting serious, well-documented clinical research. Much of the literature (materia medicas and repertories)

3.1

Empirical evidence

was compiled by particularly gifted homeopathic physicians, who compared the fruits of their many years of experience with the previous tradition and updated the growing store of homeopathic knowledge and remedies. These procedures owe their existence mainly to Hahnemann's early followers, and clearly one could not expect people in those days to adopt methodologies which were to become part and parcel of the heritage of medicine only many decades later. It is by no means an easy matter even to gain access today to the bibliographical sources so as to check on the type of documentation gathered in the construction of the vast homeopathic pharmacopoeia. Various authoritative modern homeopaths have embarked upon an updating of the homeopathic pharmacopoeia by *re-proving* many of the remedies it contains [Fuller Royal, 1991; Walach, 1993; Riley, 1994], using more modern methods.

In any event, we must refute the commonplace conviction that there is no extant documentation at all on these old homeopathic pharmacopoeias. As has been clearly shown by historical studies [Aulas and Chefdeville, 1984], at least 20 works by Hahnemann have been published, many of which in various editions updated on the basis of new experience, as well as dozens of articles and books by other experimenters who were either his coworkers or his contemporaries. The building of the edifice of homeopathy consisted in the progressive sedimentation, layer upon layer, of a vast number of contributions in the course of the nineteenth and early twentieth centuries, which, every so often, needed to be condensed by the founders of the various schools, such as Hering, Allen, Clarke, Jahr, Kent, and Vannier.

An innumerable series of articles, mostly reporting on the *provings* of new remedies or the effects of particular remedies in individual cases, were published in journals such as *Allgemeine Homöopatische Zeitung, Hygea, Biologische Medizin, Homotoxin Journal, Homöopatische Vierteljahrschrift, Proceedings of the American Institute of Homeopathy, American Homeopathic Review, Homeopathy, British Homeopathic Journal, Journal de la Societé Gallicane de Médecine Homéopathique, Annales Homéopathiques Françaises, Homéopathie Française, Cahiers de Biothérapie*, and many others with a more local readership.

Though not in themselves conclusive proof, two elements bearing witness to the essential soundness of the homeopathic approach are its longevity and its widespread use throughout the world. From a reading of various works on the subject it can be inferred, at least as regards the more commonly adopted remedies, that the materia medicas have undergone a "filtering" process on the basis of such a wealth of experience over so many years that any gross errors of indication or prescription would have been eliminated. It is hard to believe that certain remedies have continued throughout two centuries to be independently reported as being effective for certain disease situations by different schools of homeopathy in different continents. It is hard to imagine that even today fully qualified and practicing doctors with a modern university background, who are often specialists and are certainly not unaware of the existence of a placebo effect [Zala, 1994], would still continue to use a number of such remedies for certain diseases, unless they personally had found them to have a positive effect on their patients.

The use of placebo is also a current practice in homeopathy [Vithoulkas, 1980]. It is administered in the form of droplets or granules containing the diluent not treated with the active ingredient, in all those cases in which one seeks, after the first few visits, to highlight the changes (or presumed changes) in symptoms related to the patient's emotional susceptibility or to the effect of the relationship with the doctor himself. After a certain period of "treatment" with placebo, the patient is administered the remedy chosen on the basis of homeopathic principles and his or her reactions are observed. If the effects of drug and placebo were equivalent, on the basis of these procedures any homeopathic physician with a little experience should realize this.

Homeopathic treatment is also regarded as particularly effective and fast-acting in children. It is also true to say that children can be highly impressionable, but such rapid effects as those often observed in pediatric homeopathy on diseases which are not simply of a psychic or psychosomatic nature are hard to explain as being no more than a placebo effect.

Homeopathic remedies are commonly used in veterinary medicine. There are various books on the homeopathic treatment of dogs, cats, horses, and even cows. A number of experimental studies conducted in animals will be dealt with in Chapter 4. Although a certain amount of suggestion is also possible in animals, it seems somewhat unlikely that simple psychological support measures can heal an abscess in a cat, skin disorders in a horse or mastitis in a dairy cow, and that this should be observed not just once in a blue moon, but repeatedly.

As mentioned above, homeopathy became particularly popular in Europe and in the United States as a result of its successes in the course of major epidemics, as shown by newspaper reports at the time and the mortality records of hospitals [Teodonio and Negro, 1988; Haehl, 1989]. If these data are to be believed, it is most unlikely that they may have been the result of a placebo effect, not least because the same placebo effect should also have been produced by the other nonhomeopathic treatments.

Another consideration which is at variance with the placebo effect theory is the fact that when a person with a chronic disease receives a homeopathic drug, one fairly common observation is an exacerbation of the symptoms, i.e. the so-called *healing crisis* or *homeopathic aggravation* [Popova, 1991]. It is a temporary phenomenon, but may also be very intense and, according to homeopathic experience, the physician regards it as a very positive sign, which in no circumstances one should seek to suppress [Vithoulkas, 1980]. Placebo, on the other hand, usually has a symptom-improving effect. Another particularly suggestive phenomenon is the fact that one often observes the return of previously experienced symptoms in the course of homeopathic therapy, as though the therapy consisted in a "reversal" of the patient's disease history.

This phenomenon, which may sometimes be interpreted negatively by the patient, is again a very positive prognostic indicator in the resolution of complicated cases and denotes a return to past levels of disease experienced earlier in the patient's clinical history which has moved on from one form or stage of disease to another almost always of a severer nature. The reappearance of old symptoms (also called *regressive vicariation*) denotes that, under the effect of the homeopathic remedy, the patient is still capable of retracing the "false steps" he or she has taken and getting back to better levels of health. Recognition of such a phenomenon might suggest that the disease history of each individual patient is somehow related to a single pathobiological (or chronopathological) pathway and that there exists some kind of biochemical or neurohormonal "biological memory" persisting in the context of homeostatic system disorders.

3.2
Clinical
research

Certainly, all the above-mentioned considerations will hardly suffice to convince people who are used only to placing their trust in statistically significant, reproducible and strictly controlled clinical evidence. In the homeopathic literature, clinical research, as it is understood in modern medicine, has been contemplated only recently. The double-blind method is necessary to guarantee the significance of the results, but its application has often been considered impossible for ethical reasons (you cannot leave a sick person without some form of active treatment) or because it destroys the relationship of trust between doctor and patient, which is very important for the success of any therapy. Both in conventional medicine and even more so in complementary medicine, doctor, patient, and therapy cannot easily be split up into independent variables.

This problem might be overcome by performing the trial without an untreated group and comparing two groups of patients treated with different therapies, for instance conventional therapy and homeopathic therapy.

This approach might prove advantageous particularly in those fields in which patients happen to refuse conventional therapies for fear of side effects or for lack of confidence in their success. A second problem arises, however, namely the difficulty in finding physicians who have mastered both types of therapeutic strategy with a sufficient degree of skill to render any comparison reliable and significant.

Another reason (but not a justification) for the relative lack of clinical trials in homeopathy lies in the fact that it was, and is, practiced mainly on an outpatient basis by doctors working singly or in small groups. In addition to the difficulty of obtaining large enough patient samples, there is also the problem that a doctor can hardly afford to divide his patients into age- and sex-matched groups and then administer active treatment to one and placebo to the other; by so doing he could expect to lose at least half his clients (assuming the treatment really is effective). There is therefore an urgent need for double-blind trials conducted in large centers with sizeable patient samples or within the framework of programs agreed upon by groups comprising large numbers of doctors.

The most serious obstacle to clinical research in homeopathy is of a methodological nature, in that drug prescribing is based fundamentally on individual symptomatology and not so much on diagnosis of the actual disease. It is very likely that patients with the same disease, but with different histories, different vegetative reactivities, different types of constitution, and different symptom locations, will require different prescriptions. From the practical standpoint, this makes it very difficult to assess the efficacy of any single remedy for a given disease. Trials of this type, however, have been conducted, but, as we shall see, often with contrasting results.

A new approach appears to be more promising, namely, testing not the drug, but the homeopathic treatment as such. In practice, the homeopathic examination is carried out, the drug suited to each patient is prescribed, and then patients are randomized into two groups, only one of which receives the therapy opted for. By means of this system, the efficacy of the homeopathic method can be assessed in a given disease condition and one can establish statistically which drugs are often prescribed and prove efficacious in that disease.

At any rate, one point is certain: while the advocates of homeopathic therapies and natural therapies in general are largely convinced of the efficacy of these therapies on the basis of personal experience and their trust in more expert opinion leaders in homeopathy, if we wish to make any meaningful comparison between homeopathic and conventional medicine and achieve official recognition of such therapy, the conduct of methodologically correct clinical trials is absolutely mandatory. It is only in this way that convincing proof of the efficacy of any therapeutic measure, whether conventional or otherwise, can be had. A number of guidelines for clinical trials of this kind have already been suggested [Crapanne, 1985; Hornung, 1991; Haidvogl, 1994].

Although many clinical trials published to date are of low methodological quality, as acknowledged also by authoritative exponents of homeopathy [Hornung and Vogler, 1990; Hornung and Griebel, 1991], there is still a small but significant body of work reporting positive evidence in favor of the efficacy of homeopathic treatment in a number of conditions. As mentioned in the Introduction, a Dutch group [Kleijnen et al., 1991] have produced a review of 107 clinical trials in homeopathy on the basis of rigid assessment criteria of the type used for trials in the field of allopathic medicine: every trial was assigned a score resulting from the quality of the description of the patient characteristics, the number of patients included in the study population, the type of randomization implemented, the degree of clarity of the description of the methods, the adoption or otherwise of double-blindness, and the quality of the description of the results. On the basis of these criteria, 22 publications were judged to be of good quality (scores > 55/100). Fifteen of these reported positive results in favor of a homeopathic effect, in the sense that they revealed significant differences between treated and untreated (or placebo-treated) patients, whereas the other 7 yielded negative findings. In all, of the 105 trials whose results could be interpreted, 81 yielded positive results, while the remainder showed no significant difference in effect between homeopathic drugs and placebo.

Though Kleijnen et al.'s review is not comprehensive of all the studies conducted, the fact that it was published in a very authoritative journal with a very large readership prompts us to make reference to it here, indicating the scores assigned (out of a hundred) to the various studies referred to here below. An overview of the fields in which clinical trials in homeopathy have been conducted is provided in Table 1, which has been drawn up on the basis of the data reported in the above-mentioned review by Kleijnen.

This series of data leads the authors of the meta-analysis to suggest that "The evidence presented in this review would probably be sufficient for establishing homeopathy as a regular treatment for certain indications" [Kleijnen et al., 1991, p. 321].

Table 1 furnishes an estimate of the main indications and results of homeopathic therapy or at least of which sectors the investigators regard as the easiest for performing trials and obtaining significant results. We also

TABLE 1

Clinical trials in homeopathy [cited by Kleijnen *et al.*, 1991]

Diseases	Number of trials	Positive results/total
Cardiovascular disease	9	4/9
Respiratory infections	19	13/19
Other infections	7	6/7
Diseases of the gastro-intestinal system	7	5/7
Post-surgical ileus	7	5/7
Hay fever	5	5/5
Rheumatic disease	6	4/6
Trauma and/or pain	20	18/20
Psychological or mental problems	10	8/10
Other diagnoses	15	13/15

give details here of some of the more important studies, by way of examples, rather than attempting a complete review. We shall also refer to other studies not reviewed by Kleijnen *et al.* which are of historical interest or serve for later discussion as to the possible action mechanism of homeopathic remedies.

One of the first studies reported in the homeopathic literature was sponsored by the British government during World War II [Paterson, 1944; Scofield, 1984; score 41/100]. It was conducted in volunteers in whom skin burns were produced using azotized mustard gas and showed a significant improvement in subjects receiving *Mustard gas* 30c as prophylaxis (an example of isopathic treatment) or *Rhus tox* 30c (poison ivy) and *Kali bichromicum* 30c (bichromate of potash) as therapy. The study was conducted independently in two different centers (London and Glasgow) with similar results, and a double-blind placebo-controlled trial design was used.

A Scottish group [Gibson *et al.*, 1980] published a study in the *British Journal of Clinical Pharmacology* on the homeopathic treatment of rheumatoid arthritis (score 40/100) conducted at the Glasgow Homeopathic Hospital. Each patient received his or her own prescribed remedy, but half of them were treated with placebo. The results showed improvement of symptoms in 82 percent of patients treated, as against only 21 percent of those on placebo. The improvements were in terms of pain, articular index, and stiffness.

The field of rheumatic disease gives us an opportunity to see what types of controversies can be triggered by homeopathic research. For instance, a double-blind trial was conducted in patients suffering from fibrositis [Fisher, 1986; score 38/100]. The doctor had a choice between the three homeopathic drugs likely to be active in this condition (*Arnica* (mountain daisy), *Rhus tox* (poison ivy), and *Bryonia* (wild hops)). No difference was found between the groups treated with the remedy and those treated with placebo. However, the results were examined by a panel of expert homeopathic physicians who assessed the accuracy of the prescription, analyzing the match between the individual symptoms and the remedy received. On considering only the patients in this study population who had received the correct remedy according to homeopathic principles (see Chapter 2, Section 1), these showed a significant improvement compared to controls. A similar trial in fibrositis (primary fibromyalgia) was conducted in the Department of Rheumatology of St. Bartholomew's Hospital in London [Fisher *et al.*, 1989; score 45/100] and, amongst other things because it was published by the *British Medical Journal*, represents an interesting attempt to reconcile the need for a scientifically flawless protocol with the particular homeopathic methodology. The diagnosis was reached on the basis of the conventional diagnostic criteria defined by Yunus; the patients were then submitted to a homeopathic history taking and those for whom the remedy *Rhus toxicodendron* 6c (poison ivy) was indicated were included in the trial (this remedy is one of those most often prescribed for this type of disease). The trial was conducted double-blind versus placebo and with a cross-over design. After entry to the trial there was no contact between homeopath and patient. The results were positive in favor of the homeopathic treatment which brought about a reduction in pain symptoms.

A trial characterized by thoroughly negative results was conducted in osteoarthritis [Shipley *et al.*, 1983; score 50/100]. Patients suffering from this rheumatic disease were divided into three groups, one of which received *Rhus tox* 6x, one fenoprofen, and the third placebo. The results (published in *Lancet*) showed that only the group on fenoprofen had a significant improvement in symptoms as compared to the placebo-treated patients. Homeopathic physicians have responded to this experiment by pointing out that the strategy adopted was incorrect: using only one remedy for a disease instead of individualizing treatment according to the totality of the symptoms can be effective only in few conditions, and osteoarthritis is not one of them, also in view of the fact that *Rhus tox* is often prescribed in rheumatoid arthritis, but not in osteoarthritis [Ullman, 1991a]. Another objection is that it is inappropriate to compare a fast-acting drug (the antiinflammatory analgesic) and a slow-acting agent (the homeopathic medicine) [Ghosh, 1983; Scofield, 1984] over such a short time period.

Similar objections have also been made in relation to other trials [Savage and Roe, 1977 and 1978; scores 55/100 and 53/100, respectively]. These authors used a double-blind protocol to test the effect of *Arnica* 30c and *Arnica* 1M (mountain daisy) in stroke, but found no significant benefit from the treatment. However, an analysis of the results in a highly critical and objective review of homeopathic research [Scofield, 1984] showed that of the 40 patients entered into the 1977 study only three had the typical homeopathic symptom picture of *Arnica*, and these three showed good progress during homeopathic therapy. In the 1978 trial, only one patient presented typical *Arnica* symptoms and was included in the placebo group!

A double-blind study of the treatment of patients with hay fever was published in *Lancet* in 1986 [Taylor Reilly *et al.*, 1986; score 90/100]. The study compared the effects of a homeopathic preparation of 12 mixed pollens in the 30c dose with those of a placebo. The results were positive, in the sense that the patients on the homeopathic treatment had significantly fewer symptoms and used only half the amount of antihistamines compared to controls over the same period. The subject of this research was a typical example of *isopathy* (homeopathized pollens in hay fever). The report stirred up considerable controversy, not least because of the prestigious journal in which it was published.

The same group of researchers, in collaboration with statisticians and allopathic physicians, have published in the *Lancet* the findings of a study in 28 patients with severe atopic asthma (requiring daily administration of bronchodilators, steroid treatment also being needed in 21/28 cases) [Reilly *et al.*, 1994]. Without changing the basic therapy, the patients received a placebo for 4 weeks and were then randomized into two groups, one of which continuing with placebo, while the other was treated with a homeopathic preparation of the main allergen to which each patient had proven sensitive (most often, house dust mite). The patients recorded the intensity of the symptoms daily on a visual analogue scale. After another 4 weeks the data for the two groups were analyzed and active treatment was found to be superior to placebo, the difference being statistically significant.

A daily visual analogue scale of symptom intensity was the outcome measure, which revealed a favourable effect of homeopathic treatment (p=0.003). There were similar trends in the respiratory function and bronchial reactivity tests. A meta-analysis of all three trials conducted by the Reilly's group during many years of experience strengthened the evidence that homeopathy does more than a placebo (p=0.0004) [Taylor et al., 2000].

Homeopathic treatment of hay fever has also been the subject of reports by other investigators [Wiesenauer *et al.*, 1983; Wiesenauer and Gaus, 1985; scores 75/100 and 85/100, respectively]. In these cases, the type of treatment was very different: a low dilution (4x or 6x) of an extract of the plant *Galphimia glauca* was used. The results were assessed double-blind and were positive in favor of the homeopathic therapy.

The study by Wiesenauer and Gaus is also particularly interesting for another reason: this study compares *Galphimia glauca* 6x not only versus placebo but also versus *Galphimia glauca* 10^{-6}, i.e. an equivalent dose of the same drug prepared with simple dilution and not according to the homeopathic methodology. The simple dilution exhibits no activity, and, in any event, yields results no different to placebo. This observation, if confirmed (unfortunately, there are very few studies in which the problem has been tackled), would testify to the fact that by means of the particular preparation procedure used in homeopathy the drugs acquire therapeutic properties which are not attributable merely to the dose of active ingredient they contain.

Pain therapy of various kinds is one of the main fields of application of homeopathy. Among the more important trials we should mention those conducted by Brigo and coworkers in migraine [Brigo, 1987; Brigo and Serpelloni, 1991; score 68/100]. Slightly more than 100 patients with migraine underwent a classic homeopathic history taking. Sixty patients were then selected who, in the authors' opinion, offered greater guarantees of a correct choice of remedy, in other words those in whom they could be more confident that the *simillimum* had been found according to the rules of homeopathy. At that point, the patients were randomized double-blind, 30 to treatment with the homeopathic remedy (drugs such as *Belladonna* (deadly nightshade), *Gelsemium* (yellow jasmine), *Ignatia* (St. Ignatius' bean), *Cyclamen* (sowbread), *Lachesis* (venom of the bushmaster snake), *Natrum muriaticum* (sodium chloride), *Silicea* (silica), and *Sulphur* at the potency of 30c) and the other 30 to placebo. The patients periodically filled in a questionnaire on the frequency, intensity and characteristics of the pain symptoms. After the treatment, which lasted for a few months, results were compared and were found to be distinctly and significantly better in the group receiving the homeopathic remedies. On account of its precise methodology, this study has been much appreciated both by the homeopathic [Hornung, 1991; Hornung and Griebel, 1991] and nonhomeopathic communities.

A double-blind study was conducted in patients with dental neuralgic pain following tooth extraction [Albertini and Goldberg, 1986; score 38/100]. In cases such as these, where the lesion is acute and well localized it is more likely that a single treatment based mainly on local symptoms will be effective. Thirty patients were given *Arnica* 7c (mountain daisy) and *Hypericum* 15c (St. John's wort) prescribed alternately at 4 hour intervals, while 30 others were given a placebo. As many as 76 percent of the patients treated with the homeopathic remedies experienced pain relief as against only 40 percent of those on placebo.

The pain caused by a sprained ankle is significantly relieved and shortened by homeopathic treatment, administered in the form of therapy of the homotoxicological type (*Traumeel* ointment: a combination of 14 different substances in 2x-6x dilutions), according to one report in the literature [Zell *et al.*, 1988; score 80/100]. Of 33 patients treated, 24 were pain-free on treatment day 10, whereas on the same day only 13/36 on placebo had no pain. The same drug (*Traumeel*, also called *Arnica compositum* today in other pharmacopoeias) has also been experimented with in a more recent trial [Thiel and Bohro, 1991]. The authors demonstrated that the intra-articular injection of the homeopathic remedy in patients with traumatic hemarthrosis significantly reduced healing time (as compared to the group treated with placebo), assessed on the basis of objective parameters (presence of blood in synovial fluid, articular circumference, motility).

Homeopathy has also been used in the preparation for childbirth in a study by Dorfman and coworkers [Dorfman *et al.*, 1987; score 80/110]. A combination of *Caulophyllum* (blue cohosh), *Arnica* (mountain daisy), *Actea racemosa* (black snakeroot), *Pulsatilla* (windflower), and *Gelsemium* (yellow jasmine) (all 5c remedies, twice daily throughout the ninth month of pregnancy) was compared with a placebo in a double-blind study. The efficacy of the homeopathic treatment clearly emerged from the fact that the duration of labor was reduced (5.1 vs. 8.5 hours, $p < 0.001$), as was the percentage of dystocia (11.3 vs. 40%, $p < 0.01$).

In another study, *Caulophyllum* 7c was administered during the active phase of the labor in a group of healthy mothers (5 granules per hour repeated for a maximum of 4 hours). The duration of the labor (period of cervical dilatation) was significantly reduced in treated women (227 minutes versus 314 minutes) as compared to a group of labors retrospectively selected by the same criteria [Eid *et al.*, 1993]. The same result was confirmed more recently in a double-blind trial [Eid *et al.*, 1994].

As regards the action of *Arnica*, which is a remedy much used in homeopathy, there is an interesting study conducted by the Institute of Surgical Pathology of the University of Catania, which is worthy of mention [Amodeo *et al.*, 1988]. *Arnica montana* 5c was administered to patients subjected to prolonged venous perfusion, a condition which easily leads to phlebitis in the veins used. This study, which used the double-blind, placebo-controlled method, showed that *Arnica* reduced the pain symptoms, the inflammatory manifestations (hyperaemia and edema), and also the formation of hematomas. Furthermore, an improvement in blood flow (as measured by Doppler flowmetry) was also observed in the treated patients as well as a slight increase in a number of coagulation factors and in platelet aggregation.

A series of studies have revealed a positive effect of homeopathic treatment, based essentially on the use of *Opium* and *Raphanus sativus* (common radish), in shortening the time to resumption of intestinal transit postoperatively [Chevrel *et al.*, 1984; Aulagnier, 1985; scores 50/100 and 75/100, respectively]. In the wake of these reports, a multicenter study was conducted with the collaboration of homeopathic and nonhomeopathic physicians, epidemiologists, surgeons, and the French Laboratoire National de la Santé [Mayaux *et al.*, 1988; score 90/100; GRECHO, 1989]. This trial conducted in a population of 600 patients yielded negative results and led the authors to conclude that the postoperative resumption of intestinal transit should not to be regarded as an indication either for *Opium* or for *Raphanus* (used in this study at the 15c dilution).

As far as homeopathy in general is concerned, one interesting aspect is the issue raised in the Discussion regarding the individualization of the treatment; clearly, as the same two drugs were used in all cases, the classic procedure of homeopathy was not adhered to, though from the point of view of the local symptoms (gastrointestinal) the treatment was in conformity with the law of similars, inasmuch as *Opium* at high doses causes an intestinal atonia in healthy subjects and *Raphanus* a painful abdominal flatulence due to gas retention.

In conclusion, then, this report was certainly an object lesson for homeopaths: clearly, to the best of our current knowledge, inexplicable effects can be accepted only on the basis of trials conducted with impeccable methodology, using methods which, above all, are repeatable in several different independent centers. We still have a long way to go in clinical research in homeopathy, and anyone who is interested in this topic must resign himself to seeing both negative and positive studies published, as in any other field in which research is done seriously. In the case of homeopathy, particularly when the subject of the research is not homeopathic treatment as such, but a certain drug or group of drugs in a certain disease condition, the results will always be affected by variables related to the doses, administration modalities, individual sensitivities, types of pharmacopoeia. If the present tendency towards an increase in number and quality of publications is confirmed, the patient and methodical evaluation of the results, even when negative, cannot help but prove beneficial in the long run for the practice of homeopathy, if for no other reason than to avoid errors at the expense of the patients.

A randomized double-blind trial comparing homeopathic medicine with placebo in the treatment of acute childhood diarrhea was conducted in Nicaragua and published in a major American medical journal [Jacobs *et al.*, 1994]. An individualized homeopathic medicine (or placebo in the control group) was prescribed for each child in addition to the standard oral rehydration treatment. Eighteen different medicines (30c potency) were prescribed, the most common being *Podophyllum, Chamomilla, Arsenicum album, Calcarea carbonica*, and *Sulphur*. The results indicated that the treatment group (43 cases) had a statistically significant ($p < 0.05$) decrease in duration and intensity of diarrhea with respect to the control group (44 cases).

Respiratory tract infections are another sector in which homeopathic products are extensively used, and various studies have demonstrated their efficacy. One of the first was the study by Gassinger and coworkers [Gassinger *et al.*, 1981; score 58/100], which also represents a curious variant of experimental methodology. The authors compare the effect of *Eupatorium perfoliatum* 2x (boneset) with that of acetylsalicylic acid (ASA) in the common cold. Neither the subjective symptoms, nor body temperature, nor laboratory data showed any significant differences in the two groups, which led the authors to conclude that the homeopathic treatment was as effective as the allopathic treatment. Unfortunately, there was no placebo group in the study, which would have lent greater weight to the conclusions drawn.

Results similar to those obtained in this study were reported by researchers from the Medical Clinic of the University of Würzburg and from the Institute of Biometry of the University of Tübingen [Maiwald *et al.*, 1988; score 65/100]. In a simple blind randomized trial in 170 soldiers in the Germany army suffering from influenza and treated with ASA (500 mg x 3/day for the first 4 days and then once daily) or with a complex homeopathic preparation called *Grippheel* (*Aconitum* 4x (monkshood), *Bryonia* 4x (wild hops), *Lachesis* 12x (venom of the bushmaster snake), *Eupatorium perfoliatum* (boneset) 3x, *Phosphorus* 5x in tablet form x 3/day), comparison between the changes in clinical status and in subjective disorders on days 4 and 10 and between the duration of the periods off work in the two groups revealed no significant differences, leading to the conclusion that the two drugs are equieffective.

For the purposes of illustrating a typical example of the reasoning underlying combination homeopathy (or homotoxicology), we quote the conclusions of the study by Maiwald and coworkers [Maiwald *et al.*, 1988] in the part where they discuss the reasons prompting one to prefer the use of a particular homeopathic preparation for the cure of influenza (for the sake of brevity, any quotations in the text have been omitted): "The efficacy of ASA is due to its symptomatic, analgesic and antipyretic action, and to nonspecific inhibition of inflammation via blockade of prostaglandin synthesis. The use of an antipyretic in cases of influenza may also have negative effects, since the increase in body temperature inhibits proliferation of the virus. Against this antagonistic, suppressive therapy with ASA is set regulatory therapy with *Grippheel*, which stimulates the self-regulation mechanisms of the body in order to normalize the impaired functions. The prerequisite for this is therefore an intact reactivity on the part of the body. The regulatory therapy introduces, amongst other things, a para-immunity, that is to say, within a few hours it produces an increase in the nonspecific defenses which may last for a number of weeks. There is, above all, an increase in the phagocytosis index. In addition, there is stimulation of humoral factors, cell enzymes, the lymphopoietic system (especially T lymphocytes), cell-mediated cytotoxicity, monocyte lytic activity, and production or release of interferon. This activation does not leave any specific memory when the physiological functions return to normal. The use of a homeopathic preparation, which ensures such substantial efficacy with very low concentrations of active ingredients, is undoubtedly to be preferred to an antipyretic and its suppressive effects - all the more so if the effects of the homeopathic preparation and the synthetic drug prove to be of comparable efficacy in influenza" [Maiwald *et al.*, 1988, p. 581].

Ferley and coworkers [Ferley *et al.*, 1987; score 68/100; Ferley *et al.*, 1989; score 88/100] have also used homeopathic complexes in the treatment of influenza. The first of their two studies evaluated a treatment based on the methods of low-dilution combination pharmacology (a combination of 10 substances at dilutions of 1x-6x). The incidence and duration of the symptoms were no different in the group of 599 patients treated with the complex compared to 594 patients treated with placebo. The second study, on the other hand, used a unique homeopathic preparation, which, however, is very widely used, particularly in France, called *Oscillococcinum*, consisting essentially of a high Korsakovian dilution (200K) of *Anas barbariae* (duck) liver and heart extract. However strange it may seem, the study demonstrated a positive effect of the active drug treatment, in that it significantly increased the number of cures within 48 hours of diagnosis. Even more singular is the fact that the paper was published by an important nonhomeopathic journal. Probably, the soundness of the methodology and the large size of the patient sample (237 patients treated with *Oscillococcinum*, 241 with placebo) made it very hard to contest the authors' findings.

Despite the paradoxical nature of this result, modern epidemiological research appears to offer a number of rational arguments in support of its possible efficacy. Many birds today, particularly aquatic ones, are known to present asymptomatic infections due to influenza virus A, conveyed by the waters of lakes and pools in which the virus can remain viable for days or weeks. In particular, wild and domesticated ducks appear to be the natural reservoir of the virus, which is then transmitted to humans via the pig [Fields and Knipe, 1990]. It has yet to be established whether or not the liver may be a point which is certain to be infected by the virus, though this is likely in view of the intestinal site of the infection. In any event, the analogy between homeopathic empiricism and modern virological research suggests the existence of possible points of contact between the two approaches and pathways for future research.

A recent literature review of the clinical effects of *Oscillococcinum* [Vickers and Smith, 2000] showed that this medicine probably reduces the duration of illness in patients presenting with influenza symptoms. However, the Authors concluded that though promising, the data are not strong enough to make a general recommendation for its use in first-line treatment of influenza and influenza-like syndromes. Current evidence does not support a preventative effect of *Oscillococcinum* in these syndromes.

Clinical trials are more likely to be published when they are positive than when they are negative (this is true both of homeopathic and allopathic therapies). Nevertheless, even negative results have their own intrinsic importance, both in practical terms (they inhibit the use of drugs which have been shown to be ineffective) and on the conceptual plane (they oblige researchers to revise their theories). In the homeopathic field, too, this idea is now rightly beginning to gain ground [Fisher, 1990], and, where applied, bears witness to the seriousness of the researchers concerned. For example, in the influenza sector, we feel we should mention the work of Lewith and coworkers [Lewith *et al.*, 1989; score 55/100], who unsuccessfully attempted an approach to influenza therapy based on homeopathic dilutions of the influenza vaccine, and that of Wiesenauer and coworkers [Wiesenauer *et al.*, 1989; score 60/100], who demonstrated the inefficacy, in the therapy of sinusitis, of a number of remedies prepared from various combinations of *Luffa opercolata* (dishcloth gourd), *Kalium bichromicum* (bichromate of potash), and *Cinnabaris* (cinnabar) (in 3x-4x dilutions).

Lastly, to remain in the field of respiratory tract infections, we should cite a French study [Bordes and Dorfman, 1986], which is methodologically sound (score 70/100); the authors treated dry or hacking cough with a syrup based on the plant *Drosera* (sundew) and 9 other substances in 3c dilution, demonstrating an excellent effect of the treatment compared to placebo: after one week's therapy, the symptom was reduced or disappeared in 20 out of 30 patients treated as compared to only 8/30 patients on placebo. This type of therapy of dry cough is another example of how the homeopathic approach has proven capable of changing and breaking down even into very different variants. However much cough in classic homeopathy might constitute an indication for *Drosera*, Hahnemann would have been strongly opposed to a therapy, the express purpose of which was the suppression of a symptom, and above all if it were based on a mixture of many substances to be administered to all patients indiscriminately. The concern of classic homeopathy in this regard is not unfounded: on the one hand, if the aim is to suppress the symptoms, there is a risk of thwarting the reactions of natural healing (e.g. expectoration to eliminate microbial agents), and, on the other, by administering a complex therapy, one deprives oneself of the possibility of establishing, on the strength of scientifically rigorous criteria, which of the substances used is effectively responsible for any improvement observed.

The reply to these objections is based on arguments of various kinds. From the practical standpoint, if a drug works it is only logical and advantageous to administer it (the dominant criterion in allopathic pharmacology); from the logical and scientific points of view, it is possible and indeed probable that the effect of a complex of substances at low doses will not be attributable to one or more of the individual constituents, but to the synergistic action of many of them. It might also be claimed that, admitting that different patients with the same symptom (e.g. cough) need different homeopathic remedies, if we use a complex of many remedies, the likelihood increases that these will include the right one for each individual patient, whereas the other remedies in the complex will have no effect on account of their low doses.

As far as the homeopathic treatment of tumors is concerned, - a subject obviously of great interest and one upon which major problems of a scientific, economic, and ethical nature hinge, - the homeopathic literature is very cautious and, above all, presents a distinct shortage of truly significant data. The homeopathic literature in this field undeniably finds itself in considerable difficulty: on the one hand, it is claimed that homeopathic therapy, being aimed at the individual as a whole, may offer a complex of back-up measures in support of conventional therapy; on the other, criticism is often voiced particularly with regard to the use of radio- and chemotherapy, accused of being excessively toxic and thus of exerting a destructive effect on the "vital force." It frequently happens, in fact, that cancer patients, often at the terminal stage, where they have abandoned all hope or trust in conventional therapies, turn to the homeopath as the last resort. Needless to say, in such cases, in addition to the obvious ethical problems related to the administration of empirical therapies to these patients, it is liable to be difficult or even impossible to interpret the results outside the framework of evaluation in very large patient series.

Nevertheless, the problem of advanced cancer care in most cases is not solved even by conventional therapies, and experimentation with new therapeutic approaches according to precise criteria is not only legitimate but appears necessary and urgently required. For the purposes of initiating the systematic collection of the documentation on homeopathic case series in oncology an international project has been launched under the guidance of the Department of Naturopathy of the University of Berlin [Hornung and Vogler, 1990].

Homeopathy can hardly have as its objective the struggle against tumors and their cells, both as a matter of principle (curing the patient and not the disease) and on account of its therapeutic armamentarium, consisting mostly of drugs at low and very low doses. This does not mean that homeopathy has no role to play in the therapy of tumors. The recent revival of interest of medical science in immunotherapy suggests that directing attention to the host and not just to the disease may prove useful and effective. Moreover, among the drugs introduced into the homeopathic or homotoxicological armamentarium by a number of schools there is *Viscum album* (poison-weed) at low dilutions. This drug has been analyzed in both clinical and laboratory research and has been shown to be effective both as an immunostimulant and as an inhibitor of cell proliferation *in vitro* [Anderson and Phillipson, 1982; Koopman *et al.*, 1990]. The problem of conventional and nonconventional therapy of tumors will be dealt with in greater detail in Chapters 5 and 6. We shall confine our attention here to mentioning a few published studies, bearing in mind that these are not controlled clinical trials, but case reports. They are therefore of value as interesting material for discussion regarding future lines of research in this field.

Drossou [Drossou *et al.*, 1990] reports on two cases of leukemia in which, at the patient's strict behest, the only treatment was classic homeopathic therapy (administration of the *simillimum* according to Hahnemann's precepts). One patient suffering from acute myeloblastic leukemia (FAB: M4) was treated with *Thuja* 200c (arbor vitae); the therapy was then changed, when indicated, to *Mercurius cyanatus* 200c (cyanide of mercury), *Picric acid* 200c, *Natrum muriaticum* 200c (sodium chloride), *Ceanothus* (New Jersey tea), *Crotalus horridus* (rattlesnake venom), and *Ignatia* (St. Ignatius' bean) 1M. The treatment lasted 22 months, but after as little as 6 months hematocrit had reverted to normal and after one year all examination parameters were within normal limits. The patient suffered no recurrence over the following three years. Equally favorable was the homeopathic treatment of the second patient, who was suffering from chronic lymphatic (B lymphocyte) leukemia. At diagnosis this patient had 64,000 leukocytes/mm³, 86% lymphocytes. He was given *Natrum muriaticum* 200c, and then *Arnica* 30c, *Ignatia* 1M, *Zincum* 200c. Five months after the start of treatment the leukocyte count was 12,000/mm³, 25% lymphocytes. After 9 months all clinical and laboratory data were normal. The treatment lasted 21 months and no recurrence occurred over the following 3 years. This study is also of interest on account of a number of comments which the authors make in the Discussion: they assert that the homeopathic history taking revealed major psychological problems both on account of the patients' natural emotional sensitivity and owing to the type of reaction to learning the diagnosis. The homeopathic treatment solved these problems in the very first few months, along with other lesser problems such as condylomata acuminata in one patient and gastritis in the other. The authors claim to have treated many patients with leukemia, but they achieved their best results in the two cases reported, who were the only ones who opted solely for homeopathic treatment. Those patients who were receiving concomitant chemo- or radiotherapy were highly debilitated and it was difficult to identify in the symptoms the patient's particular "idiosyncrasy," since this was masked by the effects of the cytotoxic therapy.

A paper published in the journal *Thorax* [Bradley and Clover, 1989] reports on a patient suffering from small-cell lung cancer, which is notoriously a very aggressive tumor with a median survival of 6-17 weeks. The tumor was treated with radiotherapy, and the patient then refused chemotherapy, opting rather for a homeopathic cure. He was given various remedies according to his symptoms (unfortunately not specified in the report) and an extract of *Viscum album* (*Iscador*). He survived for 5 years and 7 months after diagnosis of the cancer. The authors stress the unusually long survival time and the potential importance of natural therapies in these cases, though obviously they could not attribute this result with certainty to classic homeopathic therapy, to the use of *Iscador*, or to any other single factor.

To sum up, then, we can draw the following conclusions from the clinical trials conducted to date:

a) Homeopathic treatment has proven effective in many controlled clinical trials, whereas other studies have yielded negative results, indicating that, from the experimental point of view, homeopathy can be treated like any other form of therapy. In particular, the fields of application and the limits of the homeopathic approach can be indicated.

b) The usefulness of homeopathic treatment has been explored primarily in the therapy of inflammatory and infectious syndromes, traumas, pain in general, and psychological disorders.

c) The double-blind, placebo-controlled study method can be applied and adjusted to the particular demands of homeopathic research (individualization, use of different remedies for the same disease, particular patient-physician relationship).

In the past few years a number of new reports on the clinical effects of homeopathy have appeared. Some of them gave positive or partially positive results [Hill *et al.*, 1995; Wiesenauer and Ludtke, 1996; Weiser *et al.*, 1998; 1999; Thompson *et al.*, 1998; Rastogi *et al.*, 1999; Harrison *et al.*, 1999; Chapman et al., 1999; Balzarini *et al.*, 2000; Jacobs *et al.*, 2000; Straumsheim *et al.*, 2000; Taylor *et al.*, 2000; van Haselen and Fisher, 2000; Oberbaum *et al.*, 2001; Yakir *et al.*, 2001; Jacobs et al, 2001; Stam *et al.*, 2001], others gave negative ones (no statistically significant effect over placebo) [Lokken *et al.*, 1995; Kainz *et al.*, 1996; Hart *et al.*, 1997; Whitmarsh *et al.*, 1997; Vickers *et al.*, 1998; Walach *et al.*, 1997; 2001; Goodyear *et al.*, 1998; Simpson *et al.*, 1998; Smolle, 1998; Vickers *et al.*, 1998; Ramelet *et al.*, 2000; Aabel, 2000]. The controlled clinical trials have been summarized in various reviews and meta-analyses [Melchart *et al.*, 1995; Linde *et al.*, 1997; 1998; 1999; 2001; Ernst and Pittler, 1998; Ernst and Rand, 1998; Vickers, 1999; Cucherat *et al.*, 2000; Jonas *et al.*, 2000; Linde and Jobst, 2000; Vickers and Smith, 2000; Pittler *et al.*, 2000; Long and Ernst, 2001].

The problem of possible adverse effects of homeopathic drugs has also been reviewed [Dantas and Rampes, 2000]. The authors concluded that homeopathic medicines in high dilutions, prescribed by trained professionals, are probably safe and unlikely to provoke severe adverse reactions.

Moreover, a new promising line of study that emerged in the last few years is based on prospective data collection and observational studies. This type of clinical research is increasingly utilized—also in conventional medicine—because observational studies provide the advantage of respecting with greater ease the actual methods and the conditions where therapies are applied. This is especially relevant in fields like homeopathy where the medicine is still applied in private practice and not in hospitals. Several observational studies have shown positive outcomes of homeopathic therapy, not only on clinical symptoms but also on patients' quality of life [Zorian *et al.*, 1998; Hochstrasser, 1999; Whiteford, 1999; Adler *et al.*, 1999; Attena *et al.*, 2000; Colin, 2000; Heger *et al.*, 2000; Walach and Gutlin, 2000; Muscari-Tomaioli *et al.*, 2001; Riley *et al.*, 2001].

4 *Animal Studies and Laboratory Research*

The idea that at least some of the principles of homeopathy can be subjected to experimental vetting is making headway both in the homeopathic setting and among researchers in the biological, immunological, and biochemical fields. Evidence obtained for the first time in actual experiments in animals, or in isolated organ systems, or in cells *in vitro* has been accumulating [Guillemain *et al.*, 1987; Poitevin, 1988a; Poitevin, 1988c; Bastide, 1989; Fisher, 1989; Rubik, 1989; Bellavite, 1990a; Poitevin, 1990; Bastide, 1994; Righetti, 1994; see also appendix n. 1].

The crucial role which research studies in *in vivo* and *in vitro* experimental models can play in the phase of the development of homeopathy is universally recognized. Studies of this type, in fact, free themselves of the philosophical and methodological constraints of classic homeopathy and become part and parcel of the scientific paradigm dominant today. In this context, if the research studies are conducted with correct methods and yield results which are reproducible in different laboratories, then they cannot be refuted on the basis of arguments such as the placebo effect or simply dismissed as being inexplicable.

4.1
Experiments in animals and in healthy human subjects

As in conventional research, animal models are also used in the field of homeopathy both for testing the principle of dilution/dynamization and for studying the possible mechanism of action of homeopathic remedies in a thorough and repeatable manner, as well as for discovering remedies to be used in the veterinary context.

In this chapter we report on some of the main studies conducted in this field. We wish to point out that the fact that we refer to such studies does not imply that we endorse or support them. Moreover, we are fully aware of the problems associated with certain animal studies and hope that such research be performed only when strictly necessary and avoiding inflicting unnecessary suffering or torture upon the animals.

In toxicology, an attempt has been made to investigate whether high dilutions of a toxic substance are capable of modifying either its elimination or its consequences. A number of studies have demonstrated that a seven hundredth or 7c dilution (approximately 10^{-14} M, in terms of molar concentration) of arsenic and bismuth is capable of increasing the urinary elimination of these same metals by rats intoxicated with them [Lapp *et al.*,

1955; Wurmser and Ney, 1955; Cazin *et al.*, 1987]. The arsenic had no effect on bismuth intoxication and vice versa, indicating specificity of action.

This property has not been observed with lead, in that high dilutions of this metal failed to modify the excretion kinetics of lead in rats [Fisher *et al.*, 1987]. The arsenic experiments have been repeated more recently using more updated and controlled methods [Cazin *et al.*, 1991]; the results were substantially the same: intraperitoneal injections of arsenic (as arsenic trioxide, As_2O_3, or arsenic acid, H_3AsO_3), diluted and dynamized, reduced the blood levels, and increased the excretion of arsenic in rats treated with high doses (10 mg/kg) of arsenic trioxide. In a series of dilutions tested (5c, 7c, 9c, 11c, 13c, 15c, 17c, 19c, 21c, 23c, 25c, 27c, 29c, 31c), the most active dilutions in the protective sense were 7c and 17c, and the difference versus dilutions of dynamized water alone was highly significant. It is of interest to note that the protective effect of the high dilutions was abolished if they were subjected to heating to 120 degrees for 30 minutes.

On the basis of the analogy existing on both the biological and anatomico-pathological planes between carbon tetrachloride (CCl_4) intoxication and phosphorus intoxication, the Bildet group have demonstrated the protective effect of high dilutions (7c and 15c) of phosphorus and of the 7c dilution of carbon tetrachloride on CCl_4-induced toxic hepatitis in the rat [Bildet *et al.*, 1975; Bildet *et al.*, 1984a; Bildet *et al.*, 1984b].

The effect of high dilutions of CCl_4 confirmed similar data reported in the nonhomeopathic literature, testifying to an increased resistance of the liver after treatment with low doses of a toxic agent [Ugazio *et al.*, 1972; Pound *et al.*, 1973]. It has also been reported that small doses of cadmium reduce the renal toxicity caused by that metal in the rat [Bascands *et al.*, 1990]. It is likely that a synthesis inducing mechanism (of so-called *stress proteins*) or a mechanism increasing the enzyme activity of the detoxification systems may play some role in this type of phenomenon.

According to the findings of another group of researchers (published in the form of preliminary results), the mortality of rats treated with lethal doses of a-amanitine (the poison of the mushroom *Amanita phalloides*) is significantly slowed (in the sense of protection in the early days after administration of the poison) by treatment of the rats with 15c dilutions of a-amanitine, *Phosphorus*, and rifampicin [Guillemain *et al.*, 1987]. According to these authors, the use of these substances in the therapy of liver intoxication corresponds to the homeopathic rationale of curing disease by means of small doses of the same poisonous substance, as in the case of amanitine, or of substances with similar toxicity in the more general sense of the term.

Phosphorus is known to be hepatotoxic at high doses, whereas rifampicin may be similar to amanitine in terms of mechanism of action (inhibition of enzymatic activity such as that of RNA polymerase). Further results have been reported bearing witness to a protective effect of *Phosphorus* 30c on fibrosis of the liver caused by chronic administration of CCl_4 in rats [Palmerini *et al.*, 1993]; the therapeutic effect of *Phosphorus* was also documented as a decrease in serum hepatic enzymes compared to a group of untreated rats.

In another study [Cambar et al, 1983; Guillemain *et al.*, 1984], a nephrotoxicity model was used: rats treated with 9c and 15c dilutions of *Mercurius corrosivus* (corrosive sublimate) were significantly protected, in terms of reduced mortality, against the toxicity of medium-to-high doses (5-6 mg/kg) of mercury.

A well-defined protocol of experimental carcinogenesis in rats has been utilized to test the effect of highly diluted carcinogens and tumor promoters on the development of carcinomas caused by high doses of the same agents [De Gerlache and Lans, 1991]. Briefly, a large percentage of rats which received in their diet 2-acetylaminofluorene (0.03% for 21 days) and phenobarbital (0.05% for 12 months) developed hepatocellular carcinomas after 9-20 months. Treatment of the animals with 2-acetyl-aminofluorene 9c or with phenobarbital 9c (added to the drinking water, where the final concentration was about 2×10^{-19} M) significantly reduced and delayed the development of liver tumors with respect to a control group which received only the solvent diluted and dynamized. The authors concluded that this is the first reported observation of a significant effect obtained with treatments of this nature on a large experimental basis, even if these results need further confirmation by other experimentalists to be fully demonstrative.

According to the research by Cier and coworkers [Cier *et al.*, 1966] in the mouse, the administration of *Alloxan* 9c partly inhibits the diabetogenic effect of a dose of 40 mg/kg of alloxan. This effect was obtained both with preventive and curative (i.e. after the diabetogenic injection) administration.

The observation that high dilutions (7c-9c) of bee venom (currently used in homeopathy for skin manifestations with edema, erythema, and itching) had a protective and roughly 50 percent curative effect on X-ray-induced erythema in the albino guinea-pig [Bastide *et al.*, 1975; Poitevin, 1988b; Bildet *et al.*, 1990] appears to confirm the principle of similarity of reaction which underlies homeopathy. Bee venom, which at high doses (bee stings) causes edema and erythema, is capable, at given dilutions, of curing an edema or an erythema caused by some other agent. The fact that such results are in agreement with biological studies on isolated cells, demonstrating that *Apis* 7c (crushed bee) blocks the activation of basophils *in vitro* is significant (see Chapter 4, Section 3).

Following the same line of studies, the effect of homeopathic preparations of histamine on edema of the foot in the rat, induced by the injection of inflammatory doses (0.1 mg) of histamine, has been investigated. Using this model, a small, but significant inhibitory effect of high dilutions of histamine (up to 30x), administered intraperitoneally to rats 30 minutes before and at the same time as histamine injection in the paw, was noted [Conforti *et al.*, 1993].

Another series of studies examines the action of high dilutions of silica on the production of platelet activating factor (PAF) by peritoneal macrophages in the mouse [Davenas *et al.*, 1987]. The compound was added to drinking water at the 9c dilution (corresponding to a theoretical concentration of 1.66×10^{-19} M) for 25 days. The peritoneal macrophages extracted from the mice thus treated showed a PAF production capability in response to a stimulus with yeast extracts which was 30 to 60 per cent greater than that of control macrophages (untreated mice, mice treated with NaCl in 9c dilution or with another homeopathic drug, *Gelsemium* 9c). Lower dilutions (5c) paradoxically had less effect.

Homeopathic dilutions of silica are widely used in homeopathy for the treatment of sores, chronic ulcers, and abscesses. An experimental model in animals, based on the repair of holes pierced in the ears of mice, was used by a group of investigators in Rehovot (Israel): they reported that high dilutions of silica (up to 200c), added to drinking water for 4-20 days according to the particular experiment, heal the lesions faster and bring about a greater reduction in their size than sodium chloride solutions used as a control [Oberbaum *et al.*, 1991; Oberbaum *et al.*, 1992].

Bastide's group [Doucet-Jaboeuf *et al.*, 1982; Doucet-Jaboeuf *et al.*, 1984; Bastide *et al.*, 1985; Doucet-Jaboeuf *et al.*, 1985; Bastide *et al.*, 1987; Guillemain *et al.*, 1987; Daurat *et al.*, 1988] have shown the immunostimulatory effect in mice of endogenous compounds such as thymic hormones and interferons prepared in high dilutions according to homeopathic procedures. Among the many experiments reported, particularly worthy of note are those describing the effects of high dilutions of a-b interferon ($8-16 \times 10^{-10}$ IU i.p.) and thymic hormones (8×10^{-8} pg i.p.) on parameters of humoral (number of plaque-forming cells) and cellular (allospecific cytotoxic T-cell response) immunity. The authors then suggested that to achieve good therapeutic efficacy in immunodepressed patients these immunity mediators might be used in extremely low doses [Bastide *et al.*, 1985].

From the studies conducted by this group, another interesting result emerges to illustrate one of the most significant problems of homeopathic research: the pathophysiological state of the experimental animal powerfully conditions the results of any given treatment. This prompted the investigators to assess the effect of homeopathic dilutions (from 4c to 12c) of thymus and thymuline on mice of the Swiss strain, considered immunologically normal, and mice of the New Zealand Black (NZB) strain, considered immunologically depressed. The treatment caused significant immunostimulation only in the NZB mice, whereas the Swiss mice underwent immunodepression (particularly marked with the dilutions of thymus) [Guillemain *et al.*, 1987; Daurat *et al.*, 1988].

Other findings worthy of note in the field of immunomodulatory research are those reported by Bentwich and coworkers [Weisman *et al.*, 1991; Bentwich *et al.*, 1993]. After previously demonstrating that very small amounts (6c and 7c dilutions) of KLH (hemocyanin) antigen are capable of specifically modulating the antibody response in experimental animals [Toper *et al.*, 1990], they repeated and expanded on the experiments by showing the immunomodulatory effects of homeopathic dilutions of the antigen in mice. The animals were preconditioned for 8 weeks with i.p. injections of dynamized dilutions of KLH antigen (from 10^{-14} M to 10^{-36} M) and of saline (control). They were then regularly immunized with KLH dissolved in complete or incomplete Freund's adjuvant. Serum levels of specific antibodies were determined by immunoassay and the results showed a significant increase in specific IgM response with all the preconditioning dilutions, as well as a significant increase in specific IgG response in animals pretreated with KLH 10^{-36} M. The authors conclude that extremely small amounts of antigen are enough for specific immunomodulation and, in particular, that homeopathic dilutions beyond the Avogadro constant still have some effect. The authors, however, acknowledge that in view of the vast implications of these findings, these experiments must be rigorously repeated and confirmed.

Another interesting point to emerge from the experiments in animals has to do with the importance of the chronological factor: a given treatment will be perceived differently by the organism depending upon the time of day (circadian rhythm) or the month of the year (circa-annual rhythm). This variability and its possible biological consequences have been examined by various authors [Cambar and Cal, 1982; Doucet-Jaboeuf *et al.*, 1984; Cambar and Guillemain, 1985; Guillemain *et al.*, 1987; Ibarra, 1991]. It is well known that chronobiology is today a frontier area also for conventional biomedical research [Minors, 1985; Breithaupt, 1988].

Another team of researchers have reported that homeopathic preparations of zinc in decimal dilutions (from 4x to 12x, corresponding to amounts of zinc ranging from 0.025 mg to 0.25 pg), administered to rats for seven days consecutively, significantly increased the release of histamine by peritoneal mastcells [Harish and Kretschmer, 1988].

Other data appear to indicate that two substances with similar actions can interfere with each other's effects when one of the two is used in a homeopathic dilution as an "antidote" to the other [De Caro *et al.*, 1990]. Repeated i.p. injections of isoproterenol or of the tachykinin eleidosin give rise, within the space of a fortnight, to a substantial increase in size of the salivary glands, which return to their normal size within 30 days of discontinuation of the treatment. Isoproterenol was administered i.p. as a stimulant of the glandular response (100 mg/kg for a fortnight), whereas eleidosin was given i.p. in dynamized dilutions ranging from 10^{-10} to 10^{-426} g/ml to assess whether or not it was capable of preventing the increase in size of the gland, if given earlier, or of accelerating its return to normal, if given after treatment with isoproterenol. Both responses were significantly different as compared to controls, revealing that low dynamized doses of eleidosin not only produce an action opposite to that of high doses, but also counteract the action of a substance which has similar effects on animals.

A team of American researchers have reported the results obtained with very high dilutions of mice tissues infected with *Francisella tularensis*, in practice a preparation of a nosode of tularemia [Jonas *et al.*, 1991]. They produced the dynamized dilutions from reticulo-endothelial tissue of mice infected with tularemia, obtaining three dilutions containing original tissue (3x, 7x, 12x) and three dilutions beyond the presence of original tissue (30c, 200c, 1000c). These preparations were administered orally to a group of mice, whereas another control group was treated with dilutions of ethanol. An LD_{50} or LD_{75} of *F. tularensis* was then administered and survival time and total mortality were evaluated. After 15 experiments the very high homeopathic dilutions brought about a significant increase in survival time and a significant reduction in total mortality compared to controls. The protection did not correlate with the level of dilution, number of shakings, or presence or absence of original tissue. The authors conclude: "We could not confirm our hypothesis that preparations diluted beyond the level of remaining organisms behaved identically to controls in the prophylaxis of infectious challenge. These findings should be repeated, confirmed by other investigators, and evaluated further" [Jonas *et al.*, 1991, p. 21]. A more recent report of these studies has also been published [Jonas, 1999].

Researchers from the Department of Zoology of the University of Kalyani (India) worked on radiation-induced damage [Khuda-Bukhsh and Banik, 1991; Khuda-Bukhsh and Maity, 1991]. The experimental protocol consists in irradiation of albino mice with 100-200 rad of X-rays (sublethal doses) and evaluation, after 24, 48, and 72 hours, of cytogenic damage such as frequency of chromosomal aberrations, formation of micronuclei, and the mitotic index. In this system, the possible radioprotective effects of homeopathic drugs such as *Ginseng* 6x, 30x, and 200x and *Ruta graveolens* 30x and 200x (rue), administered orally before and after irradiation, were tested. The results reported would appear to be highly significant, in the sense that the mice treated with the homeopathic remedies suffered significantly less damage than the control mice (irradiated and treated with dilutions of ethanol). Significantly, the authors, though defining this protective action as "spectacular," conclude that it is very difficult to explain the precise mechanism whereby such alterations due to the homeopathic drug may be possible at such high dilutions *in vivo* [Khuda-Bukhsh and Banik, 1991].

Interesting and sound are the studies conducted by Sukul and coworkers of the Department of Zoology of the University of Santiniketan (India) [Sukul *et al.*, 1986; Sukul, 1990; Sukul *et al.*, 1991; Sukul *et al.*, 1993]. These studies consist in numerous experiments conducted in rats, mice, and cats. Amongst other things, the authors report that the homeopathic drugs *Gelsemium* (yellow jasmine), *Cannabis indica* (Indian hemp), *Graphites* (graphite), and *Agaricus muscarius* (toadstool), administered orally (as granules dissolved in a small amount of water) to albino rats, significantly increase the catalepsis induced by motor blockade (a nervous disorder which sets in when rats are repeatedly forced to remain immobile) [Sukul *et al.*, 1986]. The effect of these drugs, in 30c and 200c dilutions, was comparable to that of well known conventional drugs such as pilocarpine and aloperidol administered in ponderal doses (5 mg/kg). The effects were assessed in comparison with rats receiving granules of lactose without active drug. The 200c dose appears to have a longer duration of action than the 30c dose.

The same research team is currently working on another interesting model which may provide important indications with regard to the mechanism of action of homeopathic remedies. In a further communication [Sukul *et al.*, 1993], the authors report that potentized homeopathic drugs applied to the tongues of rats evoke electrophysiological responses of the hypothalamic neurons. Rats kept on a high-salt diet were anesthetized and a microelectrode, connected up to an oscilloscope, was implanted in the lateral hypothalamic area to record the discharge frequency in that area. After a suitable period recording the basal tracing, a few drops of *Natrum muriaticum* (sodium chloride or common sea salt) were deposited on the tongues of the rats. The application caused marked changes (reductions) in the discharge frequency of the nerve center. This experiment suggests both that the action of the drug can be mediated by the hypothalamic nerve centers and that preconditioning with a high-salt diet makes the animal more sensitive to the remedy *Natrum muriaticum*.

Cuprum (copper) is used in homeopathic therapy as a spasmolytic agent. A French team [Santini *et al.*, 1990] have developed an animal model for assessing the possible effect of *Cuprum* on digestive motility. A 4c solution of this remedy (corresponding to roughly 10^{-10} M) was administered (0.3 ml i.p.) to mice, which then received treatment with neostigmine at ponderal doses (50 mg/kg), a drug which accelerates intestinal motility. The parameter measured was the distance travelled by phenolsulfonphthalein in the intestine. The results showed that the homeopathic treatment significantly reduces the effect of neostigmine, bringing the intestinal transit rates back to values closer to those recorded in mice not treated with neostigmine.

Homeopathy is also finding applications in veterinary medicine. For instance, there has been a report on a study conducted in dairy cows showing that the remedy *Sepia* (cuttlefish ink), at the 200c dilution, significantly reduces a number of typical postpartum complications [Williamson *et al.*, 1991] and another on a study conducted in pigs showing that various combinations of *Lachesis* (venom of the bushmaster snake), *Pulsatilla* (windflower), and *Sabina* (savin) or *Lachesis*, *Echinacea* (coneflower), and *Pyrogenium* (artificial sepsin), associated with *Caulophyllum* (blue cohosh) (all in low dilutions, from 1x to 6x) have prophylactic and therapeutic effects on infections (metritis and mastitis) of sows and on diarrhea of piglets [Both, 1987].

The development of the immune system of the chicken is stimulated by a homeopathic hormone dilution [Yubicier-Simo *et al.*, 1993; Bastide, 1994]. In this study, bursectomy was performed in chick embryos, making them immunodeficient (it is well known that the bursa of Fabricius is essential for the development of the B lymphocyte system in this animal). "*In-ovo*" administration of low doses and high dilutions of the hormone bursin (up to 10^{-30}–10^{-40} g/ml), theoretically no longer containing any molecules of the original substance, restores the immune response, as demonstrated by normal antibody production on the part of the adult animal in response to antigen stimulus (bovine thyreoglobulin). Moreover, an improvement in the response of the pituitary-adreno-cortical axis has been seen, as shown by measuring adrenocorticotropic hormone.

Some mention should be made of a number of studies published by the research group coordinated by Endler [Endler *et al.*, 1991a; Endler *et al.*, 1991b; Endler *et al.*, 1994a; Endler *et al.*, 1994b]. In these studies, two Austrian laboratories (Graz) and one Dutch laboratory (Utrecht) demonstrated that extreme dilutions (30x) of thyroxine (T_4) are capable of significantly inhibiting ($p < 0.01$) the metamorphosis of tadpoles and also the spontaneous tendency of young frogs to leave the water.

In recent years, several reports of research on animals have been published. We mention here the homeopathic regulation of inflammatory processes in rats [Lussignoli *et al.*, 1999; Bertani *et al.*, 1999] and the interesting studies on the effects of high dilutions/dynamizations of homeopathic medicines in several pathologic conditions in mice [Mitra *et al.*, 1999; Datta *et al.*, 1999; Sukul *et al.*, 1999; 2001; Kundu *et al.*, 2000] and rats [Ruiz-Vega *et al.*, 2000]. A large review of the animal research before 1998 has been also published [Wynn, 1998].

In this section, we should also mention a number of experimental studies conducted in healthy human subjects, inasmuch as they are not clinical trials as such to assess the therapeutic efficacy of a drug, but actual experiments aimed at identifying its possible mechanism of action. These experiments may also be classified within the framework of the classic homeopathic provings, which for some years now have been conducted on a double-blind, placebo-controlled basis. There are a certain number of reports of this type in the literature, showing that homeopathic drugs taken repeatedly by healthy subjects cause particular symptoms and even variations in physiological parameters detectable in the laboratory [Julian, 1979; Smith, 1979; Campbell, 1980; Bayr, 1986; Nagpaul, 1987; Koenig and Swoboda, 1987; Vakil et al., 1988]. The effect on healthy subjects would appear to be particularly pronounced in hypersensitive subjects, i.e. not all individuals respond to homeopathic test doses [Poitevin, 1988a]. More recently, others Authors were not able to show any significant difference of effects by homeopathic medicines versus placebo under double-blind experimental conditions [Goodyear *et al.*, 1998; Vickers *et al.*, 2001; Walach *et al.* 2001]. This is probably due to the fact that if drug-proving phenomena exist, they appear to be rare and require different methods to be detected. The optimal methods of provings are still a matter of discussion [Vickers *et al.*, 2000].

There have also been reports, in official hematological journals, of a paradoxical effect of acetylsalicylic acid: in healthy volunteers, homeopathic dilutions of aspirin (2 ml of 5c dilution, corresponding to approximately 0.000000002 mg by sublingual administration) caused a statistically significant reduction in bleeding time (p < 0.05) compared to placebo (distilled water) [Doutremepuich *et al.*, 1987a; Doutremepuich *et al.*, 1987b; Doutremepuich *et al.*, 1988; Doutremepuich *et al.*, 1990]. Since it is well known that aspirin causes an increase in bleeding time at pharmacological doses (50-500 mg), the findings of these studies may possibly be interpreted as a demonstration of the law of similars. Nevertheless, the mechanism whereby this happens is still unclear because, while we know that aspirin at normal doses exerts its action by inhibiting the function of platelets, in the work by Doutremepuich it is reported that "homeopathized" aspirin has no effect on platelet aggregation [Doutremepuich *et al.*, 1990].

Aubin's team [Aubin, 1984; Pennec and Aubin, 1984] have conducted pioneering studies on the cardiotoxic activity of aconitum and veratrum, both of which are substances used in homeopathy. At low dilutions (high concentrations) (10^{-5} M) aconitum caused fibrillation in the isolated perfused heart; at medium dilutions (10^{-7} M) it caused bradycardia; at high dilutions (10^{-18} M) it had no effect on the healthy heart, but on the heart pretreated with low dilutions of aconitum it had a distinct protective effect normalizing rhythm and other signs of cardiotoxicity. Similar results were obtained with veratrum [Pennec *et al.*, 1984a; Pennec *et al.*, 1984b]. These experiments appear to confirm the efficacy of high dilutions in cells and tissues somehow sensitized or predisposed by pathological situations.

4.2
Studies in isolated organs

Benveniste and coworkers [Hadji *et al.*, 1991; Benveniste, 1994] reported results obtained with an experimental model consisting in isolated perfused guinea-pig heart (Langendorf system). The coronary flow of these hearts increased with infusion of very high dilutions of histamine (above 30x), as normally occurs with the normal low dilutions. The infusion of buffer alone (control) or of a high dilution of methylhistamine (inactive histamine analogue) did not alter coronary flow. Assays were done in "blind" conditions. The vasodilatory activity of histamine in very high dilutions was destroyed by treatment at 70°C for 30 minutes or as a result of exposure to a magnetic field of 50 Hz for 15 minutes. The authors concluded that water, deprived of the solute by serial dilutions, retains a specific activity which can be suppressed by means of physical treatments which in themselves have no effect on the solute.

The isolated perfused guinea-pig heart model appears to be very effective for this type of study and to furnish reliable results. In point of fact, in two later publications [Benveniste *et al.*, 1992; Litime *et al.*, 1993], Benveniste's group reported that the system is also sensitive to immunization-dependent activation. On immunizing the animals (guinea-pigs) with ovalbumin and taking the heart for the experiment between the 9th and

20th day, an increase in coronary flow could be achieved at very high dilutions (10^{-31}–10^{-41} M) of ovalbumin.

Fragments of oat seedlings (coleoptiles) during the rapid growth phase were cultured in the presence of the vegetable growth factor indoleacetic acid. In these conditions, pretreatment with homeopathic dilutions of $CaCO_3$ (5c) caused a statistically significant increase in growth compared to coleoptiles treated with indoleacetic acid alone [Bornoroni, 1991]. Extensive studies have been carried out by the group headed by Dr. Betti at Bologna [Betti *et al.*, 1997; Brizzi *et al.*, 2000]. The studies have shown that high potencies of *Arsenicum album* (up to 45th decimal dilution/dynamization of arsenic) are capable of protecting small wheat plants from intoxication by chemical doses of arsenic.

Doutremepuich's team, who conducted the study on aspirin at high dilutions in healthy human subjects (see Chapter 4, Section 1 above), have also published reports on cultures of vascular fragments and blood platelets [Lalanne *et al.*, 1990; Lalanne *et al.*, 1991; Lalanne *et al.*, 1992; Doutremepuich *et al.*, 1993]. The platelet aggregation rate is slowed and its overall proportions reduced by the presence of fragments of vascular wall in the incubation medium. This phenomenon is well known and is probably due to the production of a number of physiological mediators. The authors cited have shown that a homeopathic preparation of high dilutions of aspirin (5c) inverts the inhibitory effect of the vascular fragments and thus, in practice, restores the previously inhibited platelet aggregation to normal; the result constitutes *in vitro* confirmation of the findings reported in healthy human subjects, where highly dilute aspirin reduces bleeding time.

We are familiar with the fact that $beta_2$-agonists (isoproterenol, salbutamol, tulobuterol) cause relaxation of tracheobronchial muscle. A report [Callens *et al.*, 1993] shows that these agents are capable of inducing relaxation of basal tone, in a model of isolated guinea-pig trachea, even at high dilutions (from 10^{-20} M to 10^{-36} M, in dynamized decimal dilutions).

4.3

Studies in
in vitro *cells*

The most significant studies have been conducted on human basophils, using the degranulation test [Benveniste, 1981; Sainte-Laudy, 1987; Cherruault *et al.*, 1989]. This test investigates the metachromatic property of these cells, using an optical microscope for the basophil count. Benveniste's team have demonstrated that this phenomenon is due to changes in membrane transport rather than to actual degranulation [Beauvais *et al.*, 1991], but here the phenomenon will be treated as *degranulation*, using the term adopted in the early studies. The first publications on the effect of high dilutions on basophils [Poitevin *et al.*, 1985; Poitevin *et al.*, 1986] report that the *in vitro* degranulation induced by various allergens (house dust mites) was inhibited by high dilutions of bee venom (*Apis mellifica* 9c and 15c). A later study [Poitevin *et al.*, 1988] examined basophils stimulated with anti-IgE serum, analyzing the effect of two products used in the homeopathic treatment of allergic syndromes, *Apis mellifica* and *Lung histamine*. These drugs yielded significant inhibition at theoretical concentrations of 10^{-9} M and 10^{-17} M. On examining the dose-effect relationship, an alternation of inhibition, inactivity, and stimulation was observed, giving rise to a *pseudosinusoidal* trend. Inhibition was then obtained with high dilutions of pure histamine, with inhibition peaks around 6–7c and 17–18c [Poitevin *et al.*, 1988; Poitevin, 1990]. Since the effects observed seem to depend on histamine and melittin (the main components of bee venom), the authors suggested as possible mechanisms of action the nonspecific blockade of IgE, or the regulation of phospholipase activity (melittin is known to activate phospholipase A2), or the negative feedback of histamine on its release.

A multicenter study under the guidance of Jacques Benveniste, conducted in collaboration with four other laboratories, has reported that human basophils are sensitive to infinitesimal doses of substances which are already known to have a stimulatory effect at ponderal doses, such as anti-IgE antibodies, calcium ionophores, or phospholipase A2. The specificity of action has been corroborated by the lack of effect of other ultradiluted substances such as anti-IgG antibodies (basophils, in fact, are activated only by anti-IgE antibodies) and phospholipase C, which has a different biochemical specificity on the membranes [Davenas *et al.*, 1988]. The dose-response curves showed that decreasing doses were accompanied first by disappearance of activity, then by its reappearance and then by various alternating activity peaks and inactivity troughs up to very high dilutions, corresponding to practically zero antibody concentrations (Figure 1). It is also reported that in order to obtain maximum activity at the infinitesimal dilutions the dilution process needed to be accompanied by vigorous succussion (10 sec. with a vortex) and that the stimulatory activity of the diluted antibody solutions persisted even after ultrafiltration through membranes with a pore size of less than 10 kDa, which should have retained the antibody out of solution.

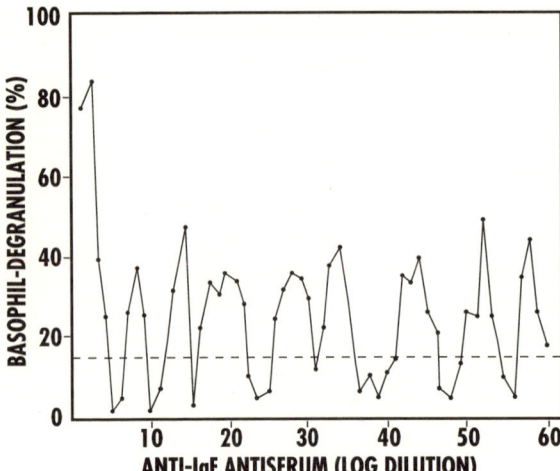

FIGURE 1 Basophil degranulation in relation to increasing dilutions of anti-IgE antibody (Reprinted with permission for Nature vol. 333, pp. 816-818; Copyright © 1988 Macmillan Magazine Limited).

Given that these experiments represent a key issue in discussions on homeopathy, they need to be examined in depth, and a number of precise points need to be made. The work of Benveniste's research team, published in the authoritative scientific journal, *Nature*, has aroused a great deal of interest as an alleged practical demonstration of the *"memory of water,"* but was fiercely criticized both on theoretical grounds (the "unbelievable" nature of the data) and on account of difficulties relating to the repeatability of the results and methodological shortcomings (a kind of inspection was organized by *Nature* in Benveniste's laboratory) [Lasters and Bardiaux, 1988; Maddox *et al.*, 1988; Pool, 1988].

Such strongly critical and sometimes downright sarcastic or ironic stances do not appear entirely justified: the concept of the "memory of water" is no more than *a metaphor denoting the hypothesis whereby the physicochemical properties of water can be modified by a solute and remain so for a certain period of time even in the absence of the solute itself.* If this were true, biology and medicine would undergo not a revolution, but certainly a significant increase in knowledge and in the related applications. It is not a matter here of postulating an "entity" (memory) which may reside in the water, conferring upon it cognitive and mnemonic properties, but of studying the physicochemical properties of water itself. In this sense, talking about memory is not so very different from talking about temperature, dielectric constants, viscosity, and other properties.

An example may serve to clarify the concept outlined here: if we take a little water and put it in the freezer, after a certain amount of time it will freeze. On removing the water from the freezer, it will be observed that the block of ice, though now exposed to room temperature, will remain a block of ice for some time. Thus, there exists in water a property which enables it to "remember" for a certain amount of time that it has been kept in the freezer. For those who find this example self-evident, we can give another: if we take a tape coated with ferric hydroxide and subject it, as it is running, to a series of differences in potential in precise succession, changes in charge occur on the magnetic substrate; the tape will remember these changes for hundreds of years. It is not the memory of water, in this case, but the memory of iron, which consists in a *particular form* that the magnetic substrate assumes on the tape.

To our mind, the attempt to repeat an experiment regarded as interesting and important is the only position which may be considered scientifically correct and useful. The Benveniste's group repeated the tests according to more reliable methodologies and more complete statistical assessments, confirming the existence of an effect of high dilutions, though not as striking as those reported in the first study published in *Nature* [Benveniste, 1991a; Benveniste *et al.*, 1991a; Benveniste *et al.*, 1991b]. The issue has therefore still to be resolved on the experimental plane.

The "Benveniste affair" is a typical example of scientific misrepresentation. Most people today simply believe that Benveniste has been proved wrong and that the issue is closed. This does not correspond to the facts [Schiff, 1995]. In the first place, if we take the trouble to read the documentation in *Nature*, we note that a panel consisting of a magician, a journalist, and an expert in statistics were invited to witness a number of experiments in the course of a week, most of which (though not all) yielded negative results, and therefore the panel produced a totally negative report based on various arguments, but largely ones which the researchers of the host laboratory had good grounds for refuting [Benveniste, 1988]. Clearly, this type of experiment will meet with reproducibility problems, due both to ignorance of the physical basis of the phenomenon and thus of the environmental and experimental factors capable of influencing it, and to the particular methodology, which is based on semiquantitative assessments using a microscope. What is quite unacceptable, however, is that a group consisting of three nonexperts in the field should feel entitled to demolish in one week more than two years' work in a laboratory which is celebrated throughout the world for its studies on mastcells.

The data reported in the above-mentioned paper in *Nature* are open to criticism of a procedural type in certain respects, but all the major lines of scientific research have had their teething problems in terms of methodology and even interpretation. The pillorying of the Benveniste group, as the editorial board of *Nature* went out of their way to do, bears all the hallmarks of a political maneuver and has precious little in common with a true scientific debate. That this is so is borne out by the fact that Benveniste's latest studies have been greeted by the scientific community with total silence. No serious criticism has been forthcoming. It is as if the new data had not even been published, and the public at large is left with the idea that the memory of water is merely a figment of the imagination. But this, as Benveniste sees it, is not a scientifically valid way of going about it: "There are only two possibilities:"—he writes in a comment—"either the data is wrong and it must be shown to be wrong; or it is right and represents a most important discovery in biology, which not only legitimizes the high dilution/agitation effect used in homeopathy, but also reaches to the core of any biological process—molecular communication. The problem therefore needs to be known and experiments need to be performed; international cooperation needs to be extended so that these important results and their implications be fully recognized" [Benveniste, 1991b]

A Dutch group have reported that they failed to reproduce the effect of high dilutions of IgE [Ovelgonne et al., 1991; Ovelgonne et al., 1992]. In their study it proved impossible to demonstrate any action of high dilutions of anti-IgE antibodies on mastcells, and the authors (one of whom had learnt the technique in Benveniste's laboratory) conclude that it is a model which is very hard to reproduce. Similar findings have also been reported by another group of investigators, who published on *Nature* [Hirst et al., 1993]. However, the latter work has been criticized for a number of methodological discrepancies by the Benveniste's team [Benveniste et al., 1994a] and also the report of Ovelgonne et al. is open to various interpretations as concerns the possible existence of "vortex-related" effects [Wiegant, 1994]. As a matter of facts, Fred Wiegant is probably right when he writes in a letter to *Nature* that in this story "the last word has not yet been spoken" [Wiegant, 1994].

A French team have investigated the effect of various homeopathic drugs, particularly homeopathically diluted histamine, on basophil degranulation (observed under the microscope) [Cherruault et al., 1989; Boiron and Belon, 1990]. The inhibitory activity of progressive centesimal dilutions was evident with activity peaks alternating with ineffective dilutions. The main activity peaks were achieved at the 7c, 17c, 28c, 39c, and 51c dilutions. All the experiments were performed blind, in the sense that the experimenter did not know which dilution he was working with. A control group received histidine dilutions, which proved ineffective, thus reducing the possibility that the results might have been artefacts.

The Sainte-Laudy and Belon group reported further data confirming the fact that high dilutions of histamine (pure histamine chloride) significantly inhibit the degranulation of basophils (sensitized with IgE antibodies to the dermatophagoid) induced in vitro by dermatophagoid extracts. In a series of 16 progressive centesimal dilutions (from 5c to 20c), the authors observed histamine inhibitory activity in dilutions of around 7c and 18c. The addition of pharmacological doses of cimetidine (an H_2-receptor antagonist) abolished the effect of all the active dilutions. The authors therefore are inclined to believe that H_2-receptors are involved in the action of the high dilutions, though they admit that "it is paradoxical to think in terms of molecular biology when theoretically there are no molecules of the effector in some of the active dilutions tested" [Sainte-Laudy et al., 1991, p. 136]. The same group showed that the activation of human basophils by IgE is strongly and significantly inhibited ($p < 0.001$) by dilutions of histamine [Sainte-Laudy and Belon, 1993]. In these experiments, two main inhibition peaks were obtained, the first with dilutions from 10^{-16} to 10^{-22} M, and the second with dilutions from 10^{-28} to 10^{-36} M. Similar findings have been recently obtained in an international cooperative study [Belon *et al.*, 1999].

Along the lines of the toxicity tests performed in animals (see above) Boiron's group [Boiron *et al.*, 1981] reported that mercuric chloride ($HgCl_2$) at minimal doses (5c) protects fibroblast cultures from intoxication by high doses of mercury. The parameter studied was the mitotic index. Others [Mansvelt and Van Amons, 1975] observed a cytotoxic effect of $HgCl_2$ on cultured mouse lymphocytes at doses from 10^{-5} to 10^{-7} M, whereas a growth inhibiting effect, without cytotoxicity, was observed at doses from 10^{-16} to 10^{-17} M. This effect, however, was not found by another group studying the action of dilutions ranging from 10^{-10} to 10^{-18} M on the same model [Kollerstrom, 1982].

We know that cadmium, an environmental pollutant, and cisplatin, a cytostatic drug used in antitumor therapies, have marked effects on the kidney tubules. It has been reported that the pretreatment of (5-day) kidney cell cultures with very low doses (10^{-16} M) of cadmium and cisplatin has a protective effect against the toxicity caused by medium-to-high doses (10^{-5}–10^{-6} M) of these substances [Delbancut *et al.*, 1993].

A Montpellier University research team has shown the effect of epidermal growth factor (EGF) on the proliferation of cells in culture (lines of human keratinocytes and fibroblasts). EGF at very low doses (10^{-19} M) and in high dilutions (10^{-45} M) caused significant effects on these cells, in the sense that it reduced the growth of the keratinocytes and stimulated that of the fibroblasts [Fougeray *et al.*, 1993].

Two papers reporting on the effect of *Phytolacca* (pokeroot) on lymphoblastic transformation appear to be of particular interest [Colas *et al.*, 1975; Bildet *et al.*, 1981]. *Phytolacca* contains a glycoprotein, the mitogenic *Pokeweed*, which is known to induce the lymphoblastic transformation of B lymphocytes in culture. *Phytolacca* has also been used empirically in homeopathy for some years now (since before its immunological action *in vitro* was known) in numerous conditions involving adenopathy, such as, for instance, infectious mononucleosis and viral disease in ORL [Mossinger, 1973; Poitevin, 1988c]. In resting lymphocytes, 5c, 7c, and 15c dilutions of *Phytolacca* have no mitogenic effect, but in lymphocytes stimulated with ponderal doses of phytohemagglutinin (PHA) they exert a 28 to 73 percent inhibitory effect on mitosis (maximum effect by the 15c dilution in one study [Colas *et al.*, 1975], and by the 7c dilution in another [Bildet *et al.*, 1981]. What emerges forcefully once again in these experiments are the concepts of biological tropism (whereby an ultradiluted solution has an activity which is directed against the same target system as the undiluted substance) and of inversion of effects (whereby the dilute solution inhibits the effect of the original substance or of a substance similar to it).

A study of the action of succussed substances on human lymphocytes stimulated with phytohemagglutinin (PHA) and on PMN granulocytes stimulated with opsonized zymosan (OZ) was conducted by a team led by Olinescu in Bucharest [Chirila *et al.*, 1990a and 1990b]. From peripheral blood of patients allergic to bee venom or immunodepressed (cancer) patients PMN granulocytes and lymphocytes were isolated, and the stimulatory index was assessed following PHA (tritiated thymidine test) for the lymphocytes, or production of O_2^- after OZ (chemiluminescence test) for the granulocytes. Before being stimulated the lymphocytes were incubated in a medium supplemented with various dilutions of bee venom and the granulocytes with various dilutions of cortisol (2c, 7c, 14c, 30c). As controls, a number of cells were supplemented with succussed or nonsuccussed distilled water. It was found that the lymphocytes of allergic patients were inhibited in their proliferative response by the high dilutions of the venom (7c, 15c, 30c). The inhibition was not observed in the controls supplemented with succussed and nonsuccussed water. The immunodepressed patients had low lymphocyte stimulatory indices, both in the presence and in the absence of dilutions of bee venom. As regards the production of O_2^- by PMN granulocytes stimulated with OZ in the presence of diluted cortisol, different responses are reported compared to controls, both stimulatory and inhibitory, though the data were not statistically significant. According to the authors, the data obtained suggest a possible effect of succussed dilutions on the structures of the cell membrane.

Other studies have also been conducted on phagocyte cells (polymorphonuclear leukocytes and macrophages). In this case, substances were tested which are used in homeopathy in situations in which there is acute inflammation with a strong polymorphonuclear component. An inhibitory effect of *Belladonna* (deadly nightshade) and of *Ferrum phosphoricum* (phosphate of iron) at dilutions of 5c and 9c has been reported on the production of oxygen free radicals (chemiluminescence) induced by opsonized zymosan [Poitevin et al., 1983]. The inhibition was highly significant and got up to approximately 30-40%, roughly the same degree of inhibition obtained with 10^{-6} M of dexamethasone and 10^{-4} M of indomethacin. Simultaneously, *Apis mellifica* (crushed bee) was tested, but no changes were found. The authors point out that there is a substantial difference in individual sensitivity to these drugs. This problem of the differing sensitivities of cells isolated from different subjects has also been stressed by others [Moss *et al.*, 1982], who investigated the effects of *Belladonna* (deadly nightshade), *Hepar sulphur* (Hahnemann's calcium sulfide), *Pyrogenium* (artificial sepsin), *Silicea* (silica), and *Staphylococcinum* on chemotaxis, obtaining contradictory results. This latter study has been criticized [Poitevin, 1988a] on the grounds that the solutions used in the tests were not sterile, which might account for the variability of the results.

It has also been reported (in a preliminary communication) that *Bryonia* 4c and 9c (wild hops) had a stimulatory effect on the oxidative metabolism of polymorphonuclear leukocytes, which may be both direct and indirect (increasing the response to chemotactic peptides) [Fletcher and Halpern, 1988].

Since in our own laboratory we currently use a method for the measurement of the functionality (in terms of production of superoxide anion and adherence) of the white blood cells, particularly the neutrophils, a similar approach has been adopted to that of Benveniste's group, attempting to activate these cells with solutions of agonists or antagonists diluted according to the homeopathic method. Our results [Bellavite *et al.*, 1991a] have been largely negative, in the sense that the cell activities undergo the influence of compounds tested in a range of dilutions from 4x to 10x, and thus in conditions in which the doses were similar to those commonly used in conventional research. It should be stressed, however, that Benveniste, too, attempted to test high dilutions on neutrophilic granulocytes and platelets, with negative results (personal communication).

Another approach to the study of the action of homeopathic drugs on cell systems in our laboratory consisted in the evaluation of the effects of homeopathic preparations on human neutrophils in culture, activated with formylated peptides [Bellavite *et al.*, 1991b; Chirumbolo *et al.*, 1993]. The results of this research, based on analysis of an extensive series of compounds and of several dilutions, can be summarized as follows:

a) *Manganum phosphoricum* 6x and 8x (phosphate of manganese), *Magnesia phosphorica* 6x and 8x (phosphate of magnesia), *Acidum citricum* 3x (citric acid, and *Acidum succinicum* 3x and 4x (succinic acid) had significant and reproducible inhibitory effects on the neutrophil's oxidative metabolism.

b) *Acidum fumaricum* (fumaric acid) and *Acidum malicum* (malic acid), both at the 4x dilution, had slightly potentiating effects.

c) *Phosphorus* and *Magnesia phosphorica* often presented inhibitory effects, in the course of the various experiments, even at very high dilutions (greater than 15x), but these effects did not always appear at the same dilutions, thus making any statistical assessment of the phenomenon a difficult matter.

These results lend themselves to multiple interpretations as to the possible reasons for the effects observed from the biochemical point of view. In the first place, they go to show that the solutions used have determined effects on blood cells at medium-high doses. Moreover, the data appear to suggest that most of the remedies tested act in such a way as to interfere with subtle regulatory mechanisms of the cell, notoriously based on ion exchanges and on phosphorylation and oxido-reduction processes. In fact, in normal cell physiology, elements of major importance in these mechanisms are phosphorus, sulphur, magnesium, manganese, calcium, and others.

Wagner's group [Wagner, 1985; Wagner, 1988; Wagner *et al.*, 1988; Wagner and Kreher, 1989], have experimentally tackled the problem of the effect, at cell level (i.e. on leukocytes), of low doses of vegetable extracts used in homeopathy and, in addition, of the unusual changes in effect observed in the dose-response curves. Among the various studies produced by the group, of particular interest are those which report that the naphthoquinones (plumbagin, alkannin, and others) and cytostatic agents (vincristine, methotrexate, fluorouracyl) at relatively high concentrations (100 mg–10 ng/ml) inhibit, whereas at very low concentrations (10 pg–10 fg/ml) they stimulate lymphoblastic transformation and granulocyte phagocytosis. Intermediate doses are ineffective. The authors have suggested that a number of antitumor effects of vegetable extracts might be explained by this dose-related double-effect mechanism.

More recent reports have shown significant effects of the homeopathic drugs in vitro on isolated duodenum [Cristea *et al.*, 1997], on osteogenesis [Palermo *et al.*, 2000], on isolated rat neurons [Jonas *et al.*, 2001], on blood leukocytes [Fimiani *et al.*, 2000], and on in vitro enzyme (uricase, glutathione transferase and cytochrome P450) activity [Dittmann and Harish, 1996; Dittmann *et al.*, 1999]. The immunoregulation concept has been proposed by others [Heine and Schmolz, 2000]

Reports have been published on various experiments on vegetable cells. These include particularly interesting papers which demonstrate that pretreatment with homeopathic dilutions of toxic substances (e.g. $CuSO_4$)

protect vegetable cells against the intoxication induced by medium-to-high doses of the toxic substance itself [Guillemain et al., 1984; Guillemain et al., 1987].

The experimental studies referred to in this section bear witness to the existence of a form of homeopathic research, about which normally very little is known. There are now many groups operating throughout the world (and above all in Europe) who have started to set themselves the task of experimentally demonstrating the truth or falsity of certain "sacred" principles of classic homeopathy, on the basis of the tenets of modern biological research. Of course, as has been done in the case of clinical research, there is no lack of critics who quite rightly subject many of the papers published—mostly in journals not ranking among the most prestigious in the field—to highly demanding methodological vetting and expose their serious shortcomings. It cannot be denied that most of what we read, particularly apropos of the effects of ultradiluted solutions, still awaits corroboration by independent research teams.

4.4
Preliminary conclusions from experimental studies

When discoveries threaten to undermine the foundations of pharmacology, or, at any rate, suggest the need for new theories, they must be corroborated by evidence which in terms of methodology and reproducibility is superior to the common standard, and not inferior to it, as, unfortunately, is all too often the case in this field. We have already mentioned the problem of how difficult it is to reproduce the spectacular results of certain laboratories. This problem, whose *raison d'etre* lies in our virtually total ignorance of the possible mechanism of action of the ultradiluted homeopathic solutions, is destined to remain the major stumbling-block in the path of all those coming to grips with this difficult and challenging area of research. If the effect of solutions which are practically devoid of molecules of the active compound exists, it is necessarily of nonmolecular type, and thus lies beyond the scope of any normal quality control of the solutions used in the experiments.

A critical review of the entire literature on research in homeopathy has been attempted in the past [Scofield, 1984] and is currently under way in certain university settings [Linde *et al.*, 1991; Linde *et al.*, 1993; Linde *et al.*, 1994]. Linde's work reviews 109 publications reporting on 106 different studies, 82 of which conducted in animals, 14 in plants, 6 in isolated organs, and 5 in cell cultures. Practically all the papers reviewed report positive results, at least at certain dilutions. In particular, the dilutions most frequently found to have demonstrable effects are 5c and 9c. According to rigorous criteria the quality standards were judged to be poor, especially on account of the shortage of information on the methods used in preparing the dilutions, on the composition of the mother tinctures and on chronobiological details. Only about 30 percent of the studies obtained a score better than 50 percent of the maximum according to the analysis by Linde and coworkers. The authors conclude that, judging only on the basis of methodologically satisfactory studies, there is distinct evidence of the efficacy of very low doses and high dilutions, but that to date too few research protocols have been reproduced by independent teams.

Needless to say, poor reliability does not mean falsification. The need for caution with regard to the reliability of research which has yet to be reproduced in different laboratories is mandatory in any case, but what we have said does not mean that part of the research conducted to date, and perhaps even a substantial part, is not valid. There remains an increasingly urgent need for experimental studies to be amplified and intensified, particularly within the framework of first-class research centers, for funds to be allocated to the teams involved in the research and for the ostracism to cease at university level in relation to anyone and anything associated with homeopathic medicine.

On the whole, then, the mounting body of laboratory experiments over recent years is beginning to provide useful information, which, alongside the more traditional and less easily controlled reports of clinical practice, enables us to draw a number of conclusions:

a) The studies cited in this section appear to demonstrate the existence of biological activity of drugs at medium and high dilutions prepared according to the standard practices of homeopathy. With reference in particular to research on high dilutions (beyond the Avogadro constant), there can be no doubt that a certain amount of difficulty or slowness emerges in reproducing results unequivocally and in a statistically significant manner.

b) Owing to the uncertainty regarding the real nature of homeopathic drugs, laboratory research has so far done very little towards clarifying its mechanism of action.

c) In many cases it would seem that there is a certain consistency between the starting hypotheses, based on experience and on the homeopathic rationale (law of similars, opposite action of high dilutions compared to the toxic effect of the substance itself) and the results achieved in animals, in healthy human subjects, and in experiments *in vitro*. A certain substance which is pharmacologically active when tested in highly diluted solutions appears to react specifically to the same biological system to which the nondiluted substance reacts [see, for example, Wurmser and Ney, 1955; Bildet *et al.*, 1984; Aubin, 1984; Bastide *et al.*, 1985; Taylor Reilly *et al.*, 1986; Doutremepuich *et al.*, 1987; Davenas *et al.*, 1988; Poitevin, 1988a; Poitevin *et al.*, 1988; Vakil *et al.*, 1988; Doutremepuich *et al.*, 1987a]. The homeopathic cure is thus thought to be due to a *biological tropism* for specific receptor systems. We can therefore postulate, though only speculatively, that the signal transmitted by the highly diluted solution is recognized specifically by the target system and processed in a particular way.

d) The reaction to the high dilution is often the opposite of that observed at low dilutions; a compound can have a protective action against the toxic effects of the same or other compounds; a pro-inflammatory agent may present anti-inflammatory effects at high dilutions [Bildet *et al.*, 1975; Bildet *et al.*, 1981; Boiron *et al.*, 1981; Bildet *et al.*, 1984; Cazin *et al.*, 1987; Guillemain *et al.*, 1987; Poitevin, 1988a; Wagner *et al.*, 1988; Bastide, 1989; Doutremepuich *et al.*, 1990; Bildet *et al.*, 1990; Delbancut *et al.*, 1993]. It should be noted, however, that this inversion of effect is not a constant feature [Mansvelt and Van Amons, 1975; Doucet-Jaboeuf *et al.*, 1984; Bastide *et al.*, 1985; Davenas *et al.*, 1988; Harish and Kretschmer 1988; Hadji *et al.*, 1991; Fougeray *et al.*, 1993], and therefore must not be considered a universal rule with regard to the action of homeopathic drugs, but merely as a possibility which comes about when suitable reactivity conditions exist in the system tested. This aspect, which is of substantial importance for the understanding of homeopathy, will be analyzed more specifically in Chapters 5 and 6 which relate the mechanism of action of the homeopathic remedy to the cybernetic complexity of cellular and systemic homeostasis.

The biological and perhaps also the therapeutic efficacy of drugs at low or very low doses might be due to the fact that the alteration of physiological systems during disease predisposes them to changes in sensitivity at specific receptor level, this being something with which classic pharmacology is also thoroughly familiar [Brodde and Michel, 1989]. The fact that a specific reactivity state should be reached for ultra-low doses to be efficient has been clearly shown also on *in vitro* model systems [Lalanne *et al.*, 1992].

The effects of homeopathic-type drugs might therefore be explained (and this explanation is meant to serve only as an initial working hypothesis) in two ways: the drug stimulates a number of biological mechanisms which are inhibited or blocked by exogenous or endogenous pathogenetic factors, or the drug inhibits a response mechanism which is activated in a disproportionate or distorted manner by the agent causing the disease. This aspect will be discussed in greater detail in Chapter 6.

Nevertheless, many studies on highly diluted solutions suggest that the type of information and signal conveyed by these solutions differs, at least in certain respects, from those known to classic biology and pharmacology. The fact that many experiments show that the effect increases, or remains stable, or oscillates between an increase and a decrease, during successive dilutions suggests that some specific type of information of a compound at homeopathic doses may be activated or amplified by the dilution and succussion process. This may therefore be interpreted as biological activity in the presence of traces of molecules or even in their absence, and on the strength of this the term *"metamolecular biology"* has been coined [Davenas *et al.*, 1988].

The precise nature of this phenomenon remains unknown, but clearly the explanation should be sought in the particular physicochemical behavior of the solvent (water, or water with various percentages of ethanol) during the dilution and succussion process. The particular characteristics of aqueous solutions of highly diluted compounds will be addressed in greater detail in Chapter 7.

4.5

Towards new paradigms

In the foregoing paragraphs we have seen that some measure of support or explanation, or at least the start of an explanation, can be found for many of the empirical observations present in the homeopathic tradition within the framework of the modern biological, biochemical, and immunological sciences. In particular, the plausibility of the law of similars and the possibility of pharmacological effects at increasingly low doses are confirmed, if not as "laws" endowed with universal validity, then at least as properties peculiar to living systems, the importance of which went unrecognized up until only very recently. From here we have still a very long way to go before we can claim that the scientific basis of homeopathy has been explained. To say that the law of similars is plausible does not mean that we have explained its mechanism of action. Moreover, the problem of the effects of very high dilutions still remains substantially unsolved.

We have seen that there are a considerable number of research studies suggesting the existence of some form of biological activity of highly diluted solutions, which is therefore of a different type from that commonly known. If the scientific community is to definitively accept this phenomenon, which would unquestionably usher in a completely new phase in the study of biology and medicine, the evidence will have to be even stronger in terms of repeatability and its applicability to various different experimental models. Nevertheless, the sum of the clinical observations (see Chapter 3) and the experimental findings (see Chapter 4) is beginning to prove so extensive and intrinsically consistent that it is no longer possible to dodge the issue by acting as if this body of evidence simply did not exist. It must be admitted, however, that there is still no model providing any satisfactory or adequate explanation as to what type of information is contained in the high homeopathic dilutions, where theoretically there is a total lack of molecules of the active ingredient.

The empirical evidence *per se* fails to provide any kind of explanatory hypothesis. At this point, then, the process of reasoning, based as ever on what is known to be scientifically certain (or at least reliable), should grind to a halt due to a lack of "fuel" or "raw material." Since, however, the aim of this book is not merely to provide an updated overview of the literature on homeopathy, but, above all, to formulate new hypotheses serving both as stimuli and guidelines for further research, the problem needs to be tackled from a broader-based viewpoint than that inspiring the individual research efforts presented. For this reason, reference will be made to a vast body of evidence and theory that science has come up with in fairly recent years. The evidence and theories discussed here are not immediately related to the study of homeopathy, but refer to the functioning of biological systems and to the physicochemical principles underlying nature. It is only in this way that a hypothesis can be constructed on sound foundations.

We have entitled this "broadening of the horizons" of the scientific viewpoint "towards new paradigms," inasmuch as any attempt to come to grips with the scientific basis of homeopathy must necessarily figure within the framework of a distinct change in our present way of conceiving science and medicine. The difficulty the academic world has in accepting homeopathy is not primarily of a scientific nature, but rather is epistemological [Attena, 1991; Chibeni, 2001]. The problem is not just the weakness of the scientific evidence, or the lack of any explanation of the mechanism of action: both of these drawbacks apply to the study of new and old conventional drugs as well. Whether a new therapy is efficacious or not is a common and thoroughly legitimate question in the modern medico-scientific setting, and in this latter context no-one would dream of protesting against drugs of very dubious efficacy being investigated or even experimented with in patients (obviously, once their nontoxicity has been proven). Moreover, medical practitioners are well aware that we do not know the precise mechanisms of action of many drugs, including some of the most common ones. Thus, the problem of the acceptance or otherwise of homeopathy lies on a different plane, where what matters is the "philosophical" conception of science (epistemology). To get a clearer idea of what this means it is worthwhile dwelling for a moment or two on the concept of a scientific paradigm.

One of the most important keys to interpretation in our present approach to the evolution of science and therefore of medicine is our view of the history of scientific theories as a discontinuous succession of paradigms. *A paradigm is a set of theoretical assumptions, experimental practices, and modes of transmitting the contents of science* [Kuhn, 1962; Arecchi and Arecchi, 1990]. It therefore constitutes a frame of reference common to scientists in a certain period, in which theories, models, methods, instruments and, above all, a certain type of language form a single, coherent whole. Seen from the inside, a paradigm may present such coherence and demonstrative strength that any contradictions prove negligible. Those who operate within the framework of a given paradigm base their efforts on a model which is accepted by all, whether it be in conceptually designing research protocols, in choosing methodologies, or in drawing conclusions from experimental results. In this way it proves much easier to obtain research funds (projects appear very logical and important to funding agencies) and to get one's work published in the leading scientific journals (the language used and the conclusions drawn come up to the expectations and understanding capability of the scientific community).

Certainly, one factor with a decisive impact on the development of a paradigm is the economic and technological situation, the evolution of which sometimes enables researchers to make veritable leaps forward in their research in quality terms. David Ruelle, for instance, a member of the French *Académie des Sciences*, writes: "Contemporary international science tends to be confused with American science. It is undoubtedly true that research (and good research) is also done elsewhere, but the United States dictate fashions and how things are done" [Ruelle, 1992, p. 75]. The predominance of North American high technology and spending power is an objective consideration which inevitably has repercussions on the way science is conducted.

The type of relationship existing between the various paradigms in a given age, or between paradigms succeeding one another in history is still a subject of heated debate among epistemologists. According to some, paradigms are struggling among themselves for a sort of supremacy, and forcibly oust one another in successive "revolutionary breaks with the past." According to others, the progressive evolution and transformation of one paradigm into another is possible without dramatic clashes or contradictions, at least on the scientific plane.

From time to time in the course of the history of medicine various different paradigms have gotten the upper hand. In primitive or pre-scientific societies the paradigm dominating the study of natural phenomena was based on philosophy or mythology; later, in western countries, with the development of anatomical techniques and physiological investigations, a more descriptive and classificatory approach was adopted (1600-1700); in the next phase, the medical world went over to a paradigm based on the cell, with the advent of cellular pathology and microbiology (1700-1800); lastly, in the wake of the enormous advances made in chemistry and biochemistry, we come to the present-day paradigm which can be defined as molecular. Molecular biology today appears to be the interpretative basis for all cellular and pathophysiological phenomena, even going so far as to embrace neuronal and psychic events. The explanation of disease processes, whether genetic or acquired, is sought and, where possible, located in mechanisms consisting in quantitative and/or qualitative modifications of particular molecules making up part of the various anatomical or physiological systems.

Today, however, in the very heyday of the molecular paradigm, we are witnessing signs of a change in tendency, or at least signs of substantial variations on the molecular theme. There are now many people who perceive the inadequacy of the molecular paradigm when it comes to coping with major health problems such as neoplastic, degenerative, autoimmune, endocrine-metabolic, and neuropsychiatric disease. This inadequacy is not quantitative, since no-one would deny the importance of making further progress in our knowledge of the molecular mechanisms involved in these diseases. The problem is another: the sheer quantity of notions, the growth of which is exponential, cannot be mastered even by the specialists in the various disciplines, and brings in its wake a progressive sub-specialization in various sectors. The pursuit of a unitary approach, capable of assuring a multidisciplinary synthesis and of defining the nature of disease processes at higher levels of organization, is proving increasingly difficult. In practice, though not in principle, this ongoing accumulation of notions and data proves inadequate as a means of furthering our understanding of complex vital phenomena and thus of the phenomena relating to health and disease. The word *complexity* is appearing with increasing frequency in scientific articles dealing with genetics, cell communication systems, and metabolism.

It makes no sense for us to react to this situation by denying the importance of the molecular approach, of which all modern biomedical practitioners are a more or less conscious expression; what makes much more sense is to respond by initiating exploration in other territories, within other paradigms, in order to see what new things they may have to offer. As often happens in operations taking place in uncharted territory, the people conducting the exploration are exposed both to the incomprehension of those who are used to keeping "both feet firmly on the ground" and to the real risk of taking the wrong path or going up blind alleys. What justifies the enterprise, from the point of view of the explorers, is basically scientific curiosity, the innate urge which prompts human beings to make new discoveries. What diminishes the foolhardiness of embarking on new and uncertain paths is the possibility of orientation and guidance provided by the scientific method, which so far has proved capable of bearing the brunt of the investigative effort, regardless of whether one is operating within the framework of one paradigm or another. The basis and origin of the experimental method is *observation*, often the product of chance or accident, but always meticulously and scrupulously recorded; this develops into a series of reasoned arguments and ideas which generate an *explanatory theory*, which in turn enables us to formulate hypotheses to be submitted to *experimental* testing. As long as experiments can be performed, we are authorized to construct hypotheses, however fanciful or outlandish these may be. Ideas and hypotheses, Karl Popper maintains, may originate in the researcher's mind perhaps as inspired guesswork or as the sudden illumination of a series of items of knowledge long imprinted on the mind, or even as the result of character traits or inclinations. What really matters is that these hypotheses can be tested and that they may be subject to invalidation.

A new paradigm enables previously inexplicable phenomena to be explained scientifically and previously unsolvable problems to be solved and therefore it becomes increasingly important, the greater the social and economic relevance of the phenomena concerned. It has been claimed that any paradigm inevitably reflects the cultural climate and economic situation of the period in which it is developed. In this day and age, when, despite the enormous scientific progress of biomedicine, an increasing number of people are turning (rightly or wrongly) to other forms of therapy, when conventional drugs are beginning to prove highly expensive both for the national health service and the patient's pocket, increasing pressure is being brought to bear for a change in attitude towards previously neglected therapies.

Homeopathy, by its very nature, presents a challenge to the molecular paradigm, or rather, to the claim the molecular paradigm sometimes makes that it is the only way of interpreting biological reality. A better place for homeopathy might be within the framework of a new paradigm emerging in medicine, which might be defined the *biophysical paradigm*. Molecules are not the only decisive factors, inasmuch as energies and information of an electromagnetic type, used so far, and only partially, for diagnostic purposes (ECG, EEG, NMR, X-rays, evoked potentials) may play a major role. The same concept has been clearly expressed by Beverly Rubik, director of the Center for Frontier Sciences at Temple University, at a recent GIRI conference: "The observations of low dose biological effects challenge the dominant paradigm of mechanical reductionism, of viewing life as a collection of biomolecules responding to molecular stimuli. The enhanced potency of very low doses as in homeopathy appears to challenge molecular theory, one of the pillars of the modern chemistry. On the other hand, it may demonstrate that something else is occurring at these very low doses that does not involve molecules" [Rubik, 1994, p. 162].

According to other views, it would be more appropriate to set homeopathy squarely within the framework of the *complexity paradigm*. In this perspective, the dynamic interrelationship between the various components of the human being, ranging from the physico-anatomical to the mental, is highlighted, as is that between human beings and their environment. The homeopathic "diagnosis" and therapy are addressed primarily at the whole person as a single unit (the homeopathic *simillimum* is at the same time an analysis and a synthesis of all the aspects of dysregulation encountered in the patient), rather than at the anatomico-functional lesion and the individual symptom. For this reason, some people see homeopathy as a form of medicine that cures the whole patient and not just the disease.

These two different interpretations of homeopathy, oriented towards biophysics and complexity, respectively, do not clash head on, but rather serve to illustrate the novelty and up-to-date topical nature of the homeopathic approach. Within the context of these two lines of thought, one should perhaps be able to view from the right perspective and perhaps even overcome the difficulties which homeopathy and other forms of so-called alternative medicine, such as those of the oriental tradition, meet with in their struggle to establish themselves and gain acceptance.

5 Complexity, Information, and Integration

The increase in biomedical knowledge which has come about over the past two decades as a result of the molecular approach has led to a further upsurge in our awareness of the extreme complexity of living systems. Human beings possess roughly 100,000 different genes and thus, theoretically, may be regarded as constructions made of a vast number of bricks of about 100,000 different types (considering proteins alone). In actual fact, these bricks are not arranged at random, but are assembled in a highly coordinated manner and, what is more, are constantly being rearranged by interaction within the system and with the environment. To this we should add our heightened awareness of the existence of numerous biological differences between individuals of the same species which make it difficult, if not impossible, to establish normal values and predict the outcome of external regulatory interventions.

In other words, the increase in knowledge of the subcomponents of the living system is accompanied by increasing difficulty in describing the unitary behavior of the system itself in scientifically precise terms and, as a consequence in the biomedical field, by an increasing awareness of the limitations of therapies based on a reductionist approach. The basic reason for this lies in the fact that the physician invariably finds himself having to apply general biological notions to a particular, unique and unrepeatable case, who reacts as a unitary being in a context with which he or she has countless interrelations.

In this connection, it is worth quoting what the Nobel Prize winner for Medicine, Alexis Carrel, one of the few top-ranking scientists to have an open mind on the study of nonconventional forms of medicine (he even edited a book on the subject), has to say: "The future of medicine is subordinate to its concept of the human being. Its greatness depends on the wealth of this concept. Rather than limit the human being to certain of his aspects, it must be all-embracing, fusing body and spirit in their essential oneness. (...) Any human individual is at the same time complexity and simplicity, oneness and multiplicity. Every individual presents a different story from all the others. He or she is a unique aspect of the universe. (...) To date we have studied ourselves only in such a way as to procure fragmentary concepts of what we are. Our analysis began right from the outset by severing the continuity of the human being and his cosmic and social environment. Then it separated the soul from the body. The body was divided into organs, cells, and fluids. And in this process of dissection, the spirit has vanished. Thus, there are many sciences, each dealing with an isolated aspect. We call them sociology, history, pedagogy, physiology, and so on. But a human being is much more than the sum of these analytical data. He should thus be considered both in his parts and as a whole, inasmuch as he reacts in the cosmic, economic, and psychological environment as a single entity and not as a multiplicity of entities" [Carrel, 1950, pp. 9–10].

Medicine may provide evidence to the effect that "a human being is much more than the sum of these analytical data," by opening its doors to the study of complexity, totality, individuality, systemic interrelation phenomena, and ecology. In this context, forms of complementary medicine such as homeopathy, acupuncture, and that vast and as yet poorly defined area known as "natural medicine" may have a role to play as a stimulus or a challenge to scientifically conceived medicine.

The need to address these problems in relation to homeopathy and its possible mode of action derives from three series of considerations:

a) Health and disease are basically determined by states of order or disorder of the body, which are an expression of the complexity of living beings.

b) The homeopathic method presents itself as an all-embracing, integrated approach to health and disease: it takes account of all the possible factors of a biological and psychological nature which characterize a given individual, seeking to grasp the essence of their interrelations. These interrelations can only be understood within a logical framework which takes due account of complexity.

c) Homeopathy claims that information is contained in the aqueous or water-alcohol solution in a "meta-molecular" form. If this is true, then it follows that such solutions are characterized by some sort of order and memory (information store). The problem of the hypothetical transfer of information from the solute to the solvent falls within the sphere of the complex behavior of liquids, and is investigated in that context. In a later section we shall see that physicists are constructing models of water in the liquid state and positing ways in which these may hypothetically store information.

To better clarify the importance of these issues for the formulation of hypotheses regarding homeopathy, we intend to examine here below a number of sectors of modern medicine in which complexity has come to play a prominent role, precisely on the basis of present-day biological and molecular knowledge.

5.1

*Complexity
of diseases*

In an initial approach to the question of complexity we can take as our starting point a reflection, which is only apparently theoretical, on the nature of disease in general. These considerations are theoretical only in appearance because *it is inevitable that the diagnostic and therapeutic approach to disease depends on the concept one has of it* in general, on the theoretical and philosophical plane, rather than in its individual details. This is all the more true for those who seek to reason and act within a holistic rather than a specialistic conceptual frame of reference.

Disease, in essence, is a disorder of structures and/or functions, with characteristic abnormalities at the cellular and molecular levels. The definition of disease inevitably depends on the standpoint (meaning not the personal opinion, but the perspective from which the matter is viewed) of those attempting to define it [Laplantine, 1986]. Today, the standpoint of modern medicine, as conceived scientifically, is represented by molecular pathology because the astonishing progress which has come about as a result of the introduction of molecular biology techniques, particularly in the analysis of proteins and nucleic acids, has led to an enormous increase in our knowledge of the molecular abnormalities (both quantitative and qualitative) present in many diseases, whether hereditary or acquired. This new molecular-based knowledge of many diseases is beginning to have significant positive repercussions in terms of diagnosis and a more rational utilization of drugs. It has been the task of the molecular approach to clarify the biological basis of disease, and this will continue to be the case for many years to come. In view of the variety of possible pathological situations at this level, it is a task which is several degrees of magnitude greater than that performed in the past by pathological anatomy at organ or cell level.

The problem of an exhaustive and satisfactory definition of the concept of disease cannot be solved merely on the basis of a knowledge of molecular biology, however detailed that may be. The great increase in the *extent* of our knowledge is not enough to guarantee an *intensive* understanding of the deeper meaning which the abnormalities observed have in the dynamics of the onset and development of a disease process. Any satisfactory description of the nature of disease necessarily entails a search for the causes (etiology) and the mechanisms (pathogenesis), or, in other words, the "why" and "how" the disease process sets in and develops. The search for causes will be successful when the causes are precise and usually confined to one or only a few physical, chemical or biological damaging factors, but encounters often insurmountable obstacles when the causes are multiple or when the disease originates from a series of causes in succession, each dependent upon the previous one. Establishing the pathogenesis requires the largest possible number of notions on the objective changes (whether anatomical, biochemical, molecular or electrophysiological), but also calls for identification of the cause-and-effect relationships and for the hierarchical ordering of phenomena in terms of space and time. Our attempt here is to outline an approach to the definition of disease based not so much and not exclusively on the molecular paradigm, but on a way of reasoning which takes account of new epistemological horizons.

Life is an expression of the complex behavior of nature. It is essentially the property of an open system in which information governs matter and energy, but without completely suppressing, and indeed often benefiting from, the chaotic element (the concepts of information and chaos will be dealt with in Chapter 5, Sections 5 and 7, respectively). Life is a metastable state: it maintains and reproduces itself as a thermodynamically far-from-equilibrium event, thanks to the exchange of energy and matter taking place between the living system and the environment [Guerritore, 1987; Guidotti, 1990]. The fact that homeostatic biological systems exist which maintain certain parameters within suitable oscillation limits does not mean that the body or its subsystems are in a state of "equilibrium," but merely that the body is well organized and knows how to channel the *flow* of matter in a manner which is productive for life itself.

For instance, it is well known that there are very substantial differences in the concentrations of ions (sodium, potassium, hydrogen, calcium, magnesium) between the various cell compartments separated by biological membranes. The cells actually make use of these differences and asymmetries to generate signals, information, and even energy. Thus, the transmission of the nerve impulse depends on the imbalance between sodium and potassium across the fiber membrane; cell division requires a transfer of hydrogen ions from the intra- to the extracellular space (alkalinization of the cytoplasm); cell movement involves an unstable alternating process of assembly and disassembly of multimeric structural proteins. The maintenance of life and health therefore consists in controlling a dysequilibrium ("controlled dysequilibrium") [Guidotti, 1990].

Clearly, the state of good health cannot be maintained indefinitely and ageing is inevitable. This problem, too, has no simple explanation, entirely attributable to molecular parameters. As the neuropharmacologist M. Trabucchi says: "The latest biomedical research has attempted to clarify the ways whereby life leaves its traces on biological structure. Some of these ways are predictable because they obey objective (or scientifically parametrized) laws, while others are unpredictable. To the former group belong the experiments, mainly conducted in animals, on the basis of which a number of environmental characteristics are reflected in simple parameters of neuronal functioning (dendritic arborization, number of synapses, etc.); to the second group belong those series of events which can be characterized by the theme of complexity, whereby enormously variable external stimuli are interpreted via various man-environment interfaces and translated into highly differentiated biological and personal realities" [Trabucchi, 1992, p. 137].

At the opposite extreme to the organization of life is death, which therefore represents the maximum disorder, dissipation of information, and increase in entropy, tending towards thermodynamic equilibrium (the concept of *entropy* in living systems will be discussed in Chapter 5, Section 8.1). Disease lies somewhere between the two, consisting in partial disorder of systems of information, energy, and matter, localized in space and time.

When reflecting upon the question of disease, one problem which immediately springs to mind is understanding which of the various events observed are primary and which secondary: not everything in the disease process is pathological, in the sense that it is damaging. Disease is disorder, but it nevertheless obeys certain laws, and thus embodies some measure of order, though this is conditioned by chance events. The homeostatic biological systems which govern health are the same that cause most pathological phenomena, when activated inadequately, excessively or unsuitably in relation to the circumstances. On the other hand, it is also true to say that many phenomena that are called pathological are biologically useful (even if they cause pain), representing a stage of transition to a state of greater vitality, energy, and resistance to pathogens (= information gain). For instance, we need only mention inflammation and immunity, both of which are pathophysiological processes which, though carrying a certain price to be paid in terms of subjective symptoms and possible organ damage, in actual fact serve the purposes of repairing, defending, and inducing a state of enhanced resistance. This enhanced resistance derives from the biological memory of past experience.

These considerations lead us to our first conclusion: judging what is useful and what is damaging, on every occasion and in every aspect of disease, is by no means easy, in that it presupposes a knowledge of the "logic" of disease and normality, a knowledge of the language of complex systems (some of these systems are inflammation, immunity, neuroendocrine organizations, subtle metabolic regulatory mechanisms) rather than of the language of molecules. Disease is a problem of molecules, but also, in a different dimension, it is a problem of cells, of physiological systems and of the human being as a whole: if the molecular disorder is not compensated for by supramolecular systems, it is the latter that are responsible for the disease, and not the molecule. Disease is a problem of the individual, but it is also a problem of the environment: the individual is often the victim of a disease greater than him- or herself (e.g. violence, pollution, epidemics, misinformation by the mass media, social alienation, loneliness), and whoever reflects upon the real nature of diseases can hardly be satisfied with a reductionist explanation which fails to go beyond the latest biochemical consequences of these problems.

Disease is thus essentially an information disorder. Genetic diseases are the most striking examples of this: the *order* of the genetic code sequence is changed, and the disorder lies in the very information store itself. Genetic disease can also be caused by a very minor transcription error in the basic cell library. Even acquired diseases, or diseases in which genetic and environmental factors are mixed (these are by far the majority) are disorders of information at a more complex level: what is altered is not just the molecular order of the DNA, but also the information order governing the supramolecular systems. In most diseases we can identify an imbalance of the homeostatic biological systems at various levels. The molecular, cellular, tissue, organic, and neuroimmunohematological systems, tend in themselves to function according to deterministically correct parameters.

For example, in inflammation, thrombosis, atherosclerosis, hyperplasias, and endocrine disorders, it often proves possible to identify not a primary defect of the system itself, but a defect in its regulation. The platelet, when it causes a thrombus, is doing its job, as are thrombin and fibrin. The macrophage, when it engulfs oxidized lipoproteins, is doing its job (scavenging), even if this then causes an accumulation of foam cells in the tunica intima of the artery. It is true that a particular genetic defect may cause the pathological event (e.g. a lack of C/S proteins in thrombosis or a lack of LDL receptors in atherosclerosis), but more often than not, in practice, such genetic defects are neither marked nor decisive. Furthermore, every disease, even if primarily genetic, depends to a large extent in its clinical course on the occurrence of regulatory imbalances, inasmuch as the system would tend to counteract every defect with an adequate compensation mechanism.

The concept of the "host" and its importance in pathology come back into the reckoning with a reappraisal in more updated terms, so that today we could talk about a neuroimmunoendocrine system, but the substance of the matter does not change: every disease has a strong component related to endogenous reactivity. It is, in fact, only after a long time and after continuous perturbations of the homeostatic biological systems that multifactorial diseases manifest themselves clinically, when the homeostatic systems have departed from the norm, adapting to a chronic situation of abnormal pathological symptoms. In practice, a substantial proportion of the diseases have as their basic mechanism an upward or downward shift in the activity of various homeostatic systems, with all the possible range of symptomatological sequelae and permanent structural abnormalities which in turn then come to form the basis for new imbalances.

A simplified block diagram of the pathophysiological events occurring in the course of a typical disease is shown in Figure 2. This diagram represents a general frame of reference, which is useful above all for illustrating the interrelationships between various steps in the disease process which integrate one another dynamically. It can be seen that if etiological agents of various kinds (chemical, physical, biological, and deficiency-related) overcome the first set of defense systems, they cause structural and/or functional biochemical damage. This damage triggers reactions on the part of the systems responsible for the conservation and restoration of biological integrity, also called *homeostatic biological systems*. These systems thus occupy a central position in the dynamic evolution of a disease: good functioning leads to repair and healing, but the homeostatic systems themselves can cause further damage, giving rise to a kind of positive pathological feedback. Obviously, if the damage, be it direct or indirect, is severe or irreversible, a no-return situation is created which may lead to death or to permanent disability (pathological state).

Most of the *signs and symptoms* of the disease stem not so much from the direct damage caused by the etiological agent as from the reactions of the body.

The block diagram in Figure 2 also shows another possible evolution of the typical pathophysiological pattern, namely *adaptation*. In a certain sense, this is an intermediate course midway between healing and the pathological state, since it represents a new state of normality adapted to the changed circumstances. For example, if there has been lung damage which has reduced the alveolar-capillary exchange surface, the homeostatic system controlling the oxygenation level will react with production of a greater number of red blood cells (polycythemia). Polycythemia is not normal in subjects who do not live at high altitude, but at the same time it cannot be regarded as a pathological state, despite constituting a long-term modification. If, for the sake of hypothesis, we succeeded in bringing about a regression of the pulmonary picture, the polycythemia would disappear. Other examples of adaptation may include cardiac hypertrophy and changes in kidney function in the course of hypertension, lymphadenomegaly in children exposed to continuous immunological stimulation, hyperinsulinemia in obese subjects, steatosis or xanthomas in certain serum lipid disorders, and many others.

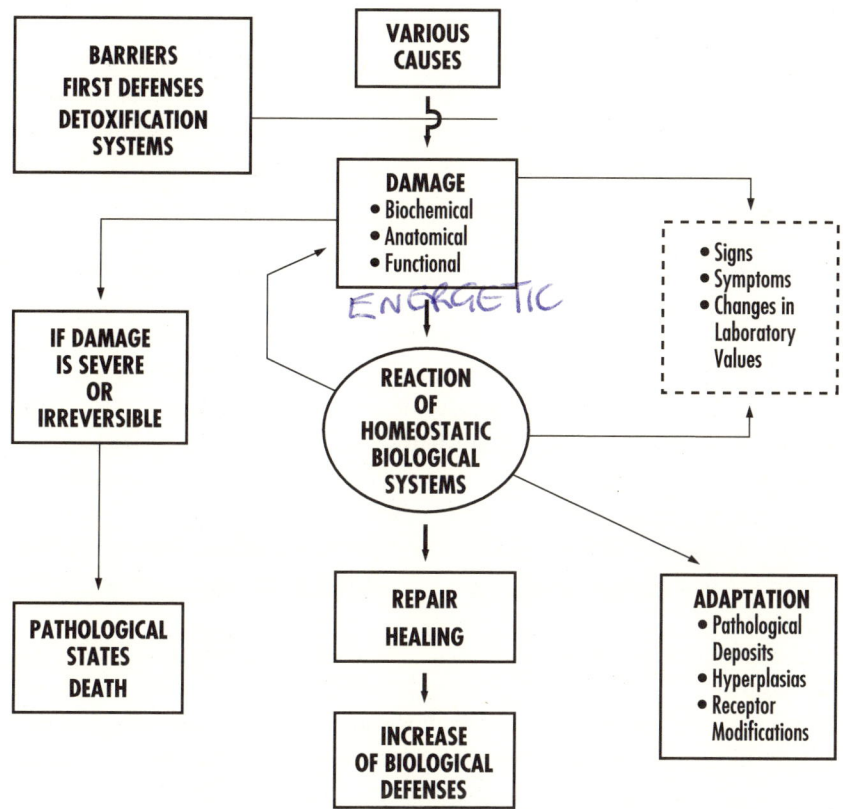

FIGURE 2 Diagram of a typical pathophysiological frame of reference representing the possible events involved in a disease. For an explanation, see text.

DISEASE

If disease is an information disorder of complex systems, to get to the heart of the matter the molecular approach, which analyzes only one aspect of information, is necessary, but not enough. New approaches, new models, and new concepts are beginning to be introduced in biology in order to overcome this hurdle. It is not enough to understand the individual elements and try to put them together according to a computer-aided or cybernetic model: no-one believes any longer that the formulation of a precise, predictive model, capable of taking account of all the variables involved in a single cell, is remotely feasible, not to mention the even unlikelier construction of exact models for the functioning of organs or systems.

Faced with this plain fact, one might be tempted to conclude that we can never describe a disease exactly and consequently that it is impossible to come up with a therapeutic measure which is completely rational and correctly oriented towards curing the disease. If this were the case, we would therefore have to settle for understanding only certain aspects of the disease (something which is certainly possible today) and opt for a therapy based on these aspects (e.g. antiinflammatory, analgesic, replacement therapy, etc.). This does not mean that these latter therapies are not useful and efficacious in many cases, or that they cannot favor definitive healing processes set in motion by the body itself. What it means is being realistically aware of the type of measure being applied and thus also understanding the reason why in many cases the current therapies are not enough to solve the problem.

If we want to capture in a single image the whole crux of the problem of information regulation in vital processes, and thus also of its pathological aspects, it may be illuminating to refer to the model of an orchestra. The orchestra is the body, and the music is its life. In the orchestra, there is a material, "molecular" part, composed of instruments with a precise structure and of musicians with their receptive, elaborative, and motor capabilities. What matters most, however, is that the orchestra plays in harmony according to a program provided by the score and at a pace dictated by the conductor.

A performance may prove unsuccessful because one of its material parts breaks (e.g. the strings of a violin, or the stool of one of the musicians), but it may also fail because the various musicians are in disaccord. The quality of the music the orchestra produces depends on conditions such as the quality of the instruments, the quality of the score, the skill of the conductor, and, above all else, the degree of unison and harmony between the members. If there should be interference due to some outside noise or disturbance, or if an orchestra is tired or distracted, there is a risk that the orchestra will play out of tune, and this risk is all the more serious, the less able the conductor is to keep the orchestra under control. If the music is seriously out of tune, or the conductor is weak, the flaw may involve the entire orchestra to the distinct detriment of the work as a whole.

This example shows us that there does not necessarily need to be a primary structural abnormality for the overall effect to be a disaster. An information disorder can also arise as a result of subtle and not immediately perceivable deviations from the norm, which are then amplified and/or stabilized by adaptation and positive feedback mechanisms. In the healthy body this orchestra plays continuously in a coordinated manner. It is difficult to say whether there is a "conductor" because all the parts, including the brain, function properly, influencing one another reciprocally. It is undeniable, however, that there is a hierarchy, whereby some systems have greater control functions and therefore may be regarded as more important from the regulatory point of view.

Apart from the example provided here, is there any way of tackling the problem of complexity rationally? Given that there is no possibility of constructing exact models of the various phenomena endowed with predictability, we have to see whether at least certain "ground rules" of behavior of complex systems can be identified, which can be used in possible attempts at modulation. As mentioned above, the study of complexity is a frontier area for science, where mathematicians, physicians, and biologists seek to break new ground. It is very likely that these studies will yield appreciable windfall gains in the biomedical area, too. One can easily imagine that substantial links will emerge between these concepts, which refer to the behavior of complex systems, and the interpretation of the mechanisms whereby complex biological systems may deviate from the state of normal homeostasis (see also Chapter 5, Sections 7 and 8).

Any approach to the definition of disease will reflect reality more closely, the more *integrated* it is, in the sense of its taking account of all the possible levels at which the pathological information disorder manifests, perpetuates, and communicates itself. What is emerging with increasing clarity and with a growing body of corroborative evidence is that order in the biological sphere is produced by an interactive network of molecules, cells, organs, and systems, made up of both *horizontal* (e.g. molecule to molecule) and *vertical* messages between systems with different levels of complexity (e.g. molecule to cell, but also cell to body, and body to environment). No biological system exists in isolation; it could never survive, since it would be overwhelmed by entropy. Thus, neither can disease be an isolated, self-sufficient event; disease is not simply an error of nature, but rather one of its "ways of being," the deeper significance of which remains largely inaccessible.

Inflammation is the response of living tissue to damage, which may be of a physical, chemical or biological nature. We are in the presence, then, of a phenomenon which is at the same time physiological and pathological and which is in some way implicated in all diseases; its comprehension on the scientific plane and its modulation on the pharmacological plane represent one of the greatest challenges to medical science.

Starting from a whole variety of endogenous and exogenous causes of noxious stimulation, a process is set in motion in which various molecular components (plasma proteins, lipids, prostaglandins, hormones, peptides, ions) and cellular components (leukocytes, platelets, macrophages, endothelial cells, neurons) take part. Though inflammation is usually a local tissue alteration, it would appear increasingly clear that various organs or systems take part directly or indirectly in its regulation.

5.2

Example of a complex biological system: inflammation

While the defensive function of inflammation as it has developed in the course of evolution is beyond doubt, an increasing amount of attention is being devoted today to diseases due to excessive activation of this patho-physiological mechanism and to the secondary damage it causes. The effector systems and the regulation mechanisms themselves turn on the host, causing a series of increasingly widespread diseases due not so much to outside causes as to malfunctioning of the inflammation and immune systems. As these same mechanisms are capable of acting both defensively and offensively, the *interpretation* of the language of inflammation (i.e. of the various messages which the systems involved exchange) is of fundamental importance for its possible control and modulation. The *language* which the inflammation systems speak tends today to become coherent through a *cybernetic model* and contains words such as "signals," "mediators," "targets," "activation," "regulation," "message" (inter- and intracellular), "priming," "desensitization," and "memory."

The inflammatory process is vital for the survival of all complex organisms and is involved in many aspects of health and disease. There can be no doubt that the inflammatory process has evolved as a basic mechanism for protecting the integrity of the organism. This protection is exerted both against possible invasion by pathogenic microorganisms present in the environment (the fight against infection) and against pathological modifications of the normal constituents of the body: for example, an inflammatory process intervenes when necrotic processes set in due to tissue anoxia, trauma or burns, when there is vascular damage and hemorrhage, when a tumor develops, when a transplant is inserted, and in tissue affected by ionizing radiation. In all these cases, the basic defensive, reparatory meaning of the inflammatory process is self-evident. This is proved by the fact that certain functional deficits or a reduction in the number of inflammatory cells easily lead to a state of high susceptibility to infection.

Since living organisms are constantly subject to stress and to aggression of various kinds, the development of more or less marked inflammatory processes is inevitable and, in a certain sense, may be regarded as a positive factor, since it contributes towards augmenting the natural defenses themselves. There are gross and painful manifestations of the inflammatory process which can quite easily be interpreted as the inevitable price to be paid if elimination of pathogens is to be achieved. These include, for instance, most of the symptoms accompanying acute infectious diseases (fever, asthenia, anorexia, pain in the infected area, exanthema). On the other hand, there are inflammatory phenomena which are frankly unjustified and thus largely damaging to the body; they include, for example, those related to autoimmunity, or to rare defects of the inflammation-inhibiting systems (e.g. hereditary angioedema), or to transplant rejection.

Midway between these two extremes lie a whole series of diseases in which the inflammation initially occurs for defensive and/or reparatory purposes, but later, for various reasons, becomes a pathogenetic mechanism which conditions—possibly to a decisive extent—the course and outcome of the disease itself. In these cases, the processes triggered off hover in a state of constant imbalance between damaging attack and defense. The inflammatory process does not succeed in fulfilling its reparatory purpose and is involved in a general *organizational disorder* of the body, with the result that its original aim is lost. It is well known that a substantial proportion of the most common diseases today can be traced back to disorders of the inflammatory process, due essentially to two mechanisms, namely either to failure to recognize its own components which are regarded as foreign, or to abnormal control of an inflammatory process, which would otherwise be suitable in terms of the molecular target (excessive amplification, nonsuppression of the process, and spread beyond the area anatomically necessary).

The basic problem is thus understanding when and how the inflammatory process strays into pathological territory. The question applies to both acute and chronic inflammation. Obviously, this is a major problem both from the conceptual and, consequently, from the clinical and therapeutic points of view. Understanding the dynamics of inflammatory processes, of the biochemical mechanisms involved in them, of the functions of the various cells involved, and of the regulatory centers responsible for centralized control constitutes one of the greatest challenges to medicine and the basic prerequisite for effective therapy.

We deal here fairly extensively with the inflammatory process because it is the main reaction and repair system for damage of any kind and must therefore occupy a central position within the framework of any hypothesis with regard to the mechanism of action of homeopathy. It has been seen, in fact, that this type of medicine has always claimed, ever since its inception, to aim at activating the endogenous reactive capability of the body ("vital force"). Some parts of this section have been taken from a previous review of the same topic [Bellavite, 1990b].

5.2.1 Basic characteristics of the inflammatory process

Inflammation (also called phlogosis) was recognized by the ancient Roman Cornelius Celsus as the process causing "*rubor, tumor, cum calore et dolore*" (redness, swelling, with heat and pain). In modern terms, it can be defined as an *integrated response of tissue and even of the entire body (when the process is sufficiently extensive) to damage caused by external or internal agents*. This series of responses consist in changes in blood vessels, circulating plasma, and cells, especially leukocytes. On a general scale, many other phenomena occur caused by remote repercussions of the originally localized process.

The view of the inflammatory reaction as a phase in a continuous process going from damage to healing or to further damage is in tune with the concepts of "*progressive vicariation*" and "*pathological metastasis*" (in the broadest sense of the term as used in conventional medicine) traditionally propounded by homotoxicology and homeopathy to suggest that there is a profound, consequential link between the various phases making up the *disease history* in a patient. The field of inflammation is an ideal subject of study for homotoxicology and natural medicine in general. Indeed, the very aim of this type of therapeutic approach is to try to use systems of care which cooperate with the natural healing process, exploiting its great intrinsic potential.

The terrain where most of the inflammatory process takes place is the connective tissue, consisting of cells of mesenchymal origin, leukocytes, afferent and efferent nerve endings, hematic and lymphatic vascular networks, fibers, and basic substance. The network of capillaries in a tissue is composed of endothelial cells resting on a thin basal membrane. The blood flow in the capillaries is determined above all by the degree of patency of the arterioles and their terminal branches which are endowed with smooth muscle with sphincter functions. At this level, the control exerted is nervous, hormonal, and also dependent upon partial oxygen pressure and pH. When a traumatic event occurs in this territory, or bacteria arrive, or toxins or irritating chemical substances are present, many biological phenomena come into operation, the most important of which are:

a) After initial contraction, the smooth muscle cells of the arterial terminal branches relax, thus allowing the entry of much more blood, which circulates in the capillary network, first rapidly and then more and more sluggishly, engorging the entire tissue (hence the old descriptors "calor" and "rubor"). An important role in this phase is played by the endothelial cells themselves, which, when activated by physicochemical changes in the surrounding environment, give rise to a series of molecules which go on to mediate further events.

b) The mast cells present in the connective tissue release their granules containing histamine and other substances, thereby causing the opening up of spaces between the endothelial cells with leakage of the fluid portion of the blood (plasma) and formation of exudate (the old "tumor," in the sense of edema, or swelling).

c) The exudate may dilute and remove microbes and toxic substances, mainly via the lymphatic network, thus contributing to activation of the immune response. The exudate may form a fibrin layer, which also constitutes a barrier to the spread of infectious pathogens. It also contains many substances which are active as mediators of the further development of the inflammation and as mediators of the amplification of the reaction. These substances include components of complement which stimulate the mast cells to release histamine (anaphylotoxins) and others which play a direct role in the killing of bacteria. Some of the mediators also stimulate sensory nerve endings, causing pain (the old "dolor") and, as discovered only fairly recently, the release by these nerve endings of neuropeptides, which in turn increase the inflammatory response.

d) We then have the action of the white blood cells in the inflammation focus, primarily granulocytes, which, in response to perceived changes in the endothelium and tissue fluids, emerge from the vessels under the influence of the bacteria themselves, cellular debris, endotoxins, fibrin fragments, activated complement, and specific cytokines such as interleukin-8.

e) In the later phases of the reaction, we also find lymphocytes, monocytes, and macrophages (chronic inflammation). Fibroblasts, as is well known, come into play in the processes of wound repair and scar formation. Among the possible consequences of inflammation there is the development of sclerosis; we need only mention the healing of wounds by second intention, cheloids, cirrhosis of the liver, pulmonary fibrosis, and atherosclerosis itself, many of whose pathogenetic elements constitute a *"response to injury."*

We are in the presence therefore of a complex series of integrated phenomena, in which the granulocytes intervene as the most active cells in the production of toxic oxygen radicals, but also as cells capable of producing a series of mediators acting as signals for other cells. We can do no more here than merely outline some of the aspects of the biochemical regulation of the inflammatory process, this being a vast and much debated topic.

The granulocytes arising in the bone marrow remain in the bloodstream only a few hours and then adhere to the endothelium and pass into the tissues to prepare the defense against possible foreign agents. The molecular mechanisms whereby cells attach themselves to one another are well known; for instance, we know that, in the vicinity of the inflammation focus, granulocytes express anchoring proteins on the outer membrane (these are of various types, including the so-called integrins) which attach themselves to specific receptors produced and expressed by the endothelium, called intercellular adhesion molecules.

A great deal is also known today about cell orientation and motility systems, which underlie the phenomena of chemotaxis and phagocytosis. Receptors have been described for dozens of different substances to which granulocytes are sensitive and which stimulate them to move and migrate in an oriented manner. It is also known that the mechanical apparatus which the cell needs in order to perform these functions is based essentially on phenomena of continuous polymerization and depolymerization of proteins of the cytoskeleton, which form organized filaments in the cytoplasm. Among the granulocyte cytotoxic and bactericidal systems a key role is played by the production of toxic oxygen radicals.

This particular type of oxygen metabolism is activated during phagocytosis or as a result of other soluble stimuli and is based on the fact that oxygen is not used to produce energy, as in all the other cells, but to produce electronically activated derivatives such as free O_2^- radicals (superoxide), OH· (hydroxyl radical), hydrogen peroxide, and other highly reactive molecules such as singlet oxygen and hypochlorous acid. Involved in the production of these latter derivatives is the enzyme myeloperoxidase. Oxygen metabolism, as described here, implies the consumption of NADPH as a donor of electrons and consumption of glucose-6-phosphate, which is necessary for the production of new NADPH [Rossi, 1986; Bellavite, 1988]. In addition to the NADPH oxidase system, several inflammation cells also produce *nitric oxide*, which has bactericidal and parasiticidal functions, as well as regulatory functions in the inflammatory process. Nitric oxide, in fact, can cause vasodilation and can also interfere with superoxide and inactivate it.

The effects of free radicals at molecular level are essentially changes in proteins (oxidation, aggregation), polysaccharides (depolymerization), lipids (peroxidation), and nucleic acids (strand break, mutations). To what extent such effects may be useful or damaging depends on the situation in which these changes occur. In fact, if the release of toxic radicals occurs in the context of a destructive action against invading pathogens or against toxins (endogenous or exogenous) or tumor cells, it may undoubtedly be regarded as useful. On the other hand, however, the same biochemical changes may be of prevalently pathological significance in other contexts such as atherosclerosis phenomena, postischemic tissue damage, pulmonary emphysema, Parkinson's disease, multiple sclerosis, shock, burns, rheumatoid arthritis, respiratory distress syndrome, and many others. Clearly, in such situations, what determines the end result of a biochemical reaction is not so much the molecule itself, or its quantity, as the *regulation* of the inflammatory process in the broadest sense of the term.

One of the most recent fields of study of the function of leukocytes in the context of inflammatory processes has to do with the regulation of their different levels of activation, which are multiple and varied. This is demonstrated both in systems in culture and in *ex vivo* cells, extracted from healthy subjects and patients suffering from various different diseases. These types of tests are not simple laboratory artefacts, but allow us to reproduce a situation which occurs *in vivo*, i.e. where the cells in a patient presenting inflammatory manifestations are *different* from the cells in a healthy person. It is also known that if we take leukocytes from a patient during a bacterial infection of a certain degree of severity, we find not only that they have grown in number, but also that they are functionally more efficient [Bass *et al.*, 1986]. In other pathological conditions, such as, for instance, in the course of viral infections or after severe burns, blood leukocytes are in a state of desensitization, and therefore present activity deficits. There may also be functional changes in leukocytes in different areas of the body in the same patient. We ourselves and other investigators have shown that leukocytes extracted from an inflammatory focus are more active in response to particular factors compared to leukocytes extracted from the bloodstream of the same subject [Briheim *et al.*, 1988; Biasi *et al.*, 1993]. The fact that the disease conditions cause changes in receptor and transduction system sensitivity in various cells of the body is well known in many fields of medicine [Brodde and Michel, 1989].

Whereas up until not so very long ago it was thought that the states of activation were essentially only two, namely, cells at rest and activated cells (e.g. in the case addressed here, cells activated to produce free radicals), today at least five different levels are known to exist:

a) Cells at rest, or inactive cells, such as, for example, young leukocytes, just produced by the bone marrow and circulating in the blood of a healthy subject.

b) Activated cells, such as young leukocytes a few seconds after coming into contact with the surface of a bacterium or of a cancer or virus-infected cell, bearing specific antibodies and complement on its surface.

c) Inactivated, or spent cells, in which the entire enzymatic and metabolic machinery has been consumed in the attack on a preponderant amount of foreign agents, with the result that it can no longer be activated by any kind of stimulus.

d) Cells specifically desensitized in relation to a number of molecules, whereas they continue to function normally or even above normal in response to the action of other stimuli.

e) Hyperresponsive or primed cells, meaning cells which in themselves are not active, i.e. do not produce free radicals, but which, once placed in contact with a stimulant, present a metabolic response which is much greater than that of normal activated cells.

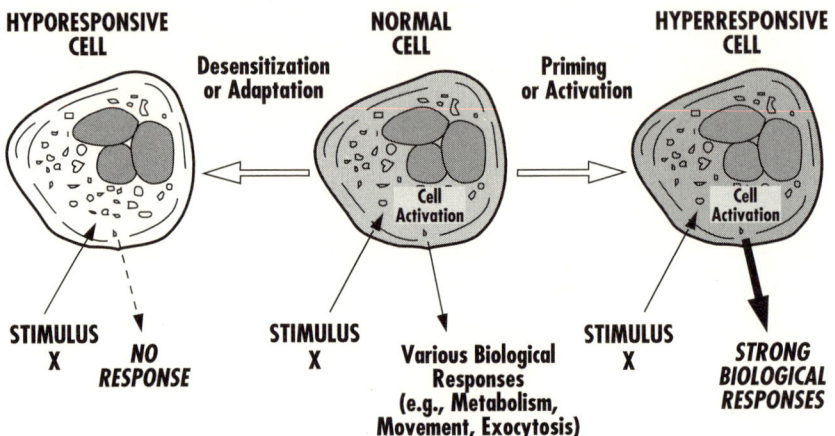

FIGURE 3 Various states of activation of a phagocytic cell. The same stimulus at the same dose (X) evokes quantitatively very different responses in cells in different sensitivity conditions.

Changes in sensitivity and in response intensity are the ways in which the inflammatory response regulation system intervenes at cell level (Figure 3). Cell priming is due to subtle molecular modifications, probably related to receptors and enzymes, but whose mechanism is still largely unknown, and which are induced by previous contact with small doses of chemotactic substances, cytokines, or bacterial products. Desensitization, on the other hand, is basically related to receptor dynamics, which may lead to loss of affinity, to down-regulation (internalization), or to uncoupling of specific receptors as a result of their excessive or prolonged occupancy. By no means extraneous to both priming and desensitization are other biological events occurring at post-receptor level, such as intracellular levels of cyclic AMP, calcium ions, sodium ions, and protons, the phosphorylation-dephosphorylation of specific proteins, the state of assembly of macromolecules, and the constitution of membrane lipids, which are in a state of constant rearrangement (cf. Chapter 5, Section 6.3).

Table 2 lists the substances which have regulatory effects at the above-mentioned levels.

Agents capable of regulating the production of free radicals by neutrophilic granulocytes	**TABLE 2**

a. Agents causing priming

1. Most cytokines, at low doses
2. Chemotactic factors, at low doses
3. Components of complement (e.g. C5a)
4. Ionophores
5. Lipids and derivatives (arachidonic acid, platelet activating factor, diacylglycerol, leukotriene B_4)
6. Bacterial endotoxins
7. Neuropeptides and tuftsin
8. Adenosine triphosphate
9. Muramyl peptide
10. Fibronectin
11. Growth hormone and insulin-like growth factor
12. Endothelin-1
13. Cytotoxic agents at very low doses

b. Agents which desensitize or inhibit

1. Repetition of medium-high doses of agonists
2. Beta-adrenergic agonists
3. Adenosine
4. Prostaglandins E_1, I_2
5. Factors produced by tumors
6. Corticosteroids
7. Bacterial toxins (e.g. pertussis)
8. Opioids
9. Contact with healthy endothelium
10. Various anesthetic and antiinflammatory drugs
11. C-reactive protein
12. Platelet-derived growth factor

The distinction between *positive* effect (priming) and agents with a *negative* effect (desensitization or inhibition) should not be made too schematically; from studies conducted in this field, the concept is emerging that the leukocytes are involved in the cybernetic information networks of inflammation in a highly sophisticated and complex way. The intensity of the response depends, for instance, on:

a) The previous condition of the cell (biochemical "memory").

b) The doses of regulatory agents, with the possibility of inverse effects: at low doses a substance acts as an activator, while at high doses it acts as an inhibitor [cf. Naum *et al.*, 1991; Bellavite *et al.*, 1993b], or, conversely, it inhibits at low doses and stimulates at high doses [Bellavite *et al.*, 1993c; Bellavite *et al.*, 1994] (see also Chapter 5, Section 6.2).

c) The coexistence of several active and antagonistic compounds (synergisms and antagonisms at receptor and transducer system level).

d) The individual's general state of health (neuro-immuno-endocrine equilibrium).

The cytokines, such as interleukin-1 (IL-1) and tumor necrosis factor (TNF), are examples of molecules which are active in a large number of cells and have endogenous inhibitors which moderate their effects. These inhibitors, which are practically *soluble* receptors for the molecules themselves or antagonists which bind competitively to their receptors, were first extracted from the urine of patients with inflammatory diseases and are actively studied today with a view to their possible use as natural anti-inflammatory drugs. There are diseases (myeloid leukemia, autoimmunity) in which an *imbalance* between the active molecule and its endogenous inhibitor can be detected [see review by Dinarello, 1991].

The free radicals produced by activated phagocytes can become a mechanism whereby molecules of the cell environment, neurohumoral mediators and bacterial products are altered, usually in the sense of oxidative inactivation. The alteration of proteins by oxygen radicals is very easy if these proteins contain methionine, a sulphurated amino acid which is particularly susceptible to oxidation. If this structural alteration involves proteins with intracellular signalling functions, there may be repercussions in terms of information: a signal protein may become inactive or may even be transformed into an antagonist of the original protein (negative feedback effect on the course of the inflammation). While, however, a number of substances have a useful effect, their oxidation may cause pathogenic effects, as is the case, for instance, with low density lipoproteins and with protease inhibitors such as alpha-1 antitrypsin and the plasminogen inhibitor.

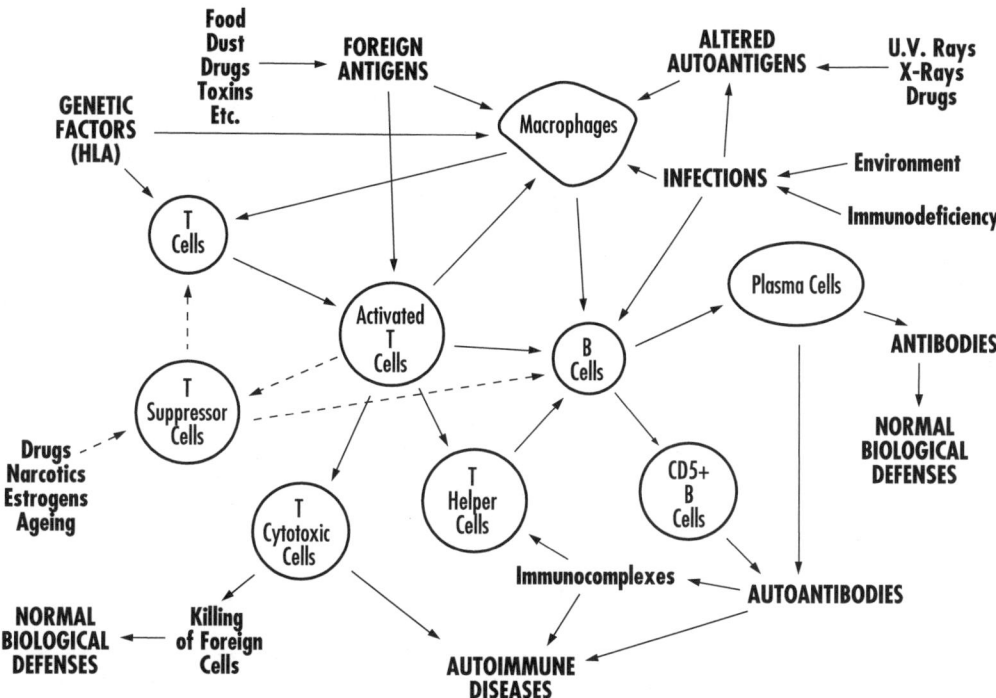

FIGURE 4 Example of an interleukocyte communications network responsible for the immune response. Depending upon the genetic or environmental factors intervening, the same network may give rise to a normal defensive response or to autoimmune disease. Solid lines: activation or transformation; dashed lines: inhibition. Based on a review from Immunology Today [Shoenfeld and Isenberg, 1989].

The complexity of the regulation of the inflammatory system is multiplied several fold if we consider the immune aspect in the strict sense of the term, where an inflammatory process with a potentially damaging action is activated by an information disorder of antigen, antibody, or some form of lymphocyte activity. Autoimmune diseases, for example, have a pathogenesis attributable to disorder in the organization of the *network* regulating the interactions between various lymphocyte subpopulations. A possible schematic representation of this network is proposed in Figure 4, which illustrates the intricate interplay between activation and inhibition, the use of various molecular messengers and the interfaces with other control systems or with systems interacting in some way with this network.

5.2.2 Relationships between the inflammation focus and the rest of the body

The inflammation focus is intimately linked to the rest of the body in various ways. The relationships are bidirectional, i.e., on the one hand, the localized inflammation is capable of influencing the entire body, and, conversely, the body influences the inflammation. The systemic effects of inflammation are currently thought to be due mainly to the production, on the part of cells involved in whatever way in the inflammation focus, of biochemical messages consisting largely of cytokines, but also of hormones such as ACTH and TSH, or of endorphins.

Table 3, which lists only a limited number of the molecules with such effects, clearly shows what a broad spectrum of changes are brought about by inflammation in the entire body. It should also be recalled that most cytokines have pleiotropic effects, i.e. they influence many types of cells, triggering a whole variety of different responses.

TABLE 3

Molecules produced by leukocytes which mediate the systemic effects of inflammation

Molecule	Effects or systems controlled
Interleukin-1	Fever Sleep T lymphocyte activation Liver protein synthesis
Tumor necrosis factor	Anti-tumor defenses Cachexia Hypotension, shock
Interleukin-2	B/T lymphocyte activation ACTH production
α,β-interferon	Antiviral activity Antiproliferative activity Fever Analgesia Adrenal activation
Colony-stimulating factors	Hematopoiesis
Endorphins	Analgesia
ACTH	Adrenal activation
TSH	Thyroid activation
Complement components	Biological defenses
Clotting factors	Fluidity of the blood and fibrinolysis

The other direction in which links are observed between inflammation and the body as a whole has to do with the effects of the neuroendocrine system on inflammation [Goetzl and Sreedharan, 1992]. This is a vast topic which proves difficult to tackle, in that it ranges from biochemistry to immunology, neurology, and psychology, i.e. fields which are clearly very distant one from another and can hardly be mastered by any single researcher or even by a single research team or institute. It had been known for some time that immune reactions can be conditioned like other physiological reactions in the classic Pavlovian manner, and that an involution of the thymus and depression of immunity occur during stress. It is now known that immune responses can be increased or suppressed by numerous situations of mental or psychological stress such as the loss of a spouse, depression, the psychological pressure of examinations or competitions, and even an infant child entrusted to a day care nursery.

The pathogenesis and clinical course of diseases ranging from the common cold to juvenile diabetes, arthritis, and hyperthyroidism are profoundly influenced by psychological stress [Vandvik *et al.*, 1989; Khansari *et al.*, 1990; Cohen *et al.*, 1991; Haggloff *et al.*, 1991; Winsa *et al.*, 1991]. Cerebral lesions in specific areas of the CNS can cause abnormal immune responses.

For a long time, however, the only link discerned between the nervous system and immunity was the pituitary-adrenocortical axis and the production of glucocorticoids. Stress induces the release of ACTH from the anterior hypophysis, which stimulates the adrenal gland to release corticosteroids, which, in turn, act as immunosuppressive agents. This is certainly true, but other mechanisms are probably involved, both because it was clearly demonstrated that even animals subjected to stress and adrenalectomized are functionally immunosuppressed, and because increasing numbers of receptors have been identified for neurotransmitters on peripheral cells as well as increasing numbers of molecules produced by the neuroendocrine system which interact with the immune system and the inflammation cells. A list of molecules of neuroendocrine origin with effects on leukocytes is given in Table 4.

As regards stress in particular, we should point out that this is an ever-present condition in human life and that, though the tendency usually is to highlight the negative aspects, it has a positive component. In fact, as emphasized by Selye (the "discoverer" of stress), there is also a constructive form of stress called "eustress" which activates the physiological responses, preparing the body to react effectively to environmental stimuli [Farné, 1990]. Figure 5 clearly illustrates this concept, showing that efficiency and state of health diminish both when stress levels are too high and when they are too low.

TABLE 4

Neuroendocrine molecules that regulate leukocyte function	
Molecule	**Effects or systems controlled**
Corticotropin releasing factor (CRF)	ACTH production
Thyrotropin releasing factor (TRF)	TSH production
Vasopressin	γ-interferon production
Vasoactive intestinal peptide (VIP)	Function inhibition
Endorphins	Function inhibition
Growth hormone	Increased proliferation Priming
Insulin-like growth factor	Priming
Substance P	Function stimulation
Angiotensin II	Proliferation inhibition
Glucocorticoids	Function inhibition Growth inhibition
Prolactin	Increased metabolism

5.2.3 Difficulties in controlling inflammation

There is a great deal of activity today in the field of studies on the molecular mechanisms of inflammation and immunity regulation. Deciphering the signals which are exchanged by cells and which are transmitted within cells for regulatory purposes goes hand in hand with the possibility of implementing specific modulation of a biological type. For example, after clarifying the important role played by interleukin-1 in activating various inflammatory phenomena, it was also discovered that there are endogenous inhibitors of interleukin-1 which have recently been proposed as a new class of antiinflammatory agents, based on a completely different action principle from the classic chemical inhibitors [Arend and Dayer, 1990; Dinarello, 1994]. Potentially, most of the cytokines known to date may eventually find therapeutic applications.

The difficulties envisaged with regard to the application of the new insights into molecular biology in medicine stem mainly from the fact that both inflammation in general and the production of toxic oxygen derivatives in particular present contradictory and apparently paradoxical aspects, in that they can be viewed either as defensive or as offensive phenomena. *At molecular level, it is by no means easy to distinguish between what is "defen-*

sive" and what is "offensive": the same biochemical mechanisms (receptors, signal molecules, enzymes such as adenylate cyclase, cyclo-oxygenase, kinase, ion pumps, oxygen radicals) are used, according to circumstances, with two different outcomes. The "defensive" or "offensive" nature of such mechanisms, like the terms "normal" and "pathological" in the more general sense, take on a clearer meaning if we abandon the molecular level and go over to considering the system at a higher level of organization (tissue, organ, body), i.e. from a broader, more all-embracing and outcome-oriented standpoint, capable of assessing the health of the individual carrier of a given disease as a whole.

On account of the substantial ambivalence of the biochemical mechanisms of inflammation, any attempt to interfere with the inflammation system at purely biochemical level so as to direct it towards the desired objective, e.g. by increasing inflammatory activity in immunodepressed or neoplastic patients, or by reducing inflammation in individuals suffering from hypersensitivity or autoimmune diseases, will also prove ambivalent.

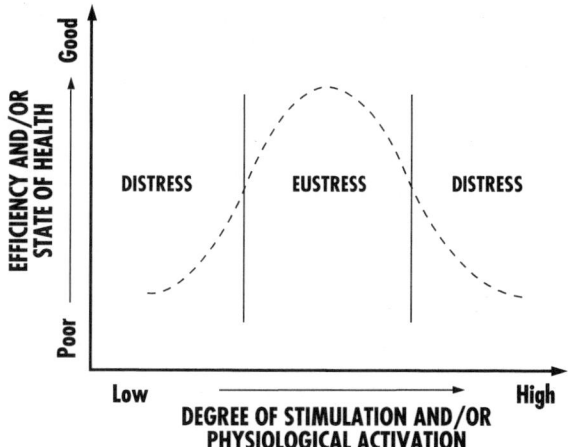

FIGURE 5 Trend of effects of stress on the state of health as a function of the degree of stimulation. Diagram taken, with modifications, from a review of the topic [Farné, 1990].

Both in the field of immunostimulation (specific and nonspecific) and in that of immunosuppression, there is no lack of pharmacological instruments (the pharmaceutical industry today can synthesize virtually any type of molecule, or produce it with genetic engineering techniques), but often they cannot be used successfully in clinical practice. Though there are sometimes "simple" cases in terms of therapeutic strategy, where it is fairly easy to understand whether it is necessary to activate or suppress certain phenomena (e.g. in cases in which the pain symptom is predominant, or in cases of transplant rejection, or in cases in which there is a precise molecular deficiency that can be corrected by replacement therapy), on many other occasions the pathophysiological picture is so complex that the outcome of some form of external modulatory intervention is utterly unpredictable. To give just a single example, it is becoming increasingly clear today that in AIDS cases we have the coexistence of immunodeficiency phenomena (T4 lymphocyte depletion) and autoimmune phenomena (attack of cytotoxic lymphocytes, even on healthy leukocytes). This coexistence theoretically precludes the possibility of utilizing both immunostimulants and immunosuppressors and prompts a search for other forms of modulation which are more specific.

We are still far from being able to construct an exact model, not only as regards inflammation control systems, but also even for a single cell. This situation should not lead to a sort of lack of trust or confidence in scientific medicine, but should spur researchers to construct new investigation approaches better geared to the problems they have to deal with. There is a conviction today that, whereas the activity aimed at investigating biological systems at molecular level (leading over the past two decades to an enormous amount of progress in theoretical and practical terms) continues unabated, we also have to start considering the importance of integration of the various new cognitive advances in a single overall picture. This can be done by studying the interrelations, or better the exchanges of information, between subsystems on the same level of complexity (e.g. information exchanges between molecules, cells, organs, individuals) and between subsystems on different levels (e.g. relationships between molecules and cells, cells and organs, organs and the central control system, individuals and society). Effectively speaking, in the field of inflammation and immunity, whereas, on the one hand, we have an immense series of publications on sequences of genes coding for various receptors, antigens, and proteins of the different types of leukocytes, on the other, we are witnessing the birth of a new discipline, namely neuroimmunoendocrinology, which embraces the tendencies to integrate knowledge in fields previously left to the various specialists. The two tendencies—analytical and synthetic—are not antithetical, but are simply jointly essential for an understanding of reality.

The neuroimmunoendocrine system is a typical complex of homeostatic biological systems which at various levels attempt to maintain the most suitable equilibrium for the survival of the body. As in all homeostatic systems, it is well known that each subsystem has its own feedback mechanisms. There are endogenous inhibitors for every major activator system, ranging from clotting to cytokines, growth factors, membrane ion flow control mechanisms, second intracellular messengers, receptor sensitivity, etc. These feedback systems are one of the decisive elements in the dynamics of the pathological process.

In diseases with a predominantly inflammatory component, a chain of changes and adaptations is generated, in which one is rarely able to clearly perceive any single defect that can be defined as decisive, i.e. the correction of which would allow the disease to be resolved. The fact is that in most diseases, if we exclude single-gene defects, the pathogenesis is multifactorial and more often than not dynamic, i.e. it continues to change as the disease progresses. We encounter external and endogenous factors, equilibria shifted in a positively reactive sense, unshifted equilibria, or pathological adaptations to situations of abnormality. Within this framework, while it is true to say that diseases heal or are cured only when the cause is removed (or when one succeeds in interfering correctly with the pathogenesis), current immunostimulatory and immunosuppressive measures are still too far from coming to grips with the basic etiological level, or even with the pathogenetic mechanism, going no further than barely touching upon the final—or almost the final—effector level.

The fact that the system tends to be self-regulating and that it is hard to distinguish between the defensive and offensive functions of inflammation makes any attempt at intervening pharmacologically a difficult task. Theoretically, the ideal drug should simultaneously activate the defensive, reparatory functions and inhibit the destructive, pain-inducing functions. Obviously, no molecule possesses such a specific integrated action, not least because the various functions are often triggered by the same biochemical mechanisms. From this viewpoint, it even appears reasonable to doubt whether the use of antiinflammatory agents (steroidal and nonsteroidal), though regarded as necessary in many situations to suppress the clinical signs and symptoms, is always scientifically justified.

One major line of pharmacological research has recently focused on the use of substances with a scavenger effect on oxygen radicals and antioxidants in the hope of being able to use them to prevent or cure toxic effects. All this research has substantially confirmed and underlined the great importance of tocopherols, carotenes, ascorbate, ceruloplasmin, cysteine, selenium, metal chelating agents, and superoxide dismutase as protective systems against free radicals. However, it is also true that, while there can be no doubt as to their biochemical and physiological functions, there is no general consensus of agreement as to the therapeutic efficacy of administration of high doses of these agents in human diseases [Dormandy, 1983; Halliwell, 1987; Southorn, 1988; Halliwell *et al.*, 1992]. This may be due to the fact that the diet normally contains a fair amount of these substances and that in any event it is difficult to demonstrate the effects of dietary supplementation in complex diseases such as those mentioned above (Chapter 5, Section 2.1). Moreover, precisely on account of the ambivalent significance of the changes induced by free radicals, any therapeutic intervention against these molecules will inevitably be of a very nonspecific type.

What we have said obviously does not mean that the current therapies in the field of inflammation and free radicals are devoid of any kind of rationale or justification, since there are, in actual fact, a vast series of molecules which have demonstrated a certain degree of efficacy "in the field," at least when it comes to resolving problems of a symptomatological nature. We merely wish to stress the need to seek more specific measures based on regulatory mechanisms located at "higher" levels which take account of the complexity of the system.

Genetic engineering has recently made available large quantities of cytokines to medical practitioners. The hope, of course, is that we shall be able to use them to stimulate the biological defenses both in immunodeficiency syndromes and in immunological cancer therapy, thus attempting to activate phagocytes, NK cells, and cytotoxic lymphocytes with interferons or interleukins (cf., for instance, Rosenberg's therapy with LAK cells). Attempts have also been made to use *tumor necrosis factor* (TNF) as a cytotoxic agent against cancer cells, and *colony stimulating factors* (CSFs) in those cases in which the production of white blood cells by the bone marrow is deficient for various reasons.

Without denying the undoubted value of, and need for, such research, it should be said, however, that the success rate to date has been below expectations and confined to very few types of tumors, particularly because these molecules have no specific effect on the target one is aiming at, but interfere with the entire network described above. Thus, we inevitably witness the occurrence of side effects, such as fever, hypotension, oliguria, weight gain, liver abnormalities, nausea, vomiting, and shock, which will be all the more severe, the higher the doses.

The problem of the side effects of drugs is clearly not confined to this sector, but in this case the risk:efficacy ratio appears highly critical. Medical practitioners faced with this problem in clinical practice are gradually coming to the conclusion that to achieve more effective use of cytokines we shall have to experiment with doses and treatment regimens, subtly exploiting synergistic effects, e.g. by administering two or more different cytokines at low doses, which in themselves do not produce side effects, but which together bring about the desired effect on a common target.

In complex systems such as inflammation and immunity, it thus proves very difficult to transpose the vast body of knowledge of cellular and molecular biology concerning the individual mechanisms involved onto the therapeutic plane. This is particularly evident in the therapy of autoimmune diseases and, generally speaking, in any type of immunomodulatory therapy [Bach, 1988; Wybran, 1988]. Faced with this situation, it is hard to see why there cannot be a reappraisal of the empirical approach as a pathway affording scope for further investigation, starting from the traditional use of phytotherapeutic and organotherapeutic preparations, as well as from homeopathic and homotoxicological experience itself (bacterial extracts, nosodes).

Complex natural preparations may prove useful precisely because they contain various different biologically active compounds which act together in a coordinated manner. The clinical and laboratory study of these compounds as possible means of modulating inflammatory phenomena is problematical, particularly on account of the difficulties encountered in standardizing and characterizing the preparations used. Despite this, the availability of highly sensitive analytical methods and the possibility of testing various biological effects in cell cultures mean that studies of this type are steadily gaining in terms of scientific rigor and are proving increasingly promising.

The possible importance of the homeopathic approach in this sector, however, goes far beyond the identification of natural preparations with a regulatory action. Homeopathy, in fact, offers itself above all as a methodology for identifying the specific remedy for each individual patient on the basis of analysis of the symptoms. Chapter 6 will show us how this methodology has adapted to face the challenge of diseases in which complexity predominates.

Cancer consists in the more or less uncontrolled growth of cells as a result of serious disorders of information contained in the cells and of information which the cells exchange with one another and with the environment. It is therefore a complex pathological phenomenon, as are the cells themselves and their regulatory mechanisms, or the human body in its entirety and in its relations with the environment.

5.3

Another example: cancer

We cannot and do not wish here to attempt a complete survey of such an enormously broad-ranging topic, but will confine ourselves to a review of the most recent advances in this field and the main lines of research, along with a number of reflections on the relationships between phenomena at molecular level and phenomena regarding the body as a whole. Cancer is one of the greatest challenges facing modern medicine, and what often happens, in practice, is that patients tend to seek the aid of "alternative" therapies as a last resort, when conventional treatments have failed to prove effective. For this reason, there is a real risk that the "alternative" therapies are applied incorrectly and to the detriment (economically and in terms of health) of the patient.

Within the framework of an extensive overview of the possible scientific basis of homeopathy, the problem of the relationship between homeopathy and tumors cannot be neglected. To get the problem into proper perspective and clear the field of common misunderstandings, it is advisable first to present a preliminary outline of our current knowledge of neoplastic disease, before going on to expound a number of considerations on the role of homeopathy. It is only in this way that we can indicate and reasonably define and delimit the fields of application of the various therapies.

The basic problem in neoplastic growth is that it is due to loss of normal control of cell proliferation and differentiation.

Each cell in the course of its life cycle, which varies in length according to the type of cell, engages in many activities which are useful both to itself and to the body, but essentially it finds itself faced with a basic choice of behavior: to undergo mitosis or to differentiate, or, in other words, to replicate or to mature. Schematically, we can go along with the simplification whereby these two possibilities are alternatives, i.e. they are mutually exclusive. This choice of behavior is often repeated several times in the life cycle of the cell and of the clone deriving from it. The decision to replicate or proliferate is typical of less specialized cells in the line of evolution both in the individual (embryo) and in the tissue (e.g. basal cells of the epidermis, bone marrow blast cells). When the result of the choice is division, the result will be two daughter cells identical to the mother cell, i.e. two fairly immature cells. When the choice is to differentiate, the cell progressively takes on the morphology and properties of a greater degree of maturity in the line of evolution of the specific tissue.

In a given tissue, then, we find cells in a state of replication and cells which progressively mature and then gradually age and die. As is well known, the mature cells of some tissues (e.g. striated muscle, nervous system) have practically no proliferative activity, whereas other cells conserve varying degrees of activity according to the functional demands and environmental stimuli. Forms of regulation of proliferative activity are particularly evident in endocrine-regulated glands and tissues. A number of cell clones in rapidly proliferating tissues (hemopoietic marrow, mucosa) conserve very substantial proliferative activity and poor differentiation, representing the germinative pool which constantly supplies the tissue with large amounts of cells.

For instance, in a population of myeloid cells such as those of normal bone marrow, there are cells (blast cells) in the proliferative phase alongside cells in the differentiation phase versus the various types of leukocytes. Even the very mature cells in a state of rapid proliferation are under strict surveillance, however, so that their activity is always in equilibrium with the disappearance rate of the mature cells and with the needs of the body in general. This control is exerted primarily by other neighboring or distant (by the endocrine route) cells by means of growth factors and differentiation factors, as well as by cell-to-cell and cell-to-matrix contacts.

These factors are fairly specific for each tissue and are often produced by the tissue cells themselves as they mature.

In tumor development this fine control is lost, and it is therefore at this level that cellular and molecular biologists have begun to understand which control mechanisms have gone missing. Both the study of the normal cell cycle and the study, more recently, of neoplastic cell genetics are rapidly revealing a picture of how the proliferative activity is regulated and what the basic differences are between normal cells and cancer cells. For instance, in a population of leukemic cells, many more cells will be found in the proliferative state and fewer (or no) differentiated, mature cells. As we are well aware, by and large, the more immature the cells are, the more malignant the tumor will be. A number of the possible reasons for this imbalance are related to the fact that leukemic cells have very little need of growth factors, or they produce them themselves in amounts in excess of their needs, or they do not produce differentiation factors. The cells in almost all tumors show a similar behavior pattern.

5.3.1 Biochemical control of cell proliferation

What are the lesions or biochemical defects leading to this type of abnormal behavior in cancer cells? The lesions clearly have to do with disorders in the cell division mechanisms and in the extracellular and intracellular signals pertaining to its control. It is therefore useful to briefly analyze the molecular and functional characteristics of these mechanisms, firstly in the normal cell, and then in the tumor cell, in order to pinpoint the essential differences.

Figure 6 illustrates a number of cellular biochemical events summarized very schematically for reasons of brevity and clarity. We may take as our starting point in this analysis the *extracellular signals* which trigger off the proliferation. In the first place, we are familiar with many growth factors, i.e. molecules mainly of a protein nature, with more or less marked tissue specificity. Many of these growth factors have been cloned and are also produced today by genetic engineering; these have added themselves to the series of traditional hormones with effects stimulating tissue growth, such as the pituitary, thyroid, and gonadal hormones. The extracellular signals can reach their intracellular targets either via membrane receptors or, after crossing the membrane, via cytoplasmic or nuclear receptors which directly regulate gene expression.

Another major line of research has highlighted the *membrane and intracellular phenomena* activated by hormones and growth factors (Figure 6). Many receptors for growth factors have the carboxy terminal portion of

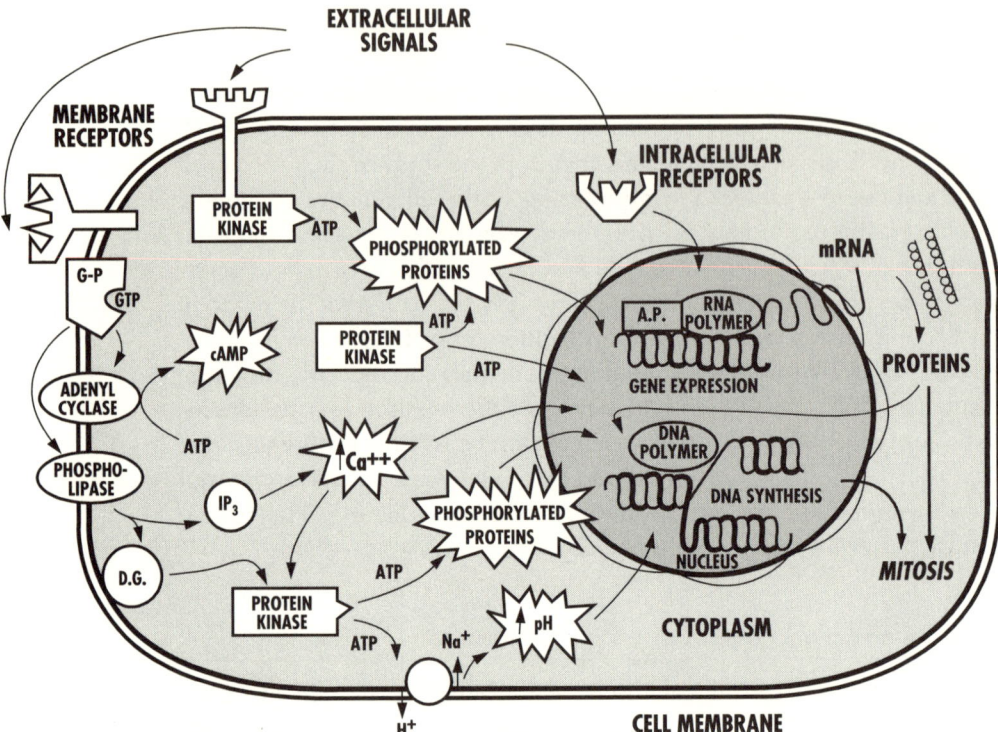

FIGURE 6 Mechanisms of transmission of the proliferative signal from the extracellular to the intracellular space. For an explanation, see text. Abbreviations: G-P: guanosine triphosphate binding protein; D.G.: diacyl-glycerol; IP$_3$: inositol 1,4,5 triphosphate; cAMP: cyclic adenosine monophosphate; ATP: adenosine triphosphate; A.P.: activator proteins, proteins which induce mRNA transcription by binding to DNA; mRNA: messenger RNA; Polymer.: polymerases, enzymes which replicate DNA or copy DNA in RNA.

the intracytoplasmic protein chain, endowed with protein-kinase activity. This means that one of the first events to occur in the cell which is starting to divide is the phosphorylation of proteins, i.e. the incorporation of phosphorus groups on particular amino acids (usually, though not exclusively, the amino acid tyrosine is involved in events related to cell proliferation and cancerogenesis).

What is the significance of protein phosphorylation? The fact is that the incorporation of phosphate in specific sites changes the electrical charges, the structure and thus the activity of the target protein, in the sense that it makes it capable of activating some kind of replication mechanism at the cytoplasmic level (e.g. movement of the cytoskeleton, protein synthesis) or at the nuclear level (e.g. gene expression, assembly/disassembly of the nuclear membrane and chromosomes during mitosis). Via other biochemical pathways, phosphorylation may also involve particular phospholipids of the cell membrane, such as phosphatidyl inositol, which play an important role in the stimulus-response coupling process.

In view of their importance, a great deal of attention has been focused upon phosphorylation processes in recent years, particularly since it was demonstrated that tumor cells contain large amounts of phosphorylated tyrosine. There are many types of protein kinases, associated directly with the receptor or activated indirectly via a series of cascade reactions schematically represented in Figure 6. These cascades are produced by G-proteins, activation of enzymes such as adenylate cyclase and phospholipase, and generation of second intracellular messengers. Among these second messengers a role of primary importance is played by cyclic adenosine monophosphate (cAMP), both because it is an activator of (type A) protein kinases and because it is itself a signal captured by proteins of the nucleus closely associated with DNA synthesis (cAMP-responsive elements).

Other important events related to activation of cell replication are Ca^{++} elevation, depolarization of the membrane, and activation of the Na^+/H^+ antiport, with a consequent increase in intracellular Na^+, alkalinization of the cytoplasm, and acidification of the external medium. It would thus appear that the acid/base equilibrium of the cell is important for regulating cell proliferation and thus for tumor growth.

A small minority of receptors, i.e. those for small hydrophobic molecules such as steroid or thyroid hormones, do not need these transduction mechanisms, since they are already inside the cell or even in the cell nucleus.

There are a whole variety of other biochemical modifications related to cell activation, including the translocation of proteins from one compartment to another, acetylation or ADP-ribosylation of proteins, formation of a broad spectrum of lipid derivatives, partial scission of macromolecules, and metabolic variations of the Krebs cycle. A number of the modifications are transient and easily reversible, while others are longer-lasting, or even permanent, thus constituting a sort of *memory* of the biological history of the cell.

The purpose of the phenomena described is to constitute a transmission system, or more precisely a transduction system, a *signal network* going from external growth factors towards the interior of the cell, i.e. towards the inside of the control center, consisting in the cell nucleus. Not all receptors activate all the intracellular signals, in that there are *preferential pathways* according to the type of receptor involved. The *network* of membrane and cytoplasmic biochemical modifications, corresponding essentially to the laws of cybernetics, receives not only activator, but also inhibitor inputs, and serves the purpose of amplifying or modulating the signal. The modification of any single element in the system has far-reaching repercussions on all the other elements [Egan and Weinberg, 1993].

At this level, the synergisms and antagonisms between factors mean that the transmission of the signal is never a drastic on/off, all or nothing matter, but rather denotes the setting up of dynamic modes of being, of conditions more or less favorable to growth, which evolve continually as the stimulation proceeds and interacts with the genetic and metabolic conditions of the cell. This interpretation accounts both for the multiplicity and variety of the biochemical mechanisms described and for the synergisms between the proliferative responses triggered by the classic growth factors and other mediators active in other systems such as inflammation and metabolism (bradykinin, thrombin, insulin, and others) [cf., for example, Pandiella *et al.*, 1989].

The membrane and cytoplasmic information network, which is overwhelmed in the case of neoplasia, carries signals at nucleus level, where they interact with specific transcriptional factors (activator proteins [A.P.], and repressor proteins [R.P.]) which in turn bind with (A.P.) or detach themselves (R.P.) from specific sequences of the DNA in a position upstream of the promotor, i.e. of the starting point of RNA polymerase. The transcription of the genes involved is thus activated, and RNA transcripts are formed, which after suitable maturation become the messengers governing the new synthesis of proteins, which, in turn, serve in various ways for cell division (DNA synthesis, formation of the mitotic spindle, etc.). Among the regulatory proteins, a place of primary importance has been accorded to the cyclines [Murray and Kirschner, 1991], and to a number of other recently discovered factors acting as enhancers or regulators for the cell cycle, in different tissues.

5.3.2 Oncogenes and proto-oncogenes

It has been common knowledge for some time now that tumor cells present abnormalities at both genetic level (mutations) and epigenetic level (biochemical and functional disorders of the gene control systems). However, it is only in the last decade that we have witnessed dramatic progress in the interpretation of the genetic and epigenetic abnormalities of cancer cells, due essentially to molecular biology techniques, which have led to the discovery of oncogenes and their products.

In point of fact, from the generic notion that cancerogenic agents cause damage to the DNA we have now homed in on the precise targets of such damage and their characterization; in practice, the defective genes in tumors have been identified. Out of all the genes present in our genome, only a few dozen can be directly involved in cancerogenesis, hence the term *oncogenes* [Hunter, 1984; Nishimura and Sekiya, 1987; Frati, 1989; Varmus, 1989].

The neoplastic cell contains one or more oncogenes in active form, i.e. expressing the information content. Generally speaking, they have been given 3-letter names deriving from the tumors in which they were initially identified.

The history of these discoveries owes a great deal to virology because it was thanks to the oncogenic viruses that investigators obtained the first evidence that particular DNA (or RNA) sequences may represent the decisive element in neoplastic transformation. In actual fact, the importance of viral oncogenes was underestimated, particularly on the strength of the argument that very few human tumors are definitely known to be of viral origin.

An enormous step forward of a conceptual nature was the demonstration, obtained by means of nucleic acid hybridization techniques, that viral oncogenes also presented homologous sequences in normal cells. The viral oncogenes (*v-onc*) made it possible to "unmask" the cellular oncogenes (*c-onc*). This means that the oncogenes present in most human tumors are not totally abnormal genes and are not genes introduced, for example, by viruses into the cell, which would thus be the victim, as it were, of a molecular parasitism, but are genes which have normal counterparts in all cells.

That is to say, oncogenes stem from the transformation of genes which are important in the functioning of all cells. These normal genes have thus been termed *proto-oncogenes*, which is perhaps something of a misnomer. The term "proto-oncogenes" is not particularly apt because it has been seen that they are beneficial, being active at various times in the cell cycle and essential for its activity and for its replication. These are genes which have been well conserved in evolution and are present practically in all eukaryote cells.

Two basic queries arise from what we have said:

a) *How does a proto-oncogene become an oncogene?*

b) *How does the oncogene cause the transformation of a normal cell into a cancer cell?*

The transformation of a proto-oncogene into an oncogene is the basic event, the *sine qua non* for the onset of cancer. Whereas it was already known on the basis of epidemiological and experimental evidence that this event is related to mutation of the genetic code induced by cancerogenic agents of various kinds, the oncogene theory has shed light on a number of aspects relating to how this can come about. One concept is very clear: the proto-oncogene becomes an oncogene as a result of the action of the cancerogenic agents. This is the *transformation* event at genetic level, which only needs to occur once to be transmitted then to all the daughter cells. For this reason, it is also called *initiation*.

The main cancerogenic agents are, as is well known, chemical substances contained in cigarette smoke, polluted air, foodstuffs, ionizing and excitatory radiation, radio-isotopes, genotoxic drugs, and viruses. Obviously, we have considered here only the general categories of cancerogenic agents, inasmuch as the molecules with cancerogenic and/or mutagenic activity amount to several hundred. The manifestation or otherwise of the transforming action of a cancerogenic agent depends on both the dose and the duration of exposure to it, as well as on factors having to do with the body, such as, for instance, the detoxification capability and the ability to eliminate the carcinogen, and the ability of cell systems to repair the DNA. It should not be forgotten, however, that many exogenous substances become mutagenic and thus cancerogenic following particular metabolic conversions which occur in the body and make them active. The common feature of cancerogenic substances is that they have a strongly electrophilic molecule (usually around carbon or nitrogen atoms), capable, therefore, of reacting with the nucleophilic centers rich in unshared electrons and present in various positions of the DNA (e.g. position 6 of guanine, the phosphoric group of the sugar-phosphate-sugar bonds).

As far as tumor pathogenesis is concerned, leukocytes may be directly involved in the genetic transformation, since they could metabolize (and thus activate) cancerogenic substances [Trush *et al.*, 1985], but, above all, because they may produce toxic oxygen radicals. It is known, in fact, that DNA mutations may originate, amongst other things, as a result of the effect of free radicals produced by leukocytes [Weitberg *et al.*, 1983; Weitzman *et al.*, 1985; Birnboim, 1986].

In this case, too, we can see the *"two faces"* of a biological phenomenon: radicals can have varying effects depending upon their quantity and upon the existence or otherwise of specific *scavenger* substances or enzymes. At high doses, radicals have a cytotoxic and thus a defensive effect, in that they cooperate in the destruction of tumor cells (particularly if the latter have not developed detoxifying systems); at low doses, oxygen radicals have no effect because they are rapidly degraded; at intermediate doses, they have both genetic effects (mutations) and epigenetic effects (activation of protein kinases and other enzymes including poly-ADP ribosyl-transferase), thus being able to behave both as cancerogenic and promoting agents [Sekkat *et al.*, 1988; Cerutti, 1991].

Lastly, many tumors are known to have defective free radical disposal systems [Casaril *et al.*, 1985; Bannister *et al.*, 1986; Vo *et al.*, 1988]. This might constitute either the basis for more effective action on the part of the anti-tumor cytotoxic surveillance systems, or, however, it may also be the cause of further damage to the genetic endowment of the neoplastic cell, with consequent activation of other oncogenes and an increase in malignancy (tumor progression process).

Thus, in the inflammatory focus (particularly of the chronic type where the histogenetic and proliferative events are more marked) and within the context of the macrophage populations infiltrating the tumor, antitumor events and cancerogenic events may co-exist in a state of unstable equilibrium. A familiar phenomenon, in fact, is the onset of dysplasia, metaplasia, and even neoplasia coming on top of chronic inflammation, particularly at bronchopulmonary, gastrointestinal, and hepatic level, these being sites where cancerogenic agents also tend to be easily localized.

The modification of the genetic information, related to the transformation of a proto-oncogene into an oncogene, may take the form of various eventualities in molecular terms:

a) Classic *point mutation*, with deletion or substitution of one or more base pairs with other erroneous base pairs, thereby obtaining a protein with a different amino acid sequence. This, for example, has been observed in connection with the first oncogenes characterized (as *src*) and in many human tumors with mutations of the *ras* proto-oncogene (some cases of carcinoma of the bladder, 10–20% of acute myeloid leukemias, approximately 30% of colorectal carcinomas, and even the majority of carcinomas of the exocrine pancreas).

b) *Translocation* of the proto-oncogene to a DNA site where it comes under the control of enhancer sequences or viral promoters ("insertional mutagenesis") or of a very active cell promotor and is thus itself activated excessively. This is the case with the *myc* oncogene in 90% of Burkitt's lymphomas and in some cases of T cell lymphomas (translocation from chromosome 8 to 14), as well as with the *bcl* oncogene in many other lymphomas (translocation from chromosome 14 to 18).

c) A particular variant of this problem related to translocation presents itself when, as a result of translocation, the oncogene undergoes *fusion with another gene*, with formation therefore of an abnormal hybrid or chimeric protein (e.g. *bcr/abl* in the classic Philadelphia chromosome of chronic myeloid leukemia, with translocation from chromosome 9 to 22, but it has been seen that this can also occur in 10–20% of cases of acute lymphatic leukemia).

d) An increase in copies of the proto-oncogene due to erroneous dupli-cation of DNA (*amplification*) or to the insertion of various copies of retroviral oncogenes (acutely transforming retroviruses). Amplification of the oncogene *myc* has been observed in sporadic cases of promyelocytic leukemia, lung cancer, and stomach cancer, whereas a particular variant of *myc*, called *N-myc* is seen to be amplified in most neuroblastomas. Ampli-fication of the *erb-B* oncogene has been described in 10-30% of cases of cancer of the breast, and this characteristic is associated with a poor prog-nosis.

In a nutshell, then, the proto-oncogene becomes an oncogene when the nucleotide sequence is altered, or when its transcription is excessively acti-vated, or when its amount is increased in terms of genetic material. The various possibilities are not mutually exclusive, but can coexist side by side.

The second important issue regarding the molecular pathology of can-cer is the role played by oncogenes in the phenotypic and behavioral trans-formation of the cell. Why are they so dangerous or damaging once activated? To answer this question the fundamental step has been to iden-tify the *products of oncogenes*. It is not enough for us to know the oncogene and its nucleotide substance to know what it does because the role of any given gene is strictly related to the protein encoded by it and to the activi-ties or functions of the protein itself. These are proteins which are local-ized on the membrane, or in the cytoplasm, or even in the nucleus itself in close contact with the DNA. More interesting even than the location is the function which the products can have in the biochemistry of the cell which produces them: in general, the products of oncogenes merely mimic the factors involved in the control of cell proliferation (see Figure 6).

A few details may be in order here: it has been seen that some proteins are very similar to the receptors for growth factors. For example, the prod-ucts of the *erb-B*, *fms*, and *kit* oncogenes present homologies with the re-ceptors for epidermal growth factor (EGF), colony-stimulating factor 1 (CSF-1), and stem cell factor (SCF), respectively. These types of recep-tors, however, are abnormal compared to those of healthy cells: the EGF receptor is truncated, i.e. it lacks the part that binds to the growth factor, and thus appears to be dysregulated; in practice, it transmits proliferative signals even in the absence of the legitimate ligand.

The proliferative signals are related essentially to the tyrosine kinase enzyme activity which these abnormal receptors have maintained and ex-press improperly. Other oncogenes (*src*, *abl*, *fps*, *mos*), too, code for protein kinases, which, however, are not associated with receptors, but whose ac-tivity has similar consequences to the previous ones. Other oncogenes produce intracellular receptors, such as, for instance, *erb-A*, whose product presents homology with the receptor for thyroid hormones. The importance of protein kinases is also strongly borne out by the fact that a number of natural inhibitors of these enzymes (such as bryostatin and genistein) can block the growth of tumor cells in suitable experimental systems [Jones *et al.*, 1990; Watanabe *et al.*, 1991]. The subject is obviously extremely broad-ranging, and research in this field is steadily expanding.

There is also a class of oncoproteins (related to the *ras* genes) of a different type, which present strong homology with the G-proteins, regarded above as important intermediaries in the transmission of the transmembrane signal. It is not hard to imagine that the quantitatively or qualitatively abnormal presence of these proteins incorporated in the membrane of a cell may alter the information system to such an extent as to impart thoroughly abnormal proliferative orders.

A further and extremely interesting aspect of oncogenesis came to light when it was seen that a number of oncogenes produced proteins homologous to growth factors (e.g. *sis* has sequences in common with platelet-derived growth factor, PDGF, and *hst* with fibroblast growth factor, FGF). In this case, the cancerogenesis mechanism is explained, at least in part, by the phenomenon of autocrine secretion: the clone of transformed cells renders itself independent of other exogenous growth factors and is self-supporting in growth; indeed, the more the cells grow, the more growth factor is available.

Finally, a different type of oncogene (the *myc, myb, fos, jun* type) have as their products proteins which are located in the cell nucleus, where they play a decisive role in the control of mitosis (e.g. the *fos* oncogene codes for the transcriptional factor A.P.-1). That this is true is also demonstrated by the fact that the respective proto-oncogenes (i.e. the "benign" versions of these nuclear oncogenes) are highly active in the rapidly growing cells of the embryo and in the blast cells of the bone marrow, as well as whenever any normal cell receives a treatment with growth factors.

In view of the fact that research in this field is booming, it is only to be expected that other properties of oncogene proteins will soon come to light. For instance, a number of studies indicated that an oncogene involved in lymphomas (bcl-2) codes for a protein which inhibits the so-called "programmed cell death" (an ancestral system which limits the cell life span): the tumor cells with this oncogene would thus have a longer life cycle than normal cells, thus explaining the increased number and selective advantage of the transformed cells.

To recapitulate: the neoplastic cell is characterized by having one or more regulation systems which are impaired qualitatively (i.e. there is an abnormal protein, albeit resembling its normal counterpart) and/or quantitatively (i.e. there is a protein overrepresented compared to normal). All this leads to the phenotypic characteristics of cancer cells.

The result could therefore be a large number and considerable variety of cellular atypia, a few examples of which are the following:

a) Abnormal phosphorylation of proteins of the cytoskeleton, producing a collapse of the structures which confer upon the cell its normal morphology.

b) Alterations of the adhesion plaques between cells, and between cell and connective tissue matrix, with possible detachment and metastatic spread.

c) Alterations of the surface characteristics with possible triggering of an immune response against the tumor.

d) Alterations of various metabolic pathways, with increased consumption of oxygen and of nutritive substances and reduced production of energy, or reduction of normal defense systems against toxic oxygen radicals and of DNA lesion repair systems, with a possible increased risk of new mutations.

e) Possible production and release of substances with effects on the cell itself (autocrine secretion) or at a distance (ectopic production of hormones).

f) As we have already said, an upheaval in the delicate system of relationships between proteins and DNA, which regulates cell division in the nucleus.

Within the framework of the molecular pathology of cancer we should not neglect to mention another major line of research relating to the existence of genes which counteract the development of the tumor. These genes are therefore called *anti-oncogenes*, or tumor-suppressor genes, or recessive oncogenes [Friend *et al.*, 1988; Vile, 1990]. They were discovered as a result of the observation that a number of tumors (retinoblastoma, Wilms' tumor, neuroblastoma, and adenomatosis of the colon, though today it would seem that it also occurs in many other cases) are associated with a lack of genes, sometimes visible as actual deletions of parts of chromosomes. If the lack of particular genes causes cancer, it has been deduced that these genes are important in inhibiting tumors. Direct proof was provided by the fact that if the deficient gene is reintroduced by genetic engineering (or formation of hybrid tumor-healthy cells), the neoplastic phenotype disappears.

Despite the fact that the importance of these genes is enormous, little is yet known about their precise function in the control of cell growth. From the study of the location of suppressor gene products and from analysis of their sequences a highly complex picture is emerging, showing that these products are involved in the control of cell proliferation in many ways [Algrain *et al.*, 1993; Bryant, 1993]. For instance, in retinoblastoma and Wilms' tumor, deficiencies of transcription factors (Rb-1 and WT1, respectively) have been described, while there have been reports of a deficiency of a membrane adhesion protein (N-CAM) in colorectal carcinoma, and of a protein associated with the cytoskeleton (merlin-schwannomin) in type 2 neurofibromatosis. It is interesting that the deletion of the gene for interferon-α has been reported in a number of leukemias [Diaz *et al.*, 1990], which suggests that this cytokine may be the product of a suppressor gene. One of the suppressor genes which has been found to be mutated in a large percentage of human malignancies (colon, breast, lung, and brain) is the p53 gene, encoding a transcriptional regulator of cell proliferation [Hollstein *et al.*, 1991].

It therefore appears that the products of anti-oncogenes are involved in the same *information network* considered above, counteracting the effects of the products of oncogenes (or of proto-oncogenes), for example by means of dephosphorylation of proteins (phosphatase) or degradation of second messengers such as cAMP (phosphodiesterase). As is observed in many other pathophysiological situations, the control of proliferation constitutes a homeostatic equilibrium between two groups of opposite factors which control one another reciprocally, and this equilibrium shifts in one direction or the other due either to an element being in excess or to a deficiency of the element counteracting it.

5.3.3 Promoting factors and neoplastic progression

After examining the mechanism of transformation at oncogene level, we may ask: *is transformation of a proto-oncogene into an oncogene enough to cause cancer?* The answer is certainly negative: the transformation of a normal cell into a neoplastic cell and the subsequent expansion of the mutated clone in the form of an actual neoplasm are hardly ever the result of a single molecular event. The experimental evidence clearly shows that the transformation of a proto-oncogene into an oncogene is not enough to bring about cancer. For a cancer to develop, starting from a transformed cell, other biological events at *epigenetic* level are necessary, related to the action of the so-called *tumor promoters* (promoting factors, also called co-cancerogenic factors).

These factors do not act directly at the level of the genetic endowment, but at the level of the whole series of reactions conditioning the expression of the genes involved in proliferation and the activity of the enzymes involved in the cell division process. To take a metaphorical leaf out of the automobile book, it could be said that, while it is the cancerogenic factor that starts up the engine (oncogene) and puts the automobile in gear (abnormal protein), it is the co-cancerogenic or promoting factors that put their foot on the accelerator to set the automobile in motion. In the absence of these factors, theoretically the cell could remain at a standstill or even degenerate and thus disappear without giving rise to any progeny. Table 5 lists a series of agents possessing possible promoting actions.

The classic promoting agents include various substances mainly of vegetable origin or resulting from chemical synthesis: phorbol esters and related diterpenes, indole alkaloids such as teleocidine, iodoacetic acid, phenol, cedarwood oil, a number of detergents, n-dodecane, and other substances. Their mechanism of action is the subject of active research and, predictably, has proved very complex and variable from type to type. The most paradigmatic co-cancerogenic factor is TPA (an active ingredient of the oil extracted from the seeds of *Croton tiglium*), which, by virtue of its hydrophobicity and its structural similarity to physiological mediators, acts by binding to protein kinase C, activating it, and then acting in synergy with other activator events considered previously. The treatment of cells with TPA causes the phosphorylation of many proteins and triggers a whole series of different metabolic responses. In itself it does not cause the onset of the neoplastic phenotype in a normal cell, but if the treatment is carried out on experimental cells or animals previously treated with a cancerogenic agent (e.g. benzopyrene, or ionizing radiation), the likelihood of onset of tumor is significantly greater than in control cells.

Another substance with a promoting action, okadaic acid, probably exerts its effects by means of inhibition of phosphatases, enzymes, which, as we have seen, constitute a sort of homeostatic equilibrium with the kinases. Low-frequency electromagnetic fields can also have a promoting effect, possibly due to interference with the intracellular homeostasis of the calcium ion [Goodman and Shirley-Henderson, 1990; Yost and Liburdy, 1992]. There are indications that exposure to low-frequency electromagnetic fields increases the risk of being affected by leukemia, though this is still subject to considerable debate [Pool, 1990; Galva, 1991].

Though the mechanism of action of various promoting agents is still under investigation, it seems clear that all they do is insert themselves in the activating information network outlined above, mimicking essentially a number of actions of physiological substances (sometimes with more marked and longer-lasting effects). For this reason it would seem logical to include many other additional agents in the table of compounds possessing promoting activity, such as hormones, growth factors, cytokines, and even neuropeptides [Malik and Balkwill, 1991; Rozengurt, 1991]. There

A number of agents which may act as tumor promoters		**TABLE 5**
Various substances:	lectins phorbol esters mezerein okadaic acid bacterial exotoxins phenol	
Hormones:	estrogens thyroid hormones insulin	
Growth factors:	PDGF (platelet-derived growth factor) EGF (epidermal growth factor) IGF (insulin-like growth factor) FGF (fibroblast growth factor) TGF (transforming growth factor) a number of other cytokines	
Neuropeptides:	bombesin vasopressin bradykinin VIP (vasoactive intestinal peptide)	
Prostaglandin E		
Low-frequency electromagnetic fields		

is evidence that even mediators with completely different "traditional" functions (catecholamines, serotonin, angiotensin) may, in certain circumstances, act as growth factors [Williams, 1991]. In this case, too, the sensitivity "status" and predisposition of the cell is of great importance, ranging from the presence of suitable receptors to the existence of conditions favoring the expression of particular transduction pathways, due to previous or concomitant conditioning by factors of a pharmacological or hormonal type. For example, a substantial series of agonist and antagonist agents which influence the intracellular level of cAMP or of protein kinase C activity may behave as growth promoters, both in normal cells and, even more so, in transformed cells. The growth of the cell clone is always conditioned to some extent by such factors, though the effects may differ greatly according to the type of cell concerned, the type of oncogene involved, and the type of receptors present. Agents which act as co-carcinogens in some cells may behave as factors inducing differentiation, and thus in practice as anticancerogenic agents in other cells.

It should be stressed that, if a promoting effect can be exerted by various endogenous substances, one factor whose importance warrants reappraisal is the *medium* in which the cancer develops. It would appear legitimate to ask oneself what *contribution* the host organism makes to the growth of the tumor, i.e. whether it may play a permissive role or even, in certain circumstances, have an incentivating function. Clearly, the tumor receives a certain amount of "help" from the host with the supply of connective tissue, the vascular network, and energy substrates, but it is likely that the help may also consist in particular biochemical mediators such as growth factors and hormones [Lang and Burgess, 1990]. As regards the latter, it has been reported that progressive tumor is associated with an increase in adrenergic tone, sensitivity and reactivity to beta-agonists, and with an accentuated metabolic effect of beta-blockers [Hyltander *et al.*, 1993].

As far as the mechanism of neoplastic promotion is concerned, it should be borne in mind that the inflammatory focus is a good *culture medium* for cells such as leukocytes, endothelial cells, fibroblasts, and even epithelial cells, thanks to the secretion of special growth factors. This is particularly true in those cases in which the inflammation does not proceed rapidly towards healing with *restitutio ad integrum*, reabsorption of exudate, inactivation of mediators due to lysis or oxidation, and cessation of leukocyte chemotaxis. In inflammation, synergisms may easily occur between substances that have demonstrable mitogenic activity, such as epidermal growth factor, insulin, insulin-like growth factor, bradykinin, endothelin, and even neuropeptides, which, as is known, are released in the site of a tissue lesion. It is therefore not unlikely that such growth factors act as accelerators of proliferation not only of normal cells, but also of those cells which form as a result of a previous or concomitant genetic transformation event.

Cancerogenic and co-cancerogenic (or promoting) factors lead to a progressive complication of the biological situation of the tumor. It has been seen that, in actual fact, several oncogenes are activated in the same cell in tumors, and that there is progression of malignancy related to the number of oncogenes activated. New mutations occur at genetic level, facilitated perhaps by a reduction of the defense and repair systems, and new impulses towards cell disorganization appear, perhaps as a result of inappropriate expression of normal genes, or of the reduced capacity of immune cells due to substances released by the tumor itself. If we examine the cells of a tumor, we find multiple biochemical atypia, and it is often difficult to establish whether they are directly related to transformation or whether they are alterations secondary to transformation.

A fundamental role in *neoplastic* progression is played by the fact that subsequent errors generate a certain degree of heterogeneity in the proliferating cell population, to such an extent that a number of clones, with

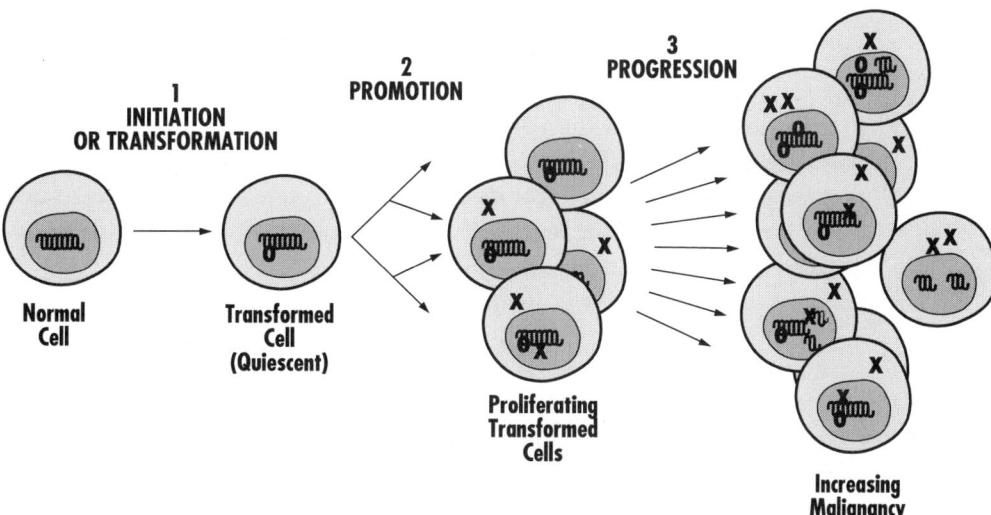

FIGURE 7 The three main stages of tumor growth. O = events at *genetic* level (changes in DNA such as mutations, insertions, deletions or translocations of oncogenes); X = events at *epigenetic* level (various biochemical changes accelerating the expression of oncogenes and genes of normal growth).

characteristics allowing greater resistance to defense systems and drugs, may gradually gain the upper hand. The malignancy of the tumor thus tends steadily to increase.

Figure 7 schematically summarizes the natural history of a tumor. The oncogene theory provides us with a unitary view of the process of cancerogenesis, where mutagenic agents, viruses, promotor agents, and endogenous regulatory factors interact at the level of receptors, transduction systems, and genetic information. In relation to this model, the growth of the neoplasm does not appear as an "all or nothing" event, but as a progressive accumulation of information errors leading the cells to increasingly pronounced levels of atypia and thus of malignancy. It is true that clinically a tumor may manifest itself suddenly, but its biological history dates back to much earlier. This concept is consistent with the theory of multistage tumor growth, already developed on the basis of solid experimental evidence back in the pre-oncogene era, and now universally accepted.

The situation *in vivo* is also complicated for many other reasons: quite apart from the major problem of immune reactions—a subject which would need to be addressed separately in view of its importance—there are many other local factors (tissue oxygenation, organ mobility, biochemical constitution of the basic substance of the connective tissue, factors relating to the compression or erosion of adjoining organs) and general factors (energy metabolism, biohumoral mediators, cachexia, hormones, drugs) which condition the progression of the tumor. Psychosocial stress or psychological or neuroendocrine characteristics similar to a *"type C personality"* (early family frustrations, denial of emotional conflicts, reduced communication with the environment, destructive fantasies, and similar) constitute *risk factors* for cancer [Invernizzi and Gala, 1989].

Tumor progression is conditioned by the tumor-host interaction, also in the sense that the tumor itself, as it grows, influences the body in various ways both via metastatic spread and through the release of soluble products, causing direct or indirect alterations to neighboring and remote organs, including the nervous system. Situations of organ damage and biohumoral disorganization of great complexity and variety are thus generated.

Given the heterogeneity of neoplastic disease and the very substantial importance of the host factor in tumor progression, it is not hard to understand why cancer therapy meets with major difficulties in practical terms as well as why treatments with all the theoretical and scientific prerequisites for efficacy often yield encouraging results in single cases, but prove to have only a poorly significant impact in statistical terms. As things stand at present, it would appear to be largely unrealistic to imagine there may be any single cure for cancer, and this goes for both conventional and unconventional therapy. This is due simply to the fact that "cancer" is an abstraction, whereas in actual fact only particular cases exist and these differ one from another. Without wanting to underrate the value of controlled clinical trials on individual treatments, it would therefore seem important to make some attempt to exploit the *individual* approach to neoplastic disease. This individualization should start on the diagnostic plane and then transfer, if possible, to the therapeutic plane.

The problem of cancer therapy and, in particular, the possible relationships between new scientific knowledge and homeopathic medicine, which is the subject matter of this treatise, will be taken up again in Chapter 6, Section 5, after illustrating the rational model we use to explain the law of similars.

5.4 Homeostasis and complexity

The complexity of pathogenetic mechanisms, stressed in the previous sections in relation to diseases in general and to a number of pathological processes (inflammation and cancer) in particular, is deeply rooted in the complexity present also in physiology and biochemistry. To make this important relationship more explicit and provide better documentary evidence of it, we shall devote the following sections to a review of a number of the general aspects of physiological homeostasis and the exchanges of biological information that regulate it. Understanding the complexity of homeostasis is a *sine qua non* for putting the action of homeopathic remedies into proper perspective.

The concept of homeostasis, first introduced by the physiologist W.B. Cannon in 1929, refers to all those activities which tend to keep the variables of a vital system constant, or, to be more precise, within acceptable

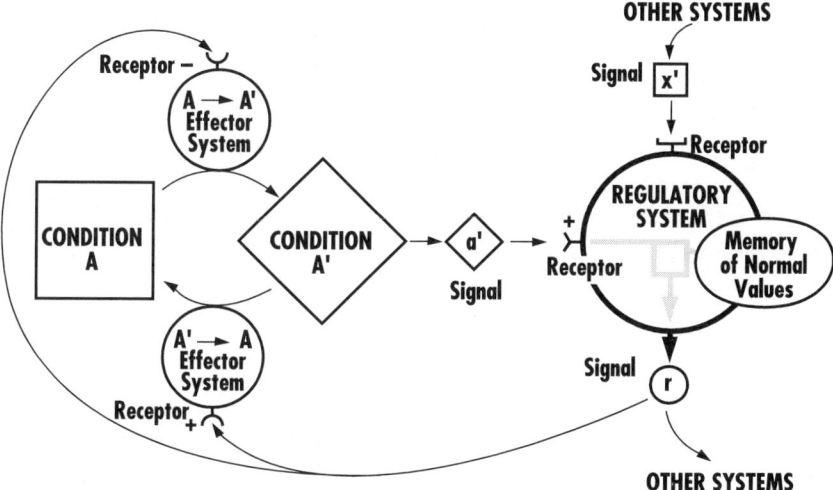

FIGURE 8 Schematic representation of a typical homeostatic system. + = stimulatory effect; - = inhibitory effect.

limits. It may be useful here to take a look at the homeostatic concept in greater detail, using a schematic model of the type illustrated in Figure 8.

A homeostatic system, in its essential make-up, consists in a *set of anatomical, biochemical, and functional elements designed to maintain a physiological variable within minimum and maximum oscillation limits.* Let us consider a *variable A-A'*, which is in a state of dysequilibrium and in conditions of reversibility due to the action of two *operator or effector mechanisms*, which may bring *A* to the level or condition *A'* and vice versa. The system, however, cannot function properly without some form of control, which is provided by a *regulation center* which receives information from *A'* in the form of a *signal a'* associated with its condition (for example, an enzyme reaction product proportional to how much of *A'* is present or to how much of *A'* is functioning). In addition to receiving *a'* signals (for which it has specific receptors), the control system somehow compares these signals with a *memory* in which the optimal value of *a'* is established. When this value is exceeded, the regulation system is activated and produces the *signal r*, which then inhibits the $A \rightarrow A'$ mechanism and/or activates the $A' \rightarrow A$ mechanism. Usually, these effector mechanisms (enzymes, membrane pumps and channels, but also antibodies or cells of various types according to the systems considered) are endowed with incorporated receptor sites for regulatory signals. The homeostatic system thus consists in a negative feedback loop, in which the information on the result of a transformation or an activity oscillation is fed back in revised and corrected form to the entry point of the cycle.

Obviously, the model outlined above is stripped down to essentials, in that if we want a more complete picture, we have to contemplate numerous variants and additions. For instance, we must be aware that there are not just negative feedback loops, but also positive loops, whereby the reaction product contributes towards accelerating the transformation. This is what occurs during the growth of a tissue or when rapid, intense functional modifications (amplification) have to be set in motion.

The model in Figure 8 should also consider the fact that condition *A* has its own control system and, above all, that the homeostatic system itself is in turn related to other systems: the signals *a'* and *r* may have effects on other control systems and on other effector mechanisms, whereas the regulatory system may have receptors for other signals and thus be influenced by these. The integrations (this is a recurrent point) are of the *horizontal* type, as between cells or between organs, or of the *vertical* type, as between molecular and cell systems, between cell systems and organs, or between organs and the body as a whole.

The essential constituents of homeostatic biological systems are therefore the following:

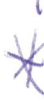

a) *Anatomical or biochemical structures* with adjustable and reversible effector functions. To mention only a few examples, these structures are represented at cell level by enzymes, membranes, contractile proteins, and at body level by the endocrine glands, vessel walls, the cell mass of a certain tissue, etc.

b) *Signal molecules* which enable nearby and remote structures to communicate, such as neurotransmitters, hormones, local chemical mediators, cytokines, physiological inhibitors, and antagonists. A particular complexity feature of the signal molecules is that their message is never wholly specific: the same molecules can be used to communicate between different systems. The same molecules can be produced by many different types of cells. The same molecules can bind to different receptors present on cells in different tissues and organs. There is thus a substantial degree of *redundancy* of biological information, which enables the system to enjoy a considerable measure of flexibility and plasticity, but at the same makes it difficult to achieve any kind of rigid schematization of the events following the production of a certain mediator in given pathophysiological conditions.

c) *Receptors* for signal molecules or for other types of messengers, endowed with specific affinity and capable of transmitting the signal to other elements of the regulation system. There are membrane receptors, intracellular receptors, and even intranuclear receptors. It should be noted that the receptors are highly *plastic*: the cells are capable of increasing (hypersensitivity, priming) or decreasing (desensitization, tolerance, adaptation, down-regulation) the number of receptors according to their needs, as well as of regulating their activity by modifying the affinity for the signal molecule. On occasion, the cells present more than one receptor for the same molecule, but with different affinities and different intracellular effects. A number of receptor properties are addressed in greater detail in Chapter 5, Section 6.3.

d) *Transduction systems*: coupling of receptor activation and production of signals or activation of effector mechanisms; variations of intracellular *second messengers*, covalent and noncovalent modifications of membrane lipids and proteins, and the opening of ion channels. The multiform characteristics of the transduction systems are too vast a topic to be dealt with here. What is beyond doubt, however, is that the level of responsiveness of a certain (control or effector) system is also controlled by such systems in the cell, that they are also modified in the course of disease, and that they are susceptible to pharmacological modulation.

e) *Elements responsible for storage of information* for a given time period: when a system undergoes a change, this may be rapidly and wholly reversible (e.g. the contraction of a muscle), but it may also be a phenomenon which leaves a more or less permanent trace. Usually, though not always, the longer-lasting changes are those which in some way involve the genetic code of the cells.

Some examples of homeostatic systems are:

a) *At cell level*: membrane transport systems, whereby concentrations of Na^+, K^+, Ca^{++}, Cl^-, H^+, are maintained in a state of dynamic dysequilibrium between the intra- and extracellular space; control of metabolism, whereby the availability of nutrients and the presence of metabolites regulate the activity of enzymes and metabolic pathways.

b) *At organ level*: regulation of blood flow in relation to the O_2 requirement; maintenance of constant numbers in cell populations and of the geometric relationships between the various parts; growth and structure of bone in relation to mechanical and gravitational stress; enzymatic induction of the detoxifying functions of the liver following introduction of toxic substances.

c) *At apparatus level*: the vegetative nervous system, for maintaining blood pressure, thermoregulation, bowel function; the endocrine system, for the control of metabolism, growth, the sexual cycle; the cardiovascular and respiratory systems; the immune system, for discriminating between endogenous and exogenous information; the hemostatic system, as an integrated system of cell and humoral mechanisms responsible for the control of the fluidity of the blood.

d) *At superior function level*: mental and emotional functions aimed at bolstering the ego (personality, character, will-power) and at facing up to variable environmental situations (e.g. survival instinct, mature handling of affectivity, decisions and frustrations).

e) *At interindividual and sociocultural level*: population density and forms of economic conditioning on various scales; cultural models, ethical values, ideologies; power systems and deviance control (laws) or incentive systems for behavior patterns accepted by the social group; learning mechanisms for past traditions and development plan forecasts; information control systems.

Of course, the more complex the system, the more complex must be the control networks responsible for guaranteeing effective and specific responses. The nervous system offers a good example of what *vertical* and *horizontal* integration mean. The neurosciences, resting mainly on molecular and cellular biology, have allowed enormous strides to be made in recent decades in our knowledge of neuronal structure, synaptic mechanisms, and signalling and modulation systems (neuromediators). From this point of view, the brain tends to be described as a "container of molecules in action" [Andreoli, 1991]. In this context, horizontal integration consists essentially in understanding the dynamics of functioning on the molecular plane: interactions between signals and receptors, between receptors and proteins of the transduction system, between ion channels and changes in potential, and so on. At the same time, however, there arises a need for vertical integration, which consists in grouping molecules and neurons in nerve *centers*, where the various cells and molecules are in charge of one or more functions. The nerve center has its own architecture and its own "language," which is composed of single molecular or electrical events, but which takes on meaning only as an integrated whole. Many centers are horizontally integrated to form a cerebral area, or a sequence of centers which confer unity upon a more complex function, as may be the case with a visual or auditory function. The nerve centers, however, are also integrated vertically in one hemisphere of the brain, in that particular functions are connected to other areas which add to sensory perception other properties such as conscience, memory, and emotionality. At this level of analysis, then, functions can be carried out which transcend the previous levels, though presupposing them as necessary elements. The organ of hearing and its nerve centers can perceive a sequence of sounds, but for these to be perceived as music a superior integration process must be realized. If we wanted to define how the brain distinguishes between music and a hotch-potch of musical notes, it would be singularly futile to look for differences in the type of enzymes phosphorylating the proteins of the cells of the cochlea, or in the type of neurotransmitters of the auditory pathways, or in the number of cells involved in the auditory area of the brain.

To proceed with this analysis, we should not neglect the fact that the hemispheres of the brain are integrated horizontally via the cerebral commissure, and vertically with the rest of the brain (where, for example, many vegetative functions reside) and then with the entire body. It is therefore essential to consider the various different levels of integration to which the different functions correspond.

Whereas there can be no doubting the complexity of the nervous system, less evident, perhaps, is the complexity at cell level. However much the cell is regarded as the basic unit of the living organism, it is fairly obvious that its organization is highly complex on account of the multiplicity of receptors, transduction routes, effector systems, and genes, all of these being elements which influence one another reciprocally. If to this we add the fact that many elements (particularly the macromolecules) are permanently subject to dynamic oscillations between activation-assembly and dectivation-disassembly, it will be understood that a precise description of what happens *in the cell as a whole* is practically impossible. Since, however, cell theory has dominated pathology for so long, today there are still people who refuse to accept such a conclusion, which mistakenly comes to be seen as conflicting with the molecular point of view.

Others, however, forcefully underline the need to develop the study of cells on a basis which is not exclusively molecular [Albrecht-Buehler, 1990]. The main argument in support of this thesis is that within the cell are concentrated and organized many structures and systems in a state of activity, the properties of which cannot be inferred only on the basis of analysis of molecules purified and studied out of context. In fact, the *proximity relationships* can be transmuted into *forms of collective behavior* of the molecules (including those of water), coherent motions, resonance phenomena, or long-ranging interactions. In other words, it is precisely the *complexity* of the systems in which many molecules interact that precludes an exhaustive description of cell functions on a purely molecular basis.

Stress has also been laid upon the importance of considering the forces generated by tension of the fibers of the cytoskeleton and of the anchoring systems of cells to the tissue matrix in cell models. These forces would appear to have an information content, in that they regulate functions such as ion transport, protein synthesis, and expression of specific genes [Ingber, 1991].

5.5
Information

In view of the importance the concept of information has taken on in our reasoning, we feel it is worthwhile devoting a special section to this topic.

It is only too clear to everyone today that information counts more than force, more than armies, and more than energy (without wishing to imply that these are not important). Companies today invest and spend more on information than on energy. Wars are won more with satellites and computers than with tanks. This information, as Maxwell's demon* has shown, has a cost in terms of energy; in a certain sense, it could be said that information *is a special type of energy required to establish order*. However, the fact that producing, transmitting and manipulating information has an energy cost does not necessarily mean that information in itself is endowed with energy, or even with mass. There are certain types of information which in themselves have only minimal energy contents, but which give rise to very precise effects in target systems. For instance, information broadcast by radio has a very low energy content, as does the information reflected by the light illuminating a text, or a word reaching our ear. Thus, it is also clear that molecules with extremely selective and specific mechanisms of action (which therefore exploit a high information content) act at very low doses (cf., for example, hormones, or antibodies, or certain toxins).

---

*Maxwell's hypothetical demon wanted to violate the second law of thermodynamics by bringing order into a gas, separating the molecules in two vessels by simply opening and closing a small gate (microscopic and friction-free) whenever a molecule approached the hole communicating between the two vessels. After a short time, the demon reasoned, without making the slightest effort I shall have trapped many molecules in one of the vessels, and will thus have pressure to exploit to perform work. He overlooked the fact, however, that, to be able to perform his trick, he needed to have information about the position and movement of the molecules he wanted to capture. It can be calculated that to acquire this information the demon had to consume more energy than he would have been able to recover from the pressure produced by the gas [Harold, 1986].

Information may also be to some extent assessed quantitatively. The information content is measured in *bits*, one bit being the amount of information necessary to be able to make a choice between two alternatives, i.e. a binary choice (yes or no). Needless to say, the more complex the system, the more information it contains and the more information is needed to describe it. For example, if 1 bit is sufficient to code between two numbers (0 and 1), 5 bits will be needed to code a number N among 32 numbers: 32 is divided into two parts and it is decided in which part the number N lies (1 bit is used). The group of 16 remaining numbers containing the number N is divided in two, and another bit is used to reduce the possibilities to 8. Proceeding in this way, we reach a situation in which only two numbers are left, and the fifth bit is used to make the final choice.

Generally speaking, the information content (I) of a system (or an event) is:

$$I = \log_2 1/p$$

where p is the probability that the system will be in this state (or that the event will occur) by chance. Thus, the information is inversely proportional to chance. The larger the number of choices possible, the less likely it is that the event will occur by chance, or that a certain system will be in a certain state by chance.

The degree of order in a given system can be estimated by calculating how many binary choices must be made to specify its structure. For example, during the synthesis of a protein, the choice of amino acid out of 20 possible candidates requires $\log_2 20$, or 4.3 bits. An entire protein of 300 amino acids requires $300 \log_2 20$, i.e. 1,300 bits, while the corresponding DNA sequence (which, for the sake of simplification, consists in 300 nucleotide triplets) requires $900 \log_2 4$, i.e. 1,800 bits of information [Harold, 1986]. The genome of a human cell has approximately 3 billion bases, corresponding to ca. 6×10^9 bits/cell, whereas if we consider the entire organization of an individual adult we get up to the astronomical figure of 10^{28} bits.

Acquiring information has a cost in terms of energy (at 27°C one bit is equivalent to 3×10^{-21} joules [Harold, 1986]). To understand how much it costs to produce information in physiology, we may consider, by way of an example, the formation and action of typical signals, namely the hormones. These molecules, produced with consumption of energy by the endocrine cell, reach the receptors (also produced with energy consumption), from which a message then departs in the form of an increase in calcium which is released from intracellular stores, dissipating the gradient which had been created by consuming energy (Ca^{++} ATPase). In a certain sense, then, the signals convey the energy of the cell, which is dissipated, i.e. they exert a form of control over the dissipation of thermodynamic gradients. This dissipation is obviously short-lasting and is followed by a new accumulation of thermodynamic gradient (at the expense, however, of energy consumption of another type, e.g. metabolic). To the energy cost account of bio-information processes we also have to charge the biosynthesis of DNA, RNA, and biochemical mediators.

The fact that information can be to some extent measured in bits does not entirely solve the problem in all its complexity because the quantity does not in itself comprise the "*meaning*" of the information. The meaning of information resides in the interaction between the information itself and the receiving system and in the result produced by this interaction. Two sequences of DNA, one of which "normal" and the other "pathological" (e.g. coding for a character that causes disease) may contain the same quantity of information, but the result is very different. Thus, a good musical score may contain the same amount of information (in the form of musical notes) as a very bad score. Accordingly, there is necessarily a qualitative element in information which cannot be quantified.

In the biological world, as stressed earlier, communicating information is essential for life: at molecular level, order is expressed in the form of a given, precise association of atoms in molecules (amino acids, proteins, lipids, nucleic acids, etc.); at cell level, order is expressed in the regularity and reproducibility of the cell organization and of biosynthesis, transport and movement processes. To impose order, i.e. to reduce the entropy of living matter, information is necessary. Information can therefore be defined as *the ability to establish order* [Harold, 1986] or, to quote Jacob's famous phrase, "*the power to direct what is done*" [Jacob, 1973].

DNA, as the main data bank of the cell, has the ability to "direct" the cell development, and at the same time to incorporate and remember information: information is stored in the DNA regarding the entire evolutionary history of the species to which the individual belongs. Of course, DNA is an important information-containing material, but it is not the only one: information is contained in *every* organized structure and in every spatiotemporal event that is not casual. While the language of the gene is fairly simple, in that it is written with only a few symbols and in a linear manner, many signals use more complex languages and symbols of various kinds. Events such as changes in transmembrane electrical potential, changes in the ratios of the various phospholipid species, the alkalinization of the cytoplasm, increases in cyclic AMP, elevations of body temperature, blood pressure, the formation of a certain complex of factors controlling the clotting of the blood, and even the emotion experienced as a result of sudden stress are signals which act in the most disparate ways. What is more, the duration of the signal is extremely important; usually signals are short-lived, since there are many control and modulation systems.

A more detailed definition of information might be the following: *information is an intrinsic function of every spatiotemporal structure, capable of being transmitted to another spatiotemporal structure and, thus, of modifying it in a specific manner.* The term *structure* in this context defines a particular configuration of particles, such as atoms, molecules or ions, but there are also structures organized on a temporal scale. A note of music, for instance, is a structure formed by vibrational waves in the air. The terms structure, order, and coherence may be regarded as synonyms.

Apropos of spatiotemporal regulation, it is interesting to note that the pure passage of time is perceived at biological level: the passage of time is signalled by "biological clocks," which induce cells to perform given functions only at certain times of the day or of the period with which the clock is associated.

Information is therefore contained not only in molecules, but also in the "way" molecules relate to the receiver systems. The quantity of the signal is very important, but so is its quality. For example, the receptor system of cells is often capable of distinguishing the *kinetics* whereby the signal is received, namely whether it is a sudden signal or a signal of slow onset, whether the concentration is stable or oscillating, whether the signal is single or accompanied by other concomitant or preceding signals, whether it is the first prompting or a repetition of something *dejà vu*. Thus, information is not merely quantitative, but essentially *spatiotemporal*. It has been suggested that one of the most important intracellular signalling systems, the increase in calcium ions, performs its function by means of pulsations, or rather oscillations of concentration, which constitute a kind of "digital code" for the various sensitive systems: for a response process to be activated, what counts is the frequency of the spatiotemporal oscillations (waves) in the calcium concentration rather than the actual amount of calcium present [Berridge and Galione, 1988; Cheek, 1991].

Single-cell measurements have shown that many hormones trigger a series of calcium *spikes* and that these spikes show a rise in frequency with increasing hormone concentrations. It has been suggested that many cell responses are controlled by *frequency-modulated* rather than *amplitude-modulated* signals, analogous to the transmission of information between neurons by changes in frequency of action potentials [Catt and Balla, 1989]. Such digitally encoded signals could more precisely regulate the cell response to changing hormone concentrations.

Calcium waves can also propagate in tissues and organs, providing a long-range signalling system, as observed in ciliated epithelial cells, in vascular endothelial cells, in hepatocytes, and in monolayers of cultured astrocytes. It has been suggested that this mechanism of cell to cell communication may contribute to the synchronization of large cell assemblies [Meyer, 1991].

In vivo, various hormones are secreted with oscillatory rhythms [Matthews, 1991]. In healthy people, insulin is secreted with pulsations that are repeated every 12-15 minutes, controlled by a pancreatic *pacemaker*, probably influenced by the vagus nerve. The insulin secreted in pulsations is metabolically more efficient in maintaining normal glucose levels, and it is significant that irregularity or even the loss of these oscillations is the earliest abnormality detectable in insulin secretion in patients with type 2 diabetes [Polonsky *et al.*, 1988; Holffenbuttel and van Haeften, 1993].

Biological communication is so important that nature has gone out of its way to find the most differentiated forms of communication (languages). To those we have already mentioned may be added others, the foremost and most obvious of which are the sense organs endowed with photoreceptors, chemoreceptors, baroreceptors, and others. This appears only too self-evident, and there is no point in dwelling on this aspect. More pertinent perhaps to our case is the problem of communication via electromagnetic waves. Light is a basic means not only of transmitting energy (sun-earth), but also of communicating; many fish communicate with light messages, and some cells in mammals also produce light (chemiluminescence), while an infinite amount of luminous information is received by the organs of sight; light would also appear to be important for establishing many biorhythms. Light, however, constitutes only a small part of the electromagnetic spectrum, and it may seem strange that nature has not learnt how to handle other types of electromagnetic fields. We shall return to this problem in Chapter 7.

In a nutshell, then, *every biochemical or biophysical system endowed with a certain degree of order acts as a vehicle for information*, which, when suitably decoded by receptor and transduction systems, may have biological consequences. The information molecules *par excellence* are the nucleic acids because they are characterized by a very substantial degree of order (cf. the arrangement of the nucleotides in very long sequences), by a major degree of complexity (cf. all the mechanisms controlling the expression of the genetic code and also its continual transformation), and by great physico-chemical stability (given its particular double-helix structure, DNA is one of the most resistant molecules, and, in addition, many systems exist for

homeostasis

repairing and remedying possible errors). Many other molecules, however, contain and transmit information: proteins, peptides, sugars, lipids, and even mineral salts and protons (H^+) serve nature as transmitters of information and thus to regulate biological systems. Leaving aside the molecular field, we also find information transmitted by frequencies, such as sound and electromagnetic waves and rhythmic, oscillatory chemical events. The more complex a system is, the more complex will be its communications strategy, which may be made up of many elements arranged in sequences and networks.

The problem of information has a close bearing on the mechanism of action of homeopathic remedies. As we shall see later (Chapter 6), the "secret" of homeopathy, in its classic form, lies precisely in the meticulous collection of information relating, on the one hand, to the remedy (cf. provings in healthy subjects) and, on the other, to the patient (every physical or mental symptom is assessed with particular reference to its extent, circadian variations, site, mode of onset, duration, association with other symptoms, and constitutional characteristics). It might be said that the bulk of the effort made in the homeopathic method is precisely in the collection and "*repertorization*" of symptoms (i.e. comparison between the patient's symptoms and symptoms caused by remedies as reported in the materia medicas). It is no accident that a major contribution to this work of data analysis and comparison is made by systems of computerized repertorization [see, for example, Van Haselen and Fisher, 1990].

In this section we shall deal in particular with a problem already raised earlier, when we talked about the difficulties in controlling homeostatic systems and pathogenetic mechanisms by means of exogenous manipulation. This problem has to do with the fact that a given type of manipulation of a biological system is not always followed by an effect proportional to the extent of the intervention implemented. This is of great importance in clinical medicine and in pharmacology, but it is obviously also of vital interest when it comes to interpreting the mechanism of action of drugs which are used at low or ultra-low doses.

5.6

Doses, target systems, and effects

The problems to be tackled here are essentially two: the first relates to the fact that the effects of a certain treatment do not always go in the direction that might appear logical, and the second has to do with the nonlinearity and nonunivocal nature of dose-response curves.

5.6.1 Apparently paradoxical effects

The complexity of homeostatic pathophysiological systems means that it is not always possible to predict the outcome of a given intervention aimed at regulating such systems. Psychiatry and the neurosciences in general represent today the main frontier where this type of problem is taken into consideration. In these disciplines, in fact, the molecular approach to pharmacology shows both its validity and its limitations. The effects of psychotropic drugs often vary very strikingly from one subject to another, not only according to whether or not the subject is sick or healthy, but also according to the type of disease and even the characteristics of the subject's personality.

Psychopharmacology is thus full of examples in which a certain treatment causes paradoxical effects. This concept is well expressed in a paper dealing with the relationships between madness and biology: "If an exogenous molecule administered to a mad person is capable of modifying his or her behavior, it is legitimate to postulate that the madness itself is related to endogenous molecules with which one thereby interferes. Corroboration of this is provided by the administration of exogenous molecules to healthy subjects with the result that their behavior is modified pathologically. In this case the molecule produces madness. These two circumstances have a long history behind them in psychopharmacology and have given rise to the two important areas known as the "therapy of madness" and as "experimental psychosis" or "drug-induced psychosis" [Andreoli, 1991, p. 52].

The nervous system is *the* complex system *par excellence*. It manifests in paradigmatic form a behavior typical of all complex systems: the effect of pharmacological manipulation depends both on the direct effect of the drug itself on cells and molecules, and on the sensitivity of the receptor or enzymatic structures, as well as on the reactions which set the system itself in motion and on the reactions secondary to endogenous reactions. This in itself does not mean that an effect is, as a rule, unpredictable, but that the *mechanism* whereby an effect is exerted cannot be interpreted merely on the basis of the direct effect on the deterministic molecular plane.

A precise example of what we have said may be the use of tricyclic antidepressants [Goodman Gilman *et al.*, 1992]. The parent molecule of the class, imipramine, was discovered by chance in 1958 in the course of a clinical trial in psychotic patients. It was noted that imipramine was relatively ineffective in calming agitated psychotic patients, but the drug proved capable of affording substantial benefit in depressed patients, who were stimulated by it. Since then these compounds have been widely used in depression. If imipramine (100–200 mg/day) is administered for a sufficiently lengthy time period to a depressed patient, the patient's spirits are raised. In some cases the effect is so pronounced that there is a real danger of generating a maniac-like excitatory effect. If, however, a dose of 100 mg of imipramine is administered to a healthy subject, the latter feels drowsy and tends to be calmer, undergoing a slight reduction in blood pressure and experiencing a "light-headed" sensation. Unpleasant anticholinergic effects occur and, sometimes, a slight change in pupil diameter. The gait may become unsteady, and the subject may feel tired and clumsy. Deterioration in performance test results may occur. These pharmacological effects are usually perceived as disagreeable and give rise to a feeling of unhappiness and increased anxiety. Repeated administration of imipramine for several days may cause intensification of these symptoms as well as difficulty in concentrating and reasoning.

Other examples of paradoxical effects of drugs can be encountered in systems other than the nervous system, such as the cardiovascular or endocrine systems, or the immune system and inflammation.

Digitalis, which is regarded today as a fully fledged hormone probably produced by the adrenal glands [*Lancet* editorial, 1991], causes depression of cardiac function in healthy subjects when administered at pharmacological doses, whereas it has a positive inotropic effect in heart failure. Conversely, adrenalin has a positive inotropic effect in healthy subjects, whereas in heart failure it has no effect, or a negative effect (when it activates the beta$_2$-adrenergic receptors, and the muscarinic and adenosine receptors are also stimulated) [Braunwald, 1991]. These changes in responsiveness are related to increases and reductions in sensitivity and in the number of specific receptors, as well as in transduction systems such as the G-proteins. Another possible example, among the many that could be mentioned with regard to the vascular system, is the fact that acetylcholine induces a vasoconstrictor effect in arteries affected by atherosclerosis, which is paradoxical, in that the drug normally causes vasodilatation [Ludmer *et al.*, 1986].

An inhibitor of nitric oxide synthase (monomethyl-L-arginine) causes a marked increase in platelet aggregation in healthy controls, presumably because it removes an endogenous feedback inhibitory mechanism. On the contrary, in hypertensive patients the same agent causes only a slight inhibition of aggregation [Cadwgan and Benjamin, 1993]. Therefore, platelets from hypertensive patients show a markedly reduced sensitivity to a drug that is effective in normal humans, suggesting that an imbalance of these control mechanisms contributes to the pathogenesis of essential hypertension.

Serotonin, which causes vasodilatation in normal arteries, induces vaso-constriction in some forms of hypertension and diabetes and in athero-sclerotic arteries. This might be an important mechanism in transient ischemic attacks [Ware and Heistad, 1993].

Japanese endocrinologists have conducted a study in 109 patients with Graves' disease (hyperthyroidism caused by autoantibodies), treated first with a conventional antithyroid treatment, and then, when this was dis-continued, with thyroid hormones (thyroxine 0.1 mg/day) long term ver-sus placebo [Hashizume *et al.*, 1991]. In the subsequent follow-up, the treated group showed a significant reduction in recurrences of hyperthy-roidism, accompanied by a progressive reduction in the autoantibody count. Treatment with thyroid hormones thus reduces activation of the thyroid in Graves' disease patients. The authors themselves found a convincing explanation of this apparent paradox: by means of an endocrine feedback mechanism, thyroxine inhibits TSH-induced thyroid stimulation and the subsequent release of receptors serving as stimuli for the production of autoantibodies.

In the field of autoimmune disease therapy, one form of therapy steadily gaining ground is that based on administration of immunoglobulins [see, for example, Kaveri *et al.*, 1991; Dwyer, 1992], i.e., in practice, of mol-ecules which are already present as pathogenetic agents. It is likely that the efficacy of this therapy depends either on competition at the level of the cell membranes suffering the immune attack or, much more probably, on the blocking action of antibodies against other antibodies (anti-idiotype antibodies) [Dwyer, 1992].

In addition, we can mention here the therapies for autoimmune diseases based on the oral administration of the same protein that caused the au-toimmunity, or of particular fragments of the same proteins ("tolerogenic epitopes") [Marx, 1991; Miller *et al.*, 1991a; Miller *et al.*, 1991b: Whitacre *et al.*, 1991; Miller *et al.*, 1992; Engel, 1992; Ku *et al.*, 1993]. It has been discovered that attacks of experimental autoimmune diseases in animals (allergic encephalitis induced by injection of a protein associated with myelin, arthritis induced by collagen, uveitis induced by a retinal protein) can be suppressed by feeding the animals the same proteins causing the attacks. These studies in animals have yielded such promising results that clinical trials have been started on "oral antigen therapy" (or specific oral tolerance induction) in patients with multiple sclerosis, rheumatoid arthritis, and uveitis [for a review see Weiner *et al.*, 1994]. The investigators con-ducting this research claim that this type of therapy induces specific im-munosuppression, based on activation of certain subsets of T lymphocytes located in the gut lymphoid tissue, which are capable of suppressing the activity of other cells of the immune system. Very recently, it has been demonstrated in animal models (mice) that the mechanism of these phenomena is determined by secretion of different cytokines according to the antigen dosage: low doses (1 mg every other day) of antigen induce active immunosuppression by the release of more transforming growth factor-β and less interleukin-4, while high doses (20 mg/day) induce anergy (lack of response) by the release of more interleukin-4 and less transforming growth factor-β [Friedman and Weiner, 1994].

It is interesting to note that the possibility that oral ingestion of antigen might modify subsequent systemic immune responses was probably recognized in ancient times by South American Indians who ate poison ivy (*Rhus toxicodendron*) leaves in an attempt to prevent contact sensitivity reactions to the plant [reported by R. Dakin, cited by Mowat, 1987].

The immune system never ceases to amaze us with its characteristics of flexibility and complexity, which physicians seek to exploit for therapeutic purposes. Up until not so very long ago, vaccinations were thought to be an excellent means of preventing infectious diseases, but that little could be done for a disease already in progress. This would seem logical, in view of the fact that the individual affected by an infectious agent is already full of antigens, and, after a short time, of specific antibodies and lymphocytes. Today, however, a different picture is beginning to emerge: vaccinations might also have a curative effect [Beardsley, 1991]. It can be postulated that this new approach to therapy by means of vaccinations (still at the experimental stage) can be justified rationally on the basis of the particular modes of functioning of the immune response.

An initial explanation lies in the fact that vaccinations can be given with antigens in a slightly different form from the natural antigen, for instance, in the form of recombinant protein or as a complex with other immunogens: the antigen therefore would be recognized by the system in a different way and would trigger off a different and possibly more effective response to the original infectious agent. Another possibility is based on the fact that different routes can be used to introduce the vaccine (oral, intramuscular, inhalatory). By modifying the administration route, compared to the route taken by the natural agent, other groups of lymph nodes or reactive centers of the immune system can be activated, and, most importantly, the surveillance cells (macrophages) can be reached via an anatomical route that they "do not expect," thereby bypassing possible blockade or adaptation mechanisms of the system which allowed the pathogen to conceal itself or survive.

Considerations of this type can hardly fail to have an impact on the debate regarding homeopathy, particularly as regards validation of the law of similars. In the sector of therapies modulating the immune system, the boundaries between allopathy and homeopathy tend to blur. *Similar substances may have opposite effects according to the doses and to the particular sensitivity of the systems with which they interact.*

We could also mention nonhomeopathic drugs which act according to a mechanism which could be regarded as an application of the law of similars. A significant example is provided by products based on extracts of *Klebsiella pneumoniae, Diplococcus pneumoniae, Haemophilus influenzae,* and similar substances, for which a substantial body of convincing literature exists [Nespoli *et al.* 1987; Capsoni *et al.,* 1988; Balsano *et al.,* 1988] and which are classed as belonging to the category of immunostimulating substances. These drugs are indicated, at low doses, for the prophylaxis and therapy of respiratory tract infections. It is interesting to note that the administration of these preparations causes, as an unwanted effect, a temporary increase in symptoms following the first few doses, which is a characteristic phenomenon reported in the literature in relation to the action of homeopathic products.

That many molecules act as "double agents" is also well known in the field of inflammation. By way of an example we can take substance P. This is an undecapeptide belonging to the family of the tachykinins and is found in many organs, such as the central nervous system, the lungs, skin, and bowels. It performs various different functions: the first function assigned to it was pain mediation, both as a neurotransmitter among the neurons of the pain pathways, and in so far as it increases the sensitivity of thermal and pressure receptors (probably by inhibiting the potassium channels of the membranes). It was later seen that substance P, even when released peripherally by the sensitive endings of type C unmyelinated fibers, mediates many inflammation phenomena. Tissues which are a prey to inflammation, as in ulcerative colitis, rheumatoid arthritis, and asthma, present a substantially increased number of receptors for substance P. On the other hand, it has also been seen that interleukin-1, one of the inflammation cell products, stimulates production of substance P by the cells of the nerve ganglia. It is in this that its role as a double agent lies: it increases sensitivity to pain, but also promotes healing of wounds by increasing the activity of leukocytes and the immune system in general. In practice, it makes the phagocytes more efficient in killing bacteria, and the lymphocytes more efficient in producing antibodies. Thus, the same mediator causes pain and heals [Skerret, 1990].

It is well known that one of the mediators of the occurrence of headache and migraine may be serotonin, inasmuch as this molecule causes vasodilatation in certain cases. On the other hand, drugs have recently been introduced which are effective in migraine and are analogues (i.e. "similar") to serotonin, acting not as antagonists, but as agonists, that is to say they have the same action as the endogenous molecule. How does it come about that a molecule similar to the mediator causing pain has a pain-relieving effect? The answer here is to be sought in the complexity of the receptors: there are at least four distinct types of serotonin receptors, and the analogue stimulates only one type, which evidently serves as a negative feedback mechanism for the pain-inducing effects of serotonin itself.

Histamine is a well known inflammatory mediator causing allergic manifestations and anaphylaxis, but histamine may have antianaphylactic action *in vivo* [Blandina *et al.*, 1987] and prevent antigenic release of histamine from cells of allergic donors [Bourne *et al.*, 1971; Lichtenstein and Gillespie, 1973; Lichtenstein and Gillespie, 1975]. These apparently paradoxical results are probably due to the existence of different histamine receptors and to the fact that stimulation of H_2-receptors causes an increase in cyclic AMP and mast cell inhibition [Masini *et al.*, 1982].

High-dose aspirin can cause hyperthermia [Goodman Gilman *et al.*, 1992], which is clearly a paradoxical effect compared to the main indication.

It has been reported, amongst other things, that onicholysis disappears during treatment with benoxaprofene, despite the fact that onicholysis figures among the possible side effects of the drug [cited by Taylor Reilly *et al.*, 1986].

Going over now to another field of research, we see that studies on tumor cells in culture have yielded apparently paradoxical, but also highly indicative results. The differentiation of leukemia cells versus more mature and thus less malignant forms can be obtained in culture not only by means of specific differentiation factors (this, however, only in a number of cell lines, obviously endowed with receptors), but also by means of agents such as lectins, or classic tumor promoters such as TPA, or low doses of cytostatic agents, or low doses of radiation [Sachs, 1986; Sachs, 1989]. Evidently, effects promoting proliferation or effects promoting maturation, and thus the arrest of proliferation, are not properties related only to the molecule used, but properties which depend on dose, receptor sensitivity, types of oncogenes active in a certain cell line, synergism or antagonism with other factors in the culture medium or produced by the cells themselves, the metabolism the substance undergoes in the cell, and other processes.

Given the complexity of the mechanisms involved in the control of cell proliferation (see also Chapter 5, Section 3.1.), it is understandable that a treatment which, according to traditional concepts, should be pro-cancerogenic may turn out to be anti-cancerogenic experimentally on changing the doses or experimental protocol. Many mitogenic agents, for example, if administered to cells in small doses over lengthy periods, desensitize the cells, almost always in a homologous manner (i.e. to themselves), but sometimes they do so in a heterologous manner (i.e. to other agents with a similar action at the transduction mechanism level) [Rozengurt, 1991]. There are also experimental animal models which show that a carcinogen at low doses can combat the onset of the cancer itself [De Gerlache, 1991] (see also Chapter 5, Section 3).

The examples mentioned here are suggestive indications of how the damaging effects of poisonous or toxic substances can transform themselves into specular therapeutic effects (or vice versa, i.e. therapeutic effects can turn into damaging effects) on changing the doses and modes of administration of the substances and the sensitivity of the system treated. This is of primary importance if we are to understand the possible mechanism of action of homeopathic remedies [Grange and Denman, 1993]. Obviously, we should stress, especially in fields such as oncology, that experimental models can illustrate certain biological phenomena which undoubtedly exist, but cannot be regarded as proof of the therapeutic efficacy of given treatments, since they often represent only particular cases in the context of biological complexity.

5.6.2 Doses

In this section we intend to consider the fact that the effects of a given treatment, aimed at modulating a given biological system, are not always proportional to the doses used. In chemistry, biology, and pharmacology, the analysis of dose-response curves is fundamental for studying the characteristics and mechanisms of action of any active compound. Such analysis provides information about the mechanisms responsible for a certain reaction. In biochemistry, for example, we can evaluate the affinity of an enzyme for a substrate or the type of inhibition of the reaction (competitive, noncompetitive) by a certain compound. In biology, such curves can be used to measure the number and affinity of receptors for a certain hormone, or active cell responses such as muscle cell contraction, enzyme secretion, and many other functions. Considering the versatility of *in vitro* studies, the effects of various doses of a certain toxic substance on the release of cytoplasmic enzymes can be measured as an index of cell mortality, or the increase in cell number as an index of proliferative activity.

In pharmacology, the production of dose-effect curves first in animals and then in man, is used to establish the correct drug dose and the so-called therapeutic interval (the difference between toxic doses and therapeutic doses).

A common conviction among nonexperts is that the higher the dose is, the greater the effect will be. This conviction is obviously wrong, in that usually the effects of a certain active substance on a certain parameter are known not to be directly proportional to the dose. In the classic dose-response curves (Figure 9) we see first of all a noneffect zone (doses below the sensitivity threshold of the system tested or of the measurement method), a certain dose at which we begin to see some effect (minimum effective dose), an exponential growth of the effect in the first part of the curve, and then a progressive slowing of growth until a plateau is reached, where the effect is maximal and further increases in dose are not followed by any quantitative increase in the parameter measured. This trend presents itself in similar forms, whether we are measuring stimulatory or inhibitory effects. The dose causing a 50% effect compared to the maximum is called ED_{50} (median effective dose), or ID_{50} (median inhibitory dose), or LD_{50} (median lethal dose, i.e. lethal for 50% of animals), according to what is being measured. By means of other mathematical operations, we can extract additional significant information from such curves, but we do not intend to discuss these possibilities here.

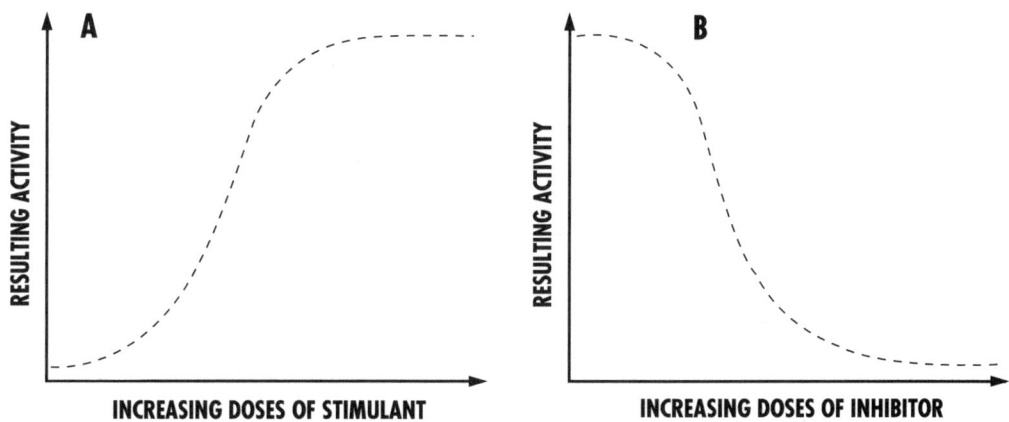

FIGURE 9 Classic dose-response curves. The curves represent the typical trend of biochemical or biological activity as a function of increasing doses of an activator compound (or enzyme substrate) (**A**) or of an inhibitor compound (**B**). The curves show an initial zone in the low-dose area where there is no effect, and then an exponential increase in the effect which later slows down until a plateau is reached (maximum activation or inhibition, which remains unchanged with further increases in dose).

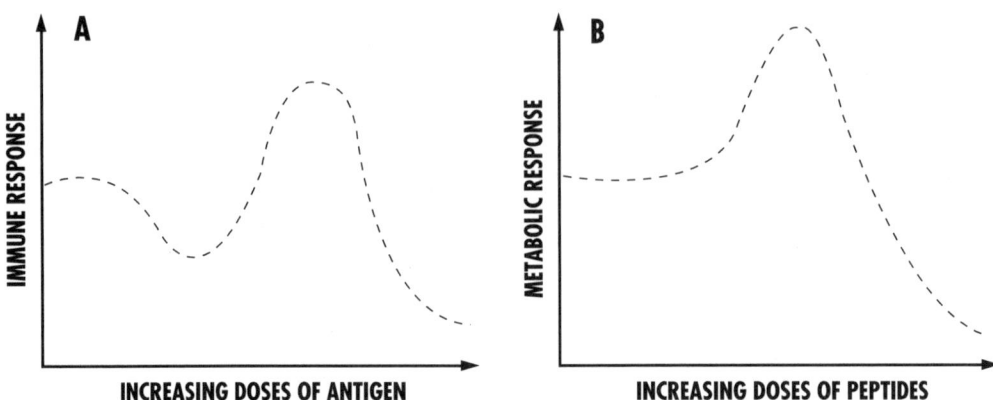

FIGURE 10 Atypical dose-response curves. Curve **A** plots the trend of the immune response to bovine albumin in mice pretreated with increasing doses of antigen. The immune response is depressed (state of *tolerance*) both in animals receiving very low doses and in animals receiving very high doses of antigen. Intermediate doses, however, cause a *greater response* [from Pontieri, 1987, with modifications]. Curve **B** plots the metabolic activity trend of human granulocytes stimulated with high doses of bacterial peptides after pretreatment with increasing doses of peptides. The graph thus shows the response to the second stimulation, which is strongly potentiated by pretreatment with low doses (*priming*) and inhibited by high-dose pretreatment (*desensitization*) [data reported in Bellavite *et al.*, 1991c, and in Bellavite *et al.*, 1993a].

These types of measurements and interpretations figure among the cornerstones of scientifically oriented medicine and clearly cannot be called into question. What appears, however, to be increasingly important in recent years is that there are many exceptions to these basic rules, with the result that they can no longer be regarded as valid in all cases. The exceptions in this case do not prove the rule, nor do they disprove it, but they narrow down its field of application to a part (at this stage it is hard to say whether or not it is the majority) of the events occurring in biology and pathology.

In this section we shall give examples of these exceptions, derived from the conventional biological and pharmacological literature and not from studies conducted for the purposes of investigating homeopathy.

Figure 10 shows two atypical dose-response curves. Curve A plots the trend of the immune response (e.g. quantity of antibodies produced) as a function of amount of antigen. At the lower doses of antigen there is a decline in the response, i.e. a desensitization, at intermediate doses an increase, and at high doses again a decline. Curve B, on the other hand, plots the metabolic activity of granulocytes stimulated with chemotactic peptides (fMLP) after pretreatment with increasing doses of the same peptides. At the lower doses we observe an increase in the response with the increase in dose, while at the higher doses it can be seen that the cell activity is depressed to the point of reaching levels which are lower than those of cells receiving no treatment at all. As can be seen from the curves, in these cases the concepts of proportionality of dose and effect clearly call for adjustment.

The reasons for these behavior patterns of biological systems are complex, relating, as they do, to the modes whereby cells, tissues, and organs regulate the degree of sensitivity at receptor, biochemical and genetic level. To cut a long story short, we can refer once again to the concepts of "priming" and "desensitization" (or adaptation), to which reference has already been made in the section on the modulation of the functions of inflammatory cells (Chapter 5, Section 2.1.)

What is meant by *priming* is a state of hyperactivation in response to a given stimulant, which characterizes a cell after it has received pretreatment with low doses of the same stimulant (homologous priming) or of other stimulants of a different type (heterologous priming). The priming is due to exposure of new receptors, to activation of the same receptors and/or to a number of changes in the intracellular communication or enzyme systems. It is worth noting that priming has been described not only at the cell level, such as in leukocytes, but also in tissue and organs, such as in the airways of allergic individuals after repeated challenge with allergens [Koh *et al.*, 1994].

What is meant by *desensitization* is a state characterized by lack of cell responsiveness to a given stimulus after the cell has received pretreatment with low, medium or high doses of the same stimulant (homologous desensitization) or of different stimulants (heterologous desensitization). Generally speaking, desensitization (whether homologous or heterologous) may be due to many mechanisms, including consumption or inactivation of receptors, decoupling of receptors from transduction systems, and deactivation of cell effector systems.

Figure 11 presents dose-response curves which document the phenomenon of priming. This event may manifest itself either as increased sensitivity to low doses (leftward shift of the dose-response curve) (Figure 11 B) or as an increase in maximum effect, doses being equal (Figure 11 A).

Figure 12 illustrates another important phenomenon which definitely plays a role in priming and in the regulation of responses to pharmacological agents in general. On subjecting the cells to increasing doses of a stimulant, effects of one type (e.g. an increase in intracellular calcium) may be recorded with very low doses, whereas effects of another type (e.g. activation of oxidative metabolism) can be obtained only with much higher

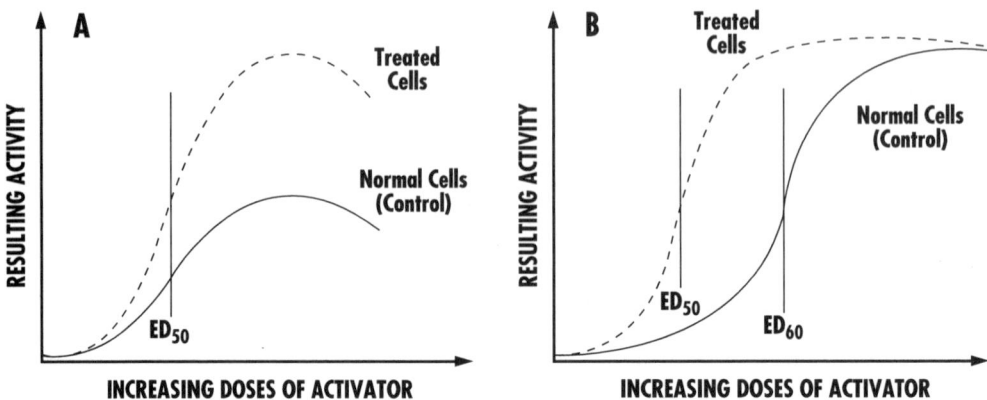

FIGURE 11 Dose-response curve illustrating the priming (or hypersensitivity) phenomenon. The solid lines plot the trends of a functional activity parameter in control cells in response to increasing doses of a stimulant. The dashed lines plot the trends for the same parameter as assessed in cells which have received a pretreatment with low doses of another stimulant. ED_{50} = dose causing 50% of maximal activation. Graph A gives an example where the dose-response curve of the pretreated cells reaches a greater height than that of the control cells, but the ED_{50} and peak activity are observed at the same doses in the two types of cells. This may indicate that the priming effect is the result of an increase in the number of receptors or of other mechanisms of post-receptor regulation. Graph B gives an example in which the dose-response curve is shifted to the left towards the low doses in the pretreated cells. This may indicate that the priming effect is the result of an increase in *affinity* (ability to bind progressively lower doses) of the receptors for the activator compound.

doses of the same stimulant. This depends on the fact that for the first type of response the occupancy of a very limited number of receptors is sufficient compared to the number necessary for triggering the second type of response. Another possibility is that the cells present more than one type of receptor for the same compound, types of receptors with different affinities (different binding intensity in relation to changes in dose), and mediators of different responses. In general (meaning that every rule in this field admits of exceptions), low doses are capable of bringing about subtle changes in cell biology, such as the assembly of colloidal proteins of the cytoskeleton, the opening of ion channels, or the exposure of a fair number of receptors. These are precisely the changes associated with priming.

Another example of the multiplicity of factors influencing receptor dynamics consists in experiments conducted in leukocytes [De Togni et al., 1985]: the same dose of a stimulant (chemotactic peptide) may give rise to very different effects according to the mode of administration. When the compound is administered all in one go, within the space of a few seconds, a very marked increase in oxygen consumption is obtained. When the compound is administered slowly, over a period of minutes, the response is very poor in terms of oxygen consumption. It has been seen that the difference in effect between the two modes of adding the compound is not due to a difference in the binding of the compound to the receptors, which exhibit the same degree of occupancy in both cases. Evidently, the receptor-transducer system perceives the molecule-to-receptor *association rate*, since, if this *rate* is high, there is no time for the counterreaction to occur which in some way disactivates the response.

In our laboratory, the adhesion of neutrophils to serum-coated surfaces was investigated in primed and normal cells. In normal cells, adhesion occurs only in the presence of suitable stimulants, such as the peptide fMLP at relatively high doses ($10^{-7}/10^{-6}$ M). However, we noted that neutrophils pre-treated with bacterial endotoxins (LPS) showed enhanced adhesion even in the absence of fMLP, and that, on addition of *low doses* of fMLP, the LPS-mediated adhesion was inhib-

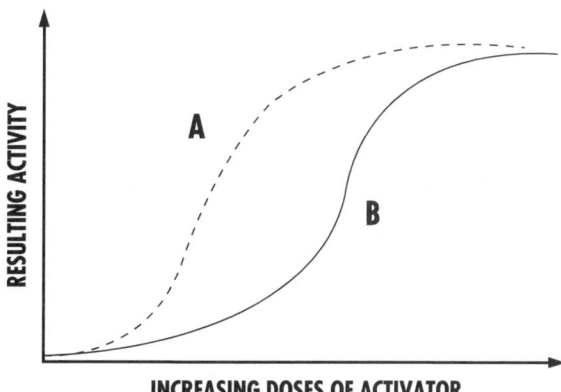

INCREASING DOSES OF ACTIVATOR

FIGURE 12 Dose-response curves plotting changes in activity of two functional parameters of the same cells as a function of increasing doses of a stimulant. Curve **A** (dashed line) plots the increase in calcium ions in the cytoplasm of activated leukocytes. Curve **B** (solid line) plots the increase in oxidative metabolism in the same cells treated with the same doses of activator (in this example, bacterial peptides). It may be noted that the increase in calcium ions sets in at much lower doses of stimulant than those needed to activate oxidative metabolism. This may indicate either that there are two types of receptors (one type with high affinity which regulates calcium flux and one with low affinity which regulates metabolism) or that only one type of receptor exists, but the occupancy of a smaller number of such receptors is sufficient to activate calcium flux.

ited [Bellavite *et al.*, 1993b; Bellavite *et al.*, 1993c]. In synthesis, the results indicated that:

a) Untreated cells show only minimal adhesion to serum-coated plastic surfaces and this adhesion is not significantly affected by low doses (1-5 x 10^{-9} M) of fMLP.

b) Fully activatory doses (5 x 10^{-7} M) of fMLP induce a significant increase in cell adhesion.

c) Pretreatment of the cells for 1 h with 1 mg/ml endotoxin augments adhesion in the absence of further stimulation.

d) Addition of very low doses of fMLP (3×10^{-9} M) inhibits the adhesion of endotoxin-treated cells.

e) High fMLP doses are additive to endotoxin in promoting adhesion.

Similar results have been recently obtained using cells which were primed *in vivo* during an inflammatory process [Bellavite *et al.*, 1994]. In conclusion, the chemotactic agent fMLP, which is considered to be an activator of neutrophil adhesion, paradoxically inhibits the same cell response at low doses when used in primed cells.

A phenomenon similar to desensitization is *tolerance*, which can be defined as the acquisition of nonreactivity of the immune system to given antigens. Tolerance is a fundamental mechanism whereby the immune system learns to distinguish the substances of the body itself from extraneous substances, though in certain conditions there may be tolerance of nonself substances (acquired tolerance). The state of tolerance may involve either B lymphocytes (antibody response) or T lymphocytes (cell-mediated response). It is possible to induce tolerance of foreign agents by exposing the body to higher doses than those which are normally immunogenic (we are dealing therefore with a lymphocyte desensitization or inactivation phenomenon) or to very low subimmunogenic doses of antigen (in this case the tolerance is due apparently to the intervention of T suppressor lymphocytes). It has been claimed that the tolerance induced by low doses bears witness to the great ability of the body to react to subliminal stimuli and may be one of the mechanisms of action of many preparations with a weak primary action [Speciani, 1991]. Other authors have proposed that the immune modulation implemented with microdoses of antigens (in some experimental models immune responses have been observed to fractions of a microgram of protein) constitutes a field in which a great deal of evidence furnished by "orthodox" science exists to support the claims of homeopathic medicine [Grange and Denman, 1993].

The examples given here above refer mainly to the field of immunity and the biology of leukocytes, but, with the necessary modifications, the same principles could also apply to the biology of platelets, liver cells, muscle, and even nerve cells.

Another example comes from the vascular pathophysiology sector. It is generally accepted that the endothelia of blood vessels produce nitric oxide, which is essentially an "endogenous nitrovasodilator." Practically speaking, this molecule is nothing other than the active component of drugs long known as vasodilators, namely amyl nitrite, trinitroglycerine, and the other nitrovasodilators [Collier and Vallance, 1991]. In this connection, it is worthwhile stressing the fact that this discovery shares certain features with the discovery of endogenous opioids (enkephalins and endorphins) and with the discovery of endogenous digitalis-like factors: the body knows how to produce many of the drugs it needs! There are clear indications that in various cardiovascular diseases there is a reduced production or increased catabolism of nitric oxide, which may thus predispose the vessels to a more marked and longer-lasting spasm and to consequent ischemia. The other side of the coin is that there may be excess production of nitric oxide in shock and hypotension.

In equilibria of this type, we would stress once again that disease changes sensitivity: when the arteries suffer endothelial damage, they produce less nitric oxide, but at the same time the underlying vascular wall becomes hypersensitive to nitrovasodilators [Moncada *et al.*, 1992]. The "sick" wall is thus more sensitive to the drug compared to the healthy wall, which would account, at least partially, for the efficacy of nitroglycerine in angina.

The existence of inverse effects on changing the dose has long been known in pharmacology, where terms such as "hormesis" and the "Arndt-Schulz law" have been used to identify positive, stimulatory effects of low doses of inhibitors or toxins, or low doses of radiation. These stimulatory effects have been detected with regard to cell vitality and growth, muscular contractility, breathing, nervous transmission, and other functions [Schulz, 1888; Towsend and Luckey, 1960; Stebbing, 1982; Calabrese et al., 1987; Furst, 1987; Sagan, 1989; Wolff, 1989; Linde, 1991; Oberbaum and Cambar, 1994; Calabrese and Baldwin, 2000].

The fact that such phenomena exist is therefore indisputable, but to date not enough attention has been paid to them, since the tendency has been to view them either as pharmacological curiosities or as simply marginal phenomena compared to the main action of the toxin or inhibitor. Within the framework of a theory which seeks to provide a rational explanation of the therapeutic effect of low doses of substances which in themselves are often poisonous, as indeed is the case in homeopathy, our traditional knowledge of hormesis takes on new and major significance [Linde, 1991; Bellavite *et al.*, 1993c]. The connection between homeopathy and hormesis has been thoroughly discussed in a review [Oberbaum and Cambar, 1994]. The authors suggest that the common basis might be the process of information in biological systems. Every toxic compound induces a series of characteristic biochemical modifications in the target. These modifications have a toxic, damaging, and even lethal effect on the system when the concentration of the agent is high. On the other hand, when the dose of the toxin is decreased, the same modifications have an "informative" effect which enables the biological system to adapt by counteracting a particular agent, using specific defense mechanisms for that agent. The adaptability of the living system indicates that it is able to recognize the aggression, and receive it as information regarding the properties of the toxin. This information helps the organism to react and reinforces its defenses.

Others have suggested that one of the most important cellular mechanisms of the hormetic effect is the production of "heat-shock proteins" or "stress proteins," a class of proteins that are coordinately synthesized after exposure to heat, radiation, heavy metals, and oxidizing agents [Smith-Sonneborn, 1993]. In fact, the same agents that have been identified as hormetic also induce the stress response, and the stress response preferentially includes the synthesis of products that repair both protein and DNA, which may stimulate growth and longevity.

In the following section we shall attempt to illustrate in greater detail some of the biological elements upon which these apparently paradoxical effects are based.

5.6.3 Receptors and transduction systems

One specific field in which the complexity of living systems can be studied and documented in laboratory systems is that of cell biology. Among the various aspects which could be adduced by way of examples, particularly significant would appear to be the studies on receptors and communication systems. These cell functions constitute a *homeostasis of signals*, made up of competitive actions, nonlinear responses, feedback loops, and spatiotemporal oscillations.

In the previous sections of this chapter and in the chapter on research in homeopathy (Chapter 4), on repeated occasions experiments were cited illustrating the following phenomena:

a) The same agent can induce opposite effects if used at different doses.

b) Two different agents can produce the same effect on the target system.

c) The same agent can determine or induce different responses in a healthy organism compared to a sick one.

d) The same agent can prove stimulatory, inhibitory or have no effect according to the mode of administration.

e) The effects of the same agent vary according to the conditions of the target system, which in turn are caused by previous or concomitant contact with other agents.

f) The effect of a certain treatment can vary according to chronobiological factors.

These are all characteristics peculiar to living systems, and are in many respects paradoxical; their general basis lies within the framework of the complexity of receptor dynamics. The topic is of cardinal importance for homeopathy because the flow of biological information depends not only on the nature of the signal (be it physical or chemical), but also on the behavior of the receptors. It is therefore advisable to briefly summarize here the recent advances made by research in this field.

Receptors are present both inside the cell and on the outer membrane (see also, for example, Figure 6).

The *intracellular receptors* are those which receive the signal in the form of molecules which cross the plasma membrane by virtue of their hydrophobicity (e.g. steroid or thyroid hormones). Once these receptors have bound the signal, they undergo activation, or a conformational change which makes them suitable for binding to specific DNA sequences or to other intermediate protein structures. In any event, eventually there will be activation of a series of genes and the triggering of a series of specific cell responses for that molecular signal.

The *membrane receptors*, on the other hand, are designed to receive molecules which do not enter the cell because of their particular size or electrical characteristics (the membrane is impermeable to small electrically charged molecules). For membrane receptors to be able to function they need a transducer, i.e. they are coupled to another transmission system which transduces the signal from the membrane to the system that has to be activated within the cell. The transducers, also called second messengers, are very important because they can intervene by modifying the signal either quantitatively (amplification, suppression) or qualitatively (altering its "meaning" in the sense of being able to re-route it towards functions other than its normal ones).

There are many types of receptors and transducers, some of which are illustrated in Figure 13. It can be seen that a type of receptors are directly coupled to an ion channel, i.e. when they bind the signal molecule they open up a passageway for the ions, which thus cross the membrane in large amounts according to their electrochemical gradient. It is worth noting that among these receptors there are some which are not activated by the signal molecule, but by variations in the electrical potential of the membrane. The signal, in this case, consists of electrons or electromagnetic fields. This can easily be explained, if we consider that almost all proteins have at least some electrically charged portion.

Other types of receptors are coupled to protein kinases, i.e. to proteins which operate a phosphorylation of other proteins, with a consumption of energy, but also with very significant consequences for the cell biology.

Phosphorylation, in fact, often constitutes a dramatic change in the physicochemical properties of the protein, with a consequent change of function (activation or deactivation of enzymes or of the receptors themselves).

The activation of protein kinases can come about as an event directly related to the receptor (see Figure 13, **2**) or with a series of intermediate steps associated with the coming into operation of other enzymes such as adenylate cyclase, phospholipase, and various ion pumps. (Figure 13, **3**). In the signalling process which forms the second messengers, G-proteins (short for GTP-binding proteins) appear to be of great importance; these proteins constitute a kind of shuttle running from the activated receptor to the other enzyme, which in turn has to be recruited into the transmission system. G-proteins are particularly important in determining the outcome of a certain signal reaching the cell. Various receptor systems contain

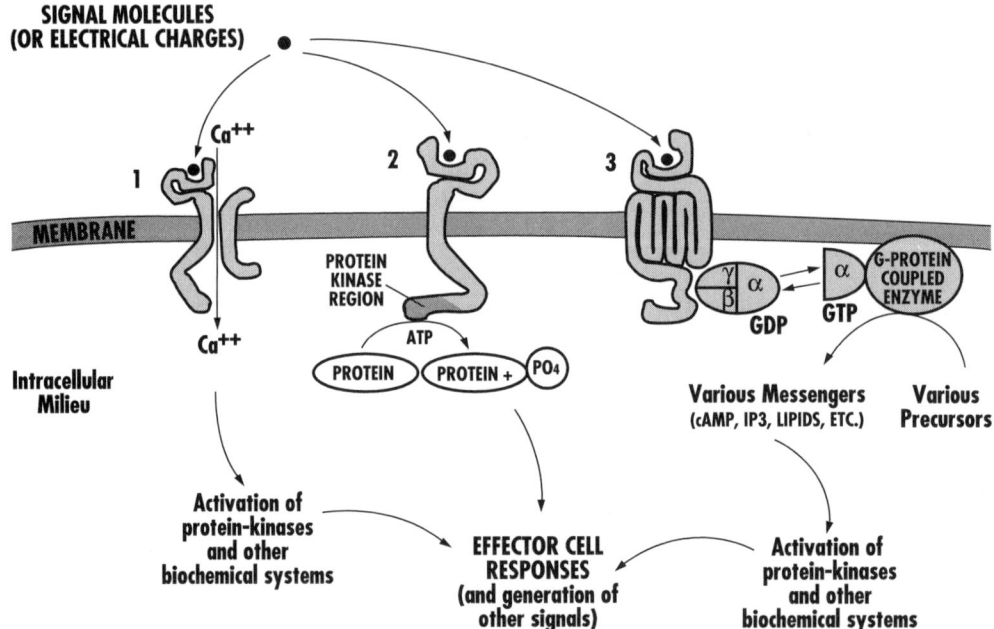

FIGURE 13 Three main functioning modes of membrane receptors. **1** = receptors directly coupled to an ion channel, which is opened (or closed) whenever interaction with a signal molecule occurs or there is a change in membrane potential; **2** = receptors directly coupled to an enzyme with protein-kinase catalytic activity (there are also those with protein-phosphatase activity), which is activated by the signal; **3** = receptors which, once they have bound the signal molecule, in turn transmit the signal—via GTP-binding proteins—to other systems such as the enzymes adenylate cyclase or phospholipase; these latter enzymes, in turn, produce other intracellular biochemical signals.

stimulatory and inhibitory G-proteins. Depending upon which of these come into action, a given signal may have opposite effects. Typical, in this connection, is the adenylate cyclase system which is coupled via G-proteins to alpha$_2$- and beta-adrenergic receptors [see, for example, Alberts *et al.*, 1989].

For reasons of simplicity, Figure 13 does not contemplate another important receptor activation mechanism, consisting in the *aggregation* of various receptors on the membrane as a result of signals constituted by macromolecules with multiple coupling sites. This aggregation can occur, as we shall see in Chapter 7, as a result of electromagnetic currents—even very weak ones—crossing the cell.

The systems for receiving and processing extracellular signals are very sophisticated and flexible, as well as being closely linked together at various levels by feedback mecha-

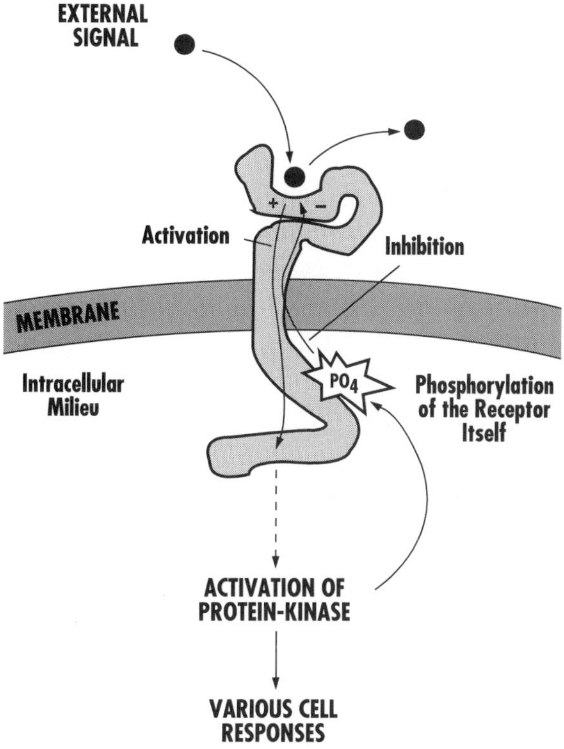

FIGURE 14 Example of how a receptor can be inactivated by a negative feedback mechanism triggered by its own activation.

nisms. The signal transducers enable the action of any single receptor to be amplified enormously, though inhibitory feedback effects are also possible. Figure 14 shows an example of how complicated the network of events resulting from signal molecule-receptor binding is. We see that, when a signals reaches the receptor, enzymes of the protein-kinase type are directly or indirectly activated, which, via the phosphorylation of proteins, trigger a series of functions. At the same time, however, the protein-kinase activity does not disdain an attack even on the very receptor from which the signal departed: the receptor is phosphorylated in a precise amino acid site, with consequent disactivation of its function. A subsequent dose of stimulant will no longer find the receptor ready to function as the "virgin" receptor did, but will find it unable to bind the stimulant itself or unable to promote phosphorylation.

This latter example explains only one of the countless possible molecular modifications associated with positive or negative variations in recep-

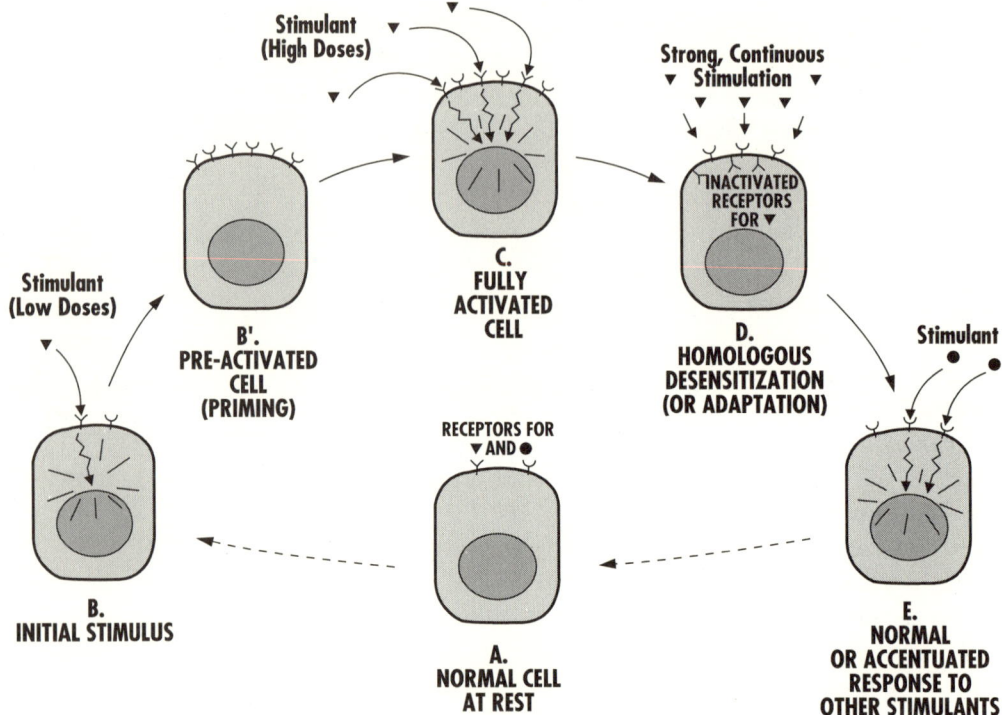

FIGURE 15 Receptor dynamics and consequent variations (potentiation or desensitization) in cell activity. For an explanation, see text.

tor sensitivity. It is well known that excessive receptor occupancy expresses itself in many cases as an effective *disappearance* of the receptors, which are *internalized* or "*sequestered*" in cell sites inaccessible to the signal molecules (so-called receptor *down-regulation* mechanism).

Another important way in which the cells and systems regulate receptor sensitivity is the so-called "*shedding*" of receptors (loss as a result of detachment and dissemination). In this case what happens is that, after cell activation, the receptors are lost because they detach themselves from the membrane, passing into the physiological fluids (blood, lymph). Consequently, in addition to cell desensitization, there is also the possibility that *soluble receptors* will bind with signal molecules outside the cell, blocking transmission of the signal. In practice, the receptor transforms itself into its opposite, namely a specific inhibitor.

To conclude this section, it may be useful to present a model of receptor dynamics which illustrates the possible oscillatory variability of cell sensitivity (Figure 15). The resting cell (*A*) has multiple receptors on the membrane, represented here for reasons of simplicity as receptors for two different types of stimulants, depicted as "triangular" and "circular" molecules. When the cell encounters a small amount of the triangular stimulant, it undergoes an initial stimulus (*B*), which, however, does not evoke any response other than an increase in receptors, both *homologous and heterologous*, i.e. for various types of molecules (*B'*). Whenever the cell encounters a greater stimulus, it presents a substantial activation of the cell response, with various specific effects (*C*). Whenever the stimulus is of considerable intensity and long-lasting, the receptors for the triangular molecule are rapidly inactivated, with the result that a state of desensitization or adaptation (*D*) comes about. Finally, if a new stimulus should arrive, produced by other molecules (depicted here as circular), the cell will be very ready to respond, since only the heterologous priming (*E*) will have persisted in it.

After a varying period of inactivity, it is possible (though not the rule) that the situation of the cell will revert to its initial state, with reappearance of the initial receptors. Another possibility is that the cell will remain "impressed" by its experience forever (memory), with modifications of gene expression, receptor expression and enzyme activities. In practice, we will have a cell which is different from the one we started with.

To these considerations should be added a related subject: that of the synergisms and antagonisms existing between substances which simultaneously occupy different cell receptors, these being aspects of major importance in physiological and pharmacological regulation. This topic, however, is perhaps among the clearest and most extensively documented areas in modern biomedical culture, and therefore there is no point in dwelling on it here any further.

The foregoing comments constitute a representative cross-section of researchers' "daily bread" in the advanced biomedical field. What has all this got to do with homeopathy? We have to proceed step by step in our analysis and thus the answer will be clearer later on (see Chapter 6). For the time being, it is important for us to have fixed the following concept firmly in the forefront of our minds: *receptor dynamics vary in physiology and pathology and are so complex that a given substance can behave as an activator or an inhibitor on the same cell or on the same organism, according to the doses of the substance itself in relation to the receptor sensitivity at a given time.*

In other words, this concept can be translated as follows: from the biological point of view, *there are no substances which are in themselves "good" (medicines) or "bad" (poisons, toxins).* Every substance is *"two-faced"* because its possible biological effect depends both on its molecular structure and dose and on the system with which it comes into contact. The quality of "goodness" or "badness," in the sense of its positive or negative effect on the homeostatic system as a whole, is "attributed" to the substance by the system with which it interacts, by its particular state of sensitivity and re-sponsiveness. Several objections to this conclusion can be raised, based on glaring exceptions (it is difficult, for instance, to see a positive role for HIV virus at any dose or in any system), but the thesis remains essentially valid as a general concept (as far as viruses are concerned, however, it is well known that they are not always pathogenetic, infecting only cells which are susceptible to them and which present suitable receptors).

5.7

Chaos and fractals

5.7.1 The "discovery" of chaos

In fairly recent times, theories explaining the dynamics of complex sys-tems have come up with a new protagonist: chaos.

The co-existence of casual phenomena alongside strictly deterministic and predictable phenomena has always been recognized, but until only fairly recently the attention of scientists was focused only on the latter. The laws of classical physics, in fact, are deterministic: if we know the state of a system at a certain moment and the laws governing its modification, we are in a position to predict its future behavior.

On the basis of the classic laws of gravity, for example, we can predict eclipses, or the trajectory of a satellite, or the motion of a pendulum. On the basis of Mendel's laws of genetics, we can predict the characters of a plant deriving from the union of two plant gametes of known character. Other natural phenomena, however, are not so readily predictable: the motion of the atmosphere, the population density of animals in a certain environment, the form of fingerprints, and the turbulence of a liquid run-ning through a pipe, elude our predictive ability. According to the classical view, one possible solution saving determinism was to ascribe failure to a dearth of information, so that all that was needed was to collect and pro-cess a sufficient amount of information on the system studied in order to get progressively closer to an exact description. As the mathematician Pierre-Simon Laplace pointed out, the laws of nature imply a rigid deter-minism and total predictability, though the incompleteness and imperfec-tions of our observations make it necessary to resort to the theory of probability. With the aid of this theory, the exploration of the physical world should have no problem developing in a progressive, linear fashion.

This "optimistic" view of the possibilities of traditional science has been modified in the course of the twentieth century, for two basic reasons: the first is the development of quantum mechanics and, in particular, the dis-covery of Heisenberg's principle of indeterminacy, whereby there is an insurmountable limit to the precision with which the position and velocity of elementary particles can be determined.

The second reason, more closely related to the question of chaos, is the discovery that systems consisting of three or more bodies may present unpredictable behavior, that does not disappear with the collection of further information about the system itself. The example cited in this connection is that of a system of hard spheres (billiard balls) which represents, in a simplified fashion, the interaction between atoms or molecules in a gas. If one billiard ball is fired against other balls, it is impossible to predict the path it will take after only a few ricochets. The nonpredictability is maintained even if we assume that the surfaces of the balls are perfectly smooth and the trajectories perfectly straight.

The reason for the unpredictability in such a simple system lies in its extreme dependence on the initial conditions. The phenomenon is known, in fact, as *sensitivity to initial conditions*. A minimal variation in the direction of incidence of the first impact is amplified on the curved surface of the ball, so that the trajectory after the first impact will be appreciably different from the expected one, and likewise after subsequent ricochets. After several impacts, the trajectories will be unpredictable. There is no instrument capable of firing the ball without the slightest imperfection (it would be a perfect instrument, but absolute perfection doses not exist in the physical world; there will always be some minor perturbation or fluctuation in the state of a physical system, though, macroscopically, this imperfection may not be apparent). For this reason, the apparently "simple" system described by the billiard-ball model has an intrinsic tendency towards chaotic behavior. The chaos does not derive from a mistake in firing the ball, or from ignorance of the laws governing trajectories and rebounds, but is a characteristic property of the system. David Ruelle, the "father" of the strange attractors and one of the world's leading experts on chaos, defines the latter as "*a temporal evolution with appreciable dependence on initial conditions*" [Ruelle, 1992, p. 77].

Another way by which the behavior of chaotic systems is exemplified is the so-called "*butterfly effect*," the principle embodied in which is conveyed by the dictum that the flapping of a butterfly's wings in Brazil may trigger off, or stop in its tracks, a tornado in Texas [Lorenz, 1979; see also Nicolis and Prigogine, 1991, p. 144 and Shinbrot *et al.*, 1993].

In this section we intend to give a brief overview of the problems raised by the "discovery" of chaos, these being topics to which we shall return later on account of their implications in the interpretative models of homeopathy presented here.

No description of complex systems in which several components interact (figuring among these without the slightest doubt are living systems) can afford to underrate chaotic phenomena, regarding them merely as factors disrupting what in other respects is a perfect theory, but any such description must find the instruments and the ways to integrate these phenomena in a theory previously regarded as adequate.

Even mathematics, once regarded as the exact science *par excellence*, has discovered chaos: there are various functions with a single variable, which, by means of an iteration process (insert the result of the first evaluation in place of the variable in the next and so on), can yield highly variable, nonperiodic results. An example is provided by the mathematical function:

$$A_{n+1} = A_n + A_n k (A_{max} - A_n)$$

where **An+1** is the value of the next cycle **n+1** which can be calculated on the basis of the value resulting from the previous cycle (**An**) added to the growth due to the cycle itself, which is equal to **An** multiplied by a coefficient of growth **k** and by a factor given by the difference between the maximum allowed (**Amax**) and **An**. An equation similar to this was described in 1845 by the mathematician B.F. Verhulst to analyze population trends [cited in the studies by Garner and Hock, 1991 and by Cramer, 1993]. We use it here to describe the time course of the value "**A**," which could be any real or imaginary parameter. What matters here is not to assign any precise value to "**A**," but to calculate its variations in successive iterative cycles, fixing an initial value and a maximum allowed value.

The additive growth (or decline) of each cycle depends on the result of the preceding cycle and is limited by the fact that there is a maximum achievable value: in fact, with the increase in the A_n trend the number to be subtracted from the maximum achievable value increases and the multiplication factor $(A_{max} - A_n)$ decreases. Consequently, it is only logical that A_{n+1} tends to increase at the beginning, but then the increase progressively declines until a plateau is reached where no further increase takes place. The formula, then, describes a fairly simple mathematical feedback. In actual fact, however, it "conceals" a very substantial measure of complexity: the results the iterative calculation allows are very different depending upon what value is assumed for the coefficient k and depending upon the initial value you start out with.

A number of such calculations are illustrated in Figure 16 in an example which assumes initial $A_n = 1$ and $A_{max} = 3$. Assuming the value of coefficient k to be fairly low compared to A_{max} (e.g. 0.1), and proceeding with the iterative calculations, the following solutions are obtained: at the beginning, as long as A_n is much lower than the maximum, the growth is effectively linear. When, however, the value starts to rise and to approach the maximum (A_n approaches A_{max}), the difference $A_{max} - A_n$ tends towards zero

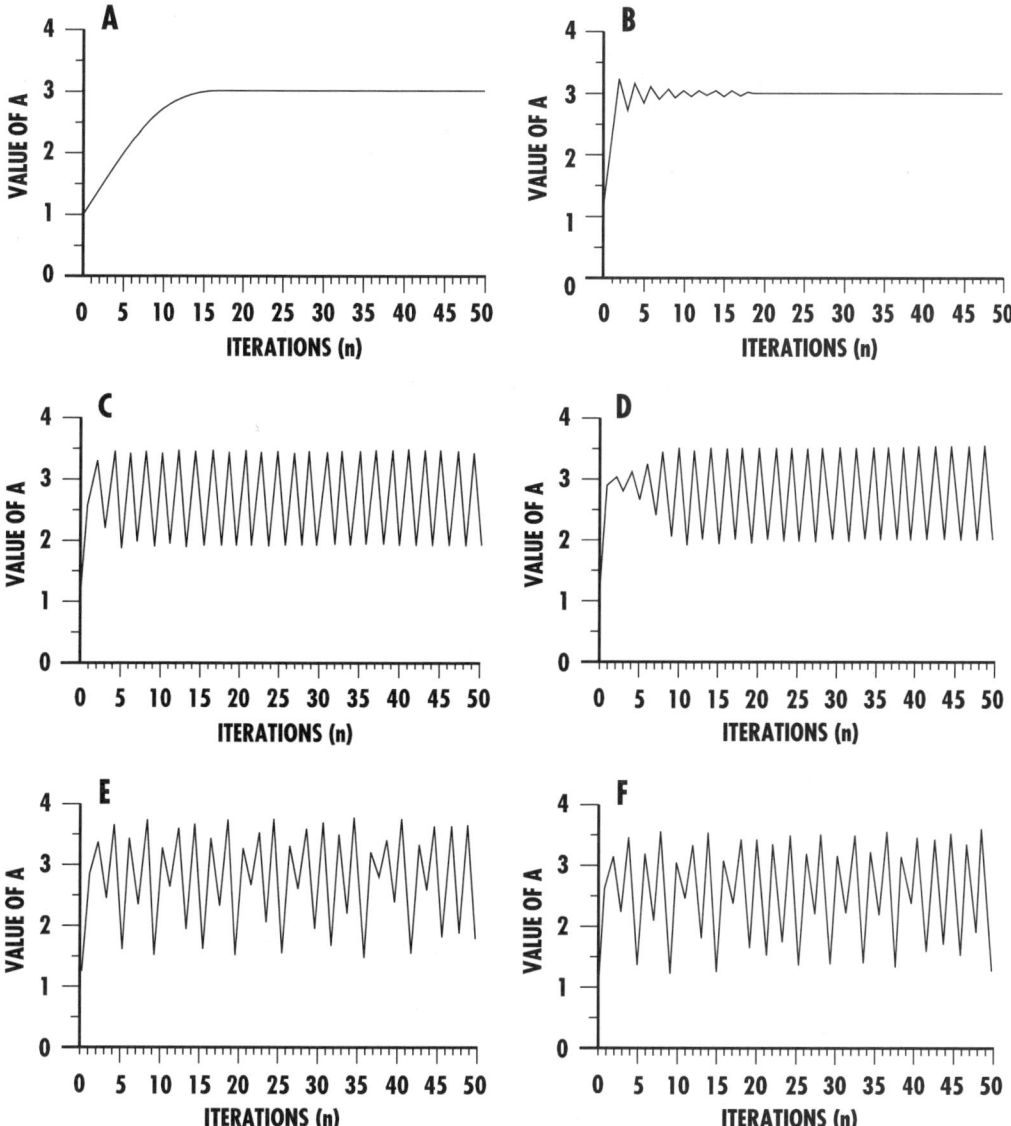

FIGURE 16 Verhulst iterations. The successive panels show variations in the parameter "A" in successive iterations of the equation $A_{n+1} = A_n + A_n k (A_{max} - A_n)$. A_{max} in all cases is assumed equal to 3.0. The (initial) A_n and k values in the various panels are as follows: panel A: $A_n = 1.0$, k = 0.1; panel B: $A_n = 1.0$, k = 0.6; panel C: $A_n = 1.0$, k = 0.8: panel D: $A_n = 1.2$, k = 0.8; panel E: $A_n = 1.0$, k = 0.88; panel F: $A_n = 1.001$, k = 0.88. For further explanations, see text.

and growth comes to a halt. Plotting the number of iterations (successive cycles) on the x axis against the value of A on the y axis, we have a growth curve which reaches the maximum asymptotically (Figure 16 A). So far there is nothing odd about the curve. If, however, we insert a coefficient of growth greater than a certain value (0.6 approx.) in the equation, we have a qualitatively different curve: at the beginning the A_{max} value is exceeded, and then subsequent iterations lead to values oscillating slightly above and below A_{max}, after which the curve stabilizes at the maximum value without any further changes (Figure 16 B). At even higher coefficients of growth, a phenomenon occurs which is called *"bifurcation"*: the function oscillates between the two fixed values which are repeated alternately in successive cycles (Figure 16 C). This oscillating function is fairly stable and is maintained even if the (initial) A_n value changes appreciably (e.g. a 20% change from 1.0 to 1.2) (Figure 16 D). On exceeding another critical k value (0.88 approx. in the example given), we have another bifurcation because the order is lost completely and an infinite number of possible solutions present themselves: practically all configurations are admitted and the oscillations of the variable A appear irregular or *chaotic* (Figure 16 E). We have entered a sphere of mathematics where chaos manifests itself in the form of totally nonperiodic results.

It is important to note that, in these conditions, in which the time trend of the A values is chaotic, the mathematical feedback is extremely sensitive to the initial conditions: on making very minor changes in (initial) A_n, for example from 1 to 1.001 (i.e. a 0.1% change) we obtain a curve which shows no difference over the first 10-15 cycles, but then diverges dramatically, with the result that after the 20th iteration the trend is completely different in the two tracings, which no longer present even a single point in common (Figure 16 F). Despite this, some basic similarities between curves 16 E and 16 F must be stressed: both are chaotic and, even more importantly, the values remain confined between two extremes, i.e. a maximum upper and a minimum lower value. Though plotting different trajectories, these point trajectories "belong" to the same area. This area may be regarded as the *attraction basin* of the function described (with the parameters k and A_{max} fixed).

On further increasing the value of k, the oscillations are increasingly high and irregular so that eventually the value of A_n may become 0 or even negative. At this point, the evolution of the function undergoes a dramatic change because the negative value of A_n produces a more negative A_{n+1} value and so on, to infinity (not shown in Figure 16). Also in this case, it can be calculated that minimal changes in initial A_n determine whether the function diverges to infinity or remains "trapped" in the attractor.

The contribution made by the physico-mathematical approach to the problem of complexity is much greater than might be imagined: while it is true to say that a living system with its thousands of subcomponents will never resemble a mechanical system with two or only a very few components and can never be described by a mathematical formula, on the other hand it is also true that the study of the complexity of "simple" systems may enable us to discover "basic rules" of behavior which are repeated in substantially identical forms in systems with a different evolutionary status. In other words, the complexity of biological systems (and their pathological aspects) may perhaps be tackled and better understood by reference to a framework common to all complex systems, i.e. to a model developed in physicochemical reference systems.

Basically, the characteristic of the equation capable of generating chaos is that it carries within it the presence of a feedback, so that the result of the calculation is used as factor for the reiteration of the calculation itself. This fact is very interesting from the biological viewpoint, in the sense that the Verhulst formula essentially describes the dynamics of a mechanism operating in living beings: as we have seen, living systems, in fact, are regulated by reaction and counterreaction cycles which constitute the so-called *homeostasis*. These "cycles" are nothing more or less than the repetition of the same operation (by analogy with mathematical iteration) in which the result of the previous cycle serves as the basis of the next one. For example, at the end of the systole-diastole cycle the heart reverts to the end-diastolic condition; at the end of a mitotic cycle the condition of the two daughter cells becomes in turn the starting condition for a new mitosis; thus, every rhythmic modification of the organism hinges upon the previous state and occurs according to fixed rules (in the analogy we have adopted, the rule is the mathematical formula). The physiological variables controlled by the homeostatic systems oscillate continually between a maximum and minimum allowed value (cf. the A_{max} values considered above), but this variability may be more or less regular or rhythmic, depending upon the initial conditions (cf. the A_n value) and upon multiple conditioning factors performing the function of coefficient "k" in the formula examined above. Now it clearly emerges that all systems endowed with these characteristics are subject to chaos and thus that this type of chaos must be regarded as a physiological phenomenon, at least within certain limits.

The chaotic behavior of billiard balls and similar systems is due to the extreme dependency on initial conditions owing to the existence of a principle which amplifies the error (the curved surface of the billiard balls). The chaotic behavior of mathematical systems is related to considering equations as nonlinear, i.e. terms appear which are not simply proportional to the variable. For an analysis of feedback in mathematical terms and its possible applications in biology, the reader is referred to the work of Nicolis and Prigogine [Nicolis and Prigogine, 1991].

The idea that deterministic systems are not always sustained by equations with regular solutions has taken a long time to come home to people [Croquette, 1991; Ruelle, 1992]. Obviously, the discovery of chaos in physical systems and in simple mathematical equations has aroused the interest of scientists, spurred on in the hope that these might afford a model for understanding the functioning of more complex systems as well. No-one would dream of denying the existence of unpredictable phenomena in systems such as meteorology, economics, the behavior of the earth's crust (earthquakes), the beating of the heart (arrhythmias), or ecology (cf. the forecasts of terrestrial temperatures or the hole in the ozone layer). This unpredictability might, however, be due only to the lack of sufficient information about the details of such systems, or to inadequacy of the experimental conditions, but if chaotic behavior is also an intrinsic characteristic of physical and mathematical systems, it can be postulated that this chaos is due to a basic principle of the physical world which cannot be ignored.

Researchers have provided an elegant demonstration of the fact that an experimental chaotic system (represented, in this case, by the oscillations of a flexible rod coupled to a magnet which generates impulses at desired frequencies) can be regulated by minimal perturbations of the system control parameters [Shinbrot *et al.*, 1993]. By slightly modifying the frequency of the impulses emitted by the magnet, the chaotic behavior of the vibrations can be made to appear and disappear. Though the mechanism utilized is fairly simple, it presents complex chaotic dynamics, thus prompting the authors to suggest that these experiments may furnish indications of a general nature about chaotic systems. Amongst other things, it is claimed that the control of chaos (in this case the appearance of periodic rhythmic oscillations) can be obtained by means of the repetition of minor corrective adjustments at intervals.

5.7.2 Attractors and fractals

Physicists and mathematicians lost no time in checking to see whether or not "laws of chaos" existed, or, in other words, whether what might have seemed to be the triumph of randomness in the deterministic domain was not actually an expression of some kind of order or regularity. Effectively speaking, this has led to the discovery and study of the so-called *strange attractors*, which, on the mathematical plane, are geometrical figures which describe the long-term behavior of a number of dynamic systems. To put it another way, an attractor is something to which the behavior of a system is attracted or whose stabilizing effect it undergoes. It therefore possesses an important property—stability. *In a system subjected to perturbations, movement tends to be towards the attractor.*

The attractor may be a single point, as for example in the trajectory of a pendulum when it reaches the stationary state (for a mathematical example of a single-point attractor, see Figure 16 A and B), or a finite number of points reflecting a periodic-type behavior (mathematical example, Figure 16 C and D), or an infinite system of points generating a figure in the form of an orbit which never repeats itself identically, as may happen in chaotic systems ("strange attractors") (mathematical example, Figure 16 E and F). It is difficult to imagine a *strange attractor* in the field of geometry because its characteristics imply that an orbit of this type must have an infinite length contained in a finite surface (the attraction area). These are therefore objects of "nonentire dimension" or *fractals* (see below) [Ruelle, 1992].

The concept of the attractor has also been analyzed in relation to pharmacology, and in particular to pharmacodynamics [van Rossum and de Bie, 1991]. In classic pharmacokinetic theory, the situation is simple because the attractor is a single point, and adequate information can be obtained by measuring a single variable such as the concentration of a drug or one of its metabolites in the blood. In the field of pharmacodynamics, which also examines the effects of drugs, the situation is more complex and the attractor can be of the chaotic or strange type. The effect induced by a drug is not a single entity, or a single modified mechanism, but a series of simultaneous changes in several variables, each of which interrelates with the others in a nonlinear manner. This implies that a dose of drug may induce unpredictable changes in a complex system, such as, for instance, the cardiovascular system. The same dose of drug can produce different effects on different occasions owing to the great sensitivity to initial conditions. It is true that the variability can be overcome by referring to the statistical mean of many observations, but the above-mentioned authors claim that, if the system is chaotic (which is something different from randomness, chance, and biological variability), the use of means is not appropriate.

Chaotic systems also present elements of regularity. For example, the equations described previously, though yielding unpredictable results at given coefficient values, do not furnish infinite solutions; the amplitude of the oscillations remains within a certain range. Moreover, in several chaotic functions, on continuing the iterations and further increasing the coefficient value, after the periods of chaos periods of order may reappear, followed by new zones of chaos and then order. There is thus a "recurrent regularity" [Hofstadter, 1991] in successive generations of transitions from chaos to order, with the reappearance of single solutions or regular oscillations which undergo cascade duplication on increasing the coefficient value. This recurrent regularity creates figures with regularity and irregularity "bands" which are repeated and resemble one another, with a fractal type pattern.

The study of the behavior of mathematical and physical systems with transitions from order to chaos and vice versa has witnessed a major upsurge with the analysis of the dynamics involved in the formation of fractal objects. Fractal geometry, in fact, is the most suitable for describing chaos and complexity [Jurgens *et al.*, 1990].

The term *"fractal"* was coined in 1975 by B.B. Mandelbrot and gained extensive notoriety in scientific circles in the early '80s [Mandelbrot, 1982]. What is meant by this term are those mathematical or geometrical entities which are endowed with a fractional dimension (from the Latin *fractus*, meaning "broken"). Many fractal figures have a repetitive configuration on changing scale, a sort of self-similarity between details and the general pattern.

Fractal shapes can be generated by the computer using algorithms (lists of instructions which specify the operations to be performed to solve a given problem) starting from mathematical functions which are suitably iterated. By means of these operations, two- or three-dimensional figures with the following characteristics appear:

a) An enormous variety of details of different shapes.

b) The presence of subtle ramifications that can be pursued in the finest detail.

c) Self-similarity, whereby, on magnifying part of the structure, details can be detected which repeat themselves on different scales of magnification.

"Eidiomatic" experiments, performed on the computer, show that figures with a fractal dimension are endowed both with a fantastic variety of shapes and with self-similarity [Dewdney, 1991]. In very complex structures such as the sets of Julia and Mandelbrot, extremely varied and fanciful details can be observed (circles, spirals, helixes, stars, various ramifications); within which other, different details can be discerned on magnifying the image (Figure 17). Within some of these particular images one finds, surprisingly, "mini-sets" very similar to the macroscopic ones from which they originated. In the close-up detail we rediscover an image

FIGURE 17 Mandelbrot set. The image is produced on a personal computer by iteration of the formula: $Z_{n+1} = Z_n^2 + C$ in the complex field, using *Fractint* software. Every point on the graph represents a complex number of the form: *x coordinate + i * y coordinate*. The x coordinate is an ordinary real number, and the y coordinate an imaginary number, i.e. a real number times *i*, where *i* is the square root of -1. C is set as a constant for each point, while Z varies with the iteration. Every black point is the set of all points C for which the value of Z is less than 2 after the indicated number of iterations; the white points represent points for which Z exceeds 2 after the indicated number of iterations. Figure **A** is the entire Mandelbrot set, the result of 18 iterations per point. In **B** we see a 20 times magnification of the detail indicated in the box shown in **A**, and in **C** a further 10 times enlargement of the boxed detail in Figure **B**. In **D** the same detail as in Figure **C** is shown with a further 5 iterations per point. In **E** with a further 30 iterations per point; and in **F** with a further 100 iterations per point. From **C** to **F** an

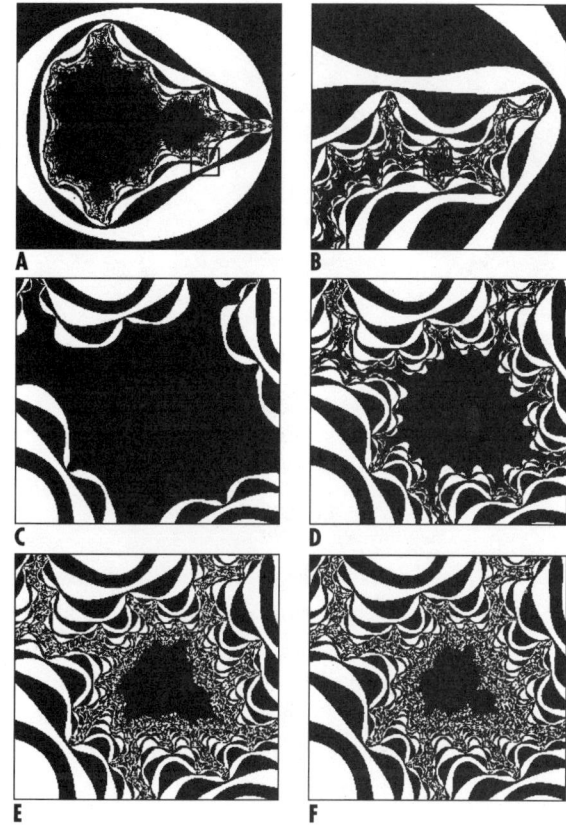

increase in the definition of the specific characteristics and details of the image is evident. In **F**, the "fragment" of the set shows a pattern similar to the "whole" (**A**).

which appeared to have been lost in the variety of details and ramifications. By increasing the number of iterations, a better definition of the fractal image is obtained (Figure 17, C—> E).

Similar figures, showing increasing definition with the increase in iterations, have been reported also by others [Garner and Hock 1991]. Interestingly, these authors outlined an analogy between this type of fractal behavior and the homeopathic concept of dilution/dynamization, in which process the information is claimed to spread and increase its "potency" in serial dilutions (see also Chapter 7, Section 4.2).

Mandelbrot and, more recently, other investigators have observed that many apparently disorderly natural objects possess this fractal property. This is having a very considerable impact in the scientific world. Despite the fact that these forms were discovered by a mathematician and are still studied mainly by mathematicians and computer scientists, fractals are useful

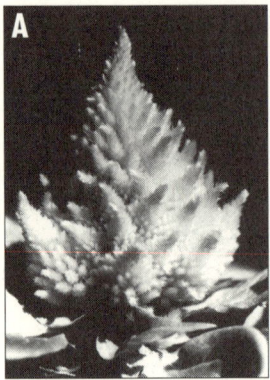 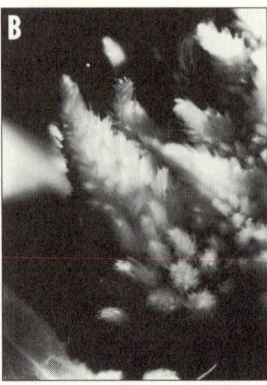

FIGURE 18 A flower (Celosia) with a fractal structure. The same pattern as in the entire flower (**A**) can be seen in a close-up of a part and in all its further subdivisions (**B**).

instruments for describing a whole variety of physical phenomena and natural forms [Sommaruga, 1992].

One example of a fractal form is a tree, whose trunk is divided into branches; the branches themselves then divide into smaller branches, twigs, and so on until you get to the leaves, which in turn present veins with multiple subdivisions.

Other examples of natural fractals are clearly illustrated by flowers (Figure 18) and snowflakes, as well as by noncrystalline molecular aggregates, viscous ramifications in unmiscible fluids, corals, electrical discharges such as lightning, the ramifications of the airways and blood vessels [Sander, 1987], the dendrites of the neurons, the Purkinje system conducting electrical signals in the heart, and the folds of the intestinal mucosa [Goldberger *et al.*, 1990]. It has also been demonstrated that, in many different physical situations, particles floating on the surface of an irregularly moving fluid display a fractal arrangement [Sommerer and Ott, 1993].

The formation and growth of such structures is well described by the laws and formulas of fractal geometry, so that today, with the indispensable aid of the computer, many objects which, on account of their complexity, formerly eluded any kind of formal or quantitative analysis can be simulated graphically. We can calculate the fractal dimension of real objects such as coastlines, mountains, clouds, etc. The human arteries have a fractal dimension of 2.7 [Jurgens *et al.*, 1990].

In the formation (= taking shape) of objects with fractal dimensions we witness a particular interaction between stochastic (random) events and events determined by the state of the physical system which is growing. This type of growth, also called *aggregation by diffusion*, very probably played a fundamental role in the birth of life on earth and continues to do so in the processes of physical and biological growth [Sander, 1986].

Aggregation by diffusion depends on the random motion of dispersed particles and on the "attraction" or "conditioning" produced by the first microaggregate, or by the temperature conditions, or by the motion of the fluid, or by other physical factors. Aggregation by diffusion produces fractal structures, fascinating geometrical shapes in which determinism and randomness, order and diversification coexist. Fractal geometry thus refers to some form of *conditioned randomness*, so much so, indeed, that some people talk about a determinism of chaos (deterministic chaos).

We are thus investigating a field which is one of the frontiers of science: identifying the "laws of disorder," or certain fundamental rules of behavior of complex systems, which reveal the way in which the chaotic system can organize itself in a broad-ranging order, at the same time maintaining a certain degree of randomness. This randomness, discovered even within the atom [Gutzwiller, 1992], remains as an uneliminable factor in ontogenetic and philogenetic evolution, a factor which, coupled to information capable of generating order, constitutes a means of continuously generating novel forms and novel diversities. Fractal geometry tends to reveal that "hidden order" which is not always apparent in natural objects. This order is believed to be represented precisely by what has been termed *scale invariance symmetry* [Sander, 1986].

5.7.3 Boolean networks and self-organization

A peculiar property of complex systems is the ability to evolve in the course of time. This is observed both in the biological development of any organism (ontogenesis) and in the development of living species in general throughout history (evolution). In the classic Darwinian theory of evolution, the emergence of increasingly complex species is the fruit of *random variability* and *selection*, which operate to the advantage of those species which, by virtue of characteristics acquired by chance mutations, better succeed in adapting to increasingly difficult environmental conditions and in surviving the competitive struggle for vital space and food. This well-known concept of natural selection and the survival of the fittest in evolution has also been applied on a molecular and cellular scale as well as in embryology. The classic view of the origin of order and diversification of biological species—based on natural selection—has recently been contested on the basis of mathematical studies and computer models showing that, alongside natural selection, other mechanisms are involved, which have been grouped together under the term *self-organization* [Kauffman, 1991; Kauffman, 1993].

As a result of the laws of chaos, nonlinear dynamic systems can easily present transition from order to disorder and vice versa, following even only minimal perturbations in control parameters or in the energy flow across such systems (cf. butterfly effect, dissipative systems, see also Chapter 5, sections 8.1 and 8.2). Nevertheless, in these cases, we are invariably in the presence of changes somehow induced from the outside. There may, however, also be a phenomenon whereby the complex, disorderly system spontaneously "crystallizes" in an orderly state. From disorder to order thanks to *an intrinsic original property* of the system itself and with no input of outside energy; quite rightly, this phenomenon has been termed *anti-chaos*.

The mathematical models of self-organization were initially developed with the aim of explaining how the cell genome is organized. The genome can be viewed as a complex computer in which there is a data memory (information stored in the DNA for approximately 100,000 different proteins), but also the parallel processing of some of this information (a few hundred or a few thousand data units simultaneously). What is more, many of these protein data units influence the genome itself in its activity, in multiple control sites. In this way, many genes are "coupled" with the functioning of others, influencing one another reciprocally, and constituting a *network*. The coordinated and sequential behavior of this network is the basic factor responsible for the functioning and differentiation of the cell, with the result that a liver cell is different from a heart muscle cell and performs different functions, despite containing the same genetic information, being composed of the same elementary materials (amino acids, sugars, lipids, carbohydrates), and obeying the same "general functioning rules" (biochemical reactions).

We cannot go into any detail here about the mathematical parallel processing systems constructed to explain self-organization; such details can be found in the literature cited. We will confine our attention here to the essential notions. To describe the behavior of a great many elements coupled together (network), each of which may be in an active or an inactive state, we resort to the use of models based on stochastic Boolean networks (after the logician George Boole). In such a network, formed by a number of elements N, the behavior of each element (active or inactive) is determined by the input variables which connect ("AND" variable) or disjoin ("OR" variable) it from the behavior of the other elements. Each element can have a number of inputs according to choice. If the number of inputs is K, the possible combinations of the two variables (AND + OR) will be 2^K. Networks of this type are called NK networks because they contain a number of elements N, each of which has K inputs, and *stochastic* because the choices AND and OR and the number of inputs of each individual element are selected at random at the start. Since the elements are connected, by activating (AND) or disactivating (OR) one element in the network, we can observe the evolution of the states of the network in subsequent cycles. For the sake of simplicity, each passage from one state to another is implemented by synchronous modification of all the elements involved. The system passes from one state to another in a deterministic manner and then, in view of the fact that the possible combinations are not infinite, however complex the network, it will always end up sooner or later by finding itself in a state previously formed, thus resuming the cycle of transformations. The cycles of states which Boolean networks pass through in the course of time are called *dynamic attractors*, and each network, if left to its own devices, will sooner or later finish up in one of these attractors and will stay there.

Experiments can be performed on these mathematical systems, introducing *perturbations*, some of which modify the network only locally and for a short time, until it resumes its original cycle, returning to the same attractor. Other perturbations, on the other hand, are not absorbed; these destabilize the network and force it towards another attraction basin, whence it can no longer return to the previous one. Experiments can also be performed by modifying the *structure* of the network itself, altering the number of elements N, or the number of inputs K for each element. It can be observed that the attractors are modified accordingly. When the number N is equal to K (N = K), we have the maximum disorder, and the system is totally chaotic and unpredictable. Chaotic behavior patterns can also be observed when K < N, provided that K is equal to or greater than 3. If K = 2, the properties of stochastic Boolean networks are such that a tendency towards spontaneous collective order is easily manifested. In practice, groups of elements are formed which are interconnected so that not every perturbation causes them to shift towards the attractor. It is as if there were a kind of homeostatic behavior in the system, and this is one of the main reasons why such networks tend to simulate a number of properties of biological systems.

The basic reason for the birth of spontaneous collective order in stochastic Boolean networks lies in the fact that a "frozen core" forms randomly in these networks, that is to say a set of elements which are blocked, by the crossfire of opposing control elements, in a certain active or inactive state. This core creates uniform, interlaced "walls," which are propagated to a broader zone, "infiltrating" themselves into the system. As a consequence, one orderly zone isolates itself from other elements which remain variable and disorderly. Since, in these networks where K = 2, there is not much communication (in other words, the system is not very *connected*), the modifications described remain confined to islands, which do not communicate with one another, but are homogeneous aggregates, distinct from the rest. By suitably modifying the values of parameters N and K, moments of transition can be found between order and disorder, changes in size of the "frozen islands" can be observed, and so on. With an increase in the number of inputs K (and thus of connections), the well organized and rigid frozen components "melt" and the network gains in complexity and dynamism.

These mathematical models, endowed with great flexibility, are used to simulate the natural selection and the self-organization capabilities of complex systems. Networks can be designed, for example, which simulate the human genome, assuming the number N equal to 100,000 (i.e. the estimated number of genes) and the coefficient K equal to 10 (i.e. the number of inputs, or controls, which every gene is subject to). Or we can simulate cell populations, on the basis of an empirical knowledge of the number of cells and the signals (e.g. hormones) which they exchange. In such networks, which "hover" between order and disorder, alterations to an element (appropriately called "mutations") can be introduced (for example, by changing it from active to inactive), and one can observe what happens in the evolution of the system. In some cases, the Boolean networks adapt to the mutation with minimal adjustments, as in a homeostatic system; in other cases, the mutations cause cascades of impressive alterations, substantially modifying the structure of the network and the shapes and sizes of the islands.

Using similar methods, it has been possible to calculate approximately how long the life cycle of a cell should be for it to pass through all the forms of expression of its genes (i.e., in mathematical terms, to pass through the entire attractor and return to the starting point). The results obtained (from 370 to 3700 minutes) closely match the data provided by experimental observations of the mitotic cycle. It has also proved possible to calculate, on the basis of the possible attractors in a genome, how many cell types are feasible (a cell type, in fact, distinguishes itself from the others precisely because it activates some genes and represses others). These estimates, too, have been found to correspond to experimental findings in organisms of increasing complexity, from bacteria to the human being. Lastly, the models also allow us to predict the stability of the cell types and the effect of genetic mutations, which is of considerable importance in the study of tumors.

In conclusion, then, thanks to this interesting type of mathematical approach, it has proved possible to gain deeper insights into complex systems and the relationships between stochastic phenomena and the birth of order. Above all, this kind of approach has been able to demonstrate a phenomenon which has been of undoubted importance in evolutionary theory, namely that microscopic order may originate *at random* from the chaos of multiple interconnected elements; this initial core may give rise *spontaneously* to macroscopic order in the form of islands of order or cycles of modifications which are repeated according to cycles described by the attractors. This theory, therefore, amplifies (rather than replacing) that of natural selection and that of dissipative structures (see Chapter 5, Section 8.1.) to explain biological order.

5.7.4 Chaotic systems in medicine

The models of chaos and interconnected networks can be applied to physiology and pathology. The pathogenesis of many diseases, at least in the initial phases, are characterized by communication defects arising in the complex networks of integrated systems, such as those considered in other sections of this book (control of cell proliferation, immune system, equilibrium between pro- and antiinflammatory factors, etc.), for which models can be created like the Boolean networks. In a network in which many homeostatic systems (molecular, cellular, systemic) are interconnected, the information of the entire system "passes through" cycles (attractors) which have variable, fluctuating spatiotemporal forms, but which can always be traced back, in states of normality, to a harmonic pattern where the whole is viewed in its entirety, aimed at the survival of the organism with the least possible consumption of energy. If one or more elements in these networks lose their information connections, i.e. something snaps in the homeostatic system itself, or the flow of information is cut off between different systems, a pathological process occurs precisely because chaos is generated, or rather the chaotic system goes over to another attractor, as was seen to be possible in the Boolean models. According to these models, the new attractor, regarded as "pathological" in the case in question, may be preserved even if the initial perturbation (loss of connection) is only temporary (in pathology, one could speak of a *tendency towards chronicity*).

What is certain is that chaotic dynamic patterns are normally present in the homeostasis of networks with multiple crossed components such as cytokines, neuropeptides, the endocrine system, idiotype-anti-idiotype networks, and immune HLA-receptor equilibrium.

The rate of enzymatic activities oscillate when two enzymes compete for the same substrates, and small changes in the concentrations can lead to changes in the frequencies and amplitudes of oscillations, causing them to become chaotic if previously harmonic or to become harmonic if previously chaotic [Cramer, 1993].

Analysis of temporal variations in hormone levels in healthy subjects has revealed chaotic situations in this sector, too [Nugent *et al.*, 1994].

We have already mentioned that chaos is not in itself negative, since it is an element of flexibility and a generator of diversity. Oscillations of the control parameters of the various physiological systems are the norm in biology and in medicine. If, however, the coordination is lost, i.e. the *connectivity* of the system as a whole and in relation to the rest of the body, certain subcomponents may oscillate in an excessive, unpredictable and pointless manner, thus generating localized disorders which may, however, be amplified (the amplification of fluctuations is a typical behavior of chaotic systems). Oscillation thus becomes disorder and takes on the aspect of disease, in that it causes the emergence of substantial symptoms and damage. It is as if chaos were amplified and formed "nuclei" of pathological interrelations between cells or systems, also involving the connective system; these nuclei then in some way isolate themselves from the global control system and prove self-maintaining.

Mental disease, too, often originates from, and is then consolidated by, the loss of ability to communicate with one's fellow human beings.

There are many ways in which an integrated system loses complexity and connectivity, some of which are listed here by way of examples (basically, all pathology could be viewed in this light):

a) Reduction of the number of cell elements involved (cf., for example, processes of senile atrophy or atrophy due to cellular anoxia).

b) Loss of number or sensitivity of receptors when they are occupied for too long or too intensely (cf. what was said in the section on receptors), or when they are directly attacked by the disease (e.g. myasthenia gravis), or when they are genetically defective (e.g. familial hypercholesterolemia).

c) Lack of production of the signal (e.g. anatomical defect or endocrine glandular disease) or its interception en route (interruption of nerves, presence of autoantibodies to the signal protein).

d) Defect of intracellular signal transduction mechanisms (from the receptor to the intracellular space): we need only mention, for example, the action of bacterial toxins which put G-proteins out of action, or the adaptation of the G-proteins themselves in cardiac failure, or the action of many pharmacologically active substances such as calcium antagonists or agents which elevate cyclic AMP. Many oncogenes act precisely on these delicate proliferation control pathways.

e) Distortion or suppression of homeostatic responses by ingestion of excess alcohol, or by overmedication with enzyme inhibitors, antibiotics, anaesthetics, narcotics, and similar drugs.

Other applications of the theory of chaos have been described in cardiology. For example, it has been reported [Goldberger *et al.*, 1990] that the

heart rate of a healthy individual varies over time with an intrinsically chaotic periodicity and not, as was believed in the past, according to a normal
sinus rhythm influenced only by the homeostatic systems. On observing
these variations according to different time scales (minutes, ten minute
periods, and hours), we see similar fluctuations reminding us of a fractal
behavior in the temporal rather than in the spatial domain. Obviously,
these are not arrhythmias, but oscillations in normal rhythm. The electroencephalogram also shows similar chaotic patterns as normal aspects of its
functioning [Freeman, 1991].

The above-mentioned authors claim that the physiological systems with
intrinsically chaotic dynamics have functional advantages, in that they are
more flexible and adaptable to variations in conditions and demands on
the part of an environment in a state of continual change. In other words,
it might be said that *a chaotic system can be more easily modulated than a system
presenting a greater measure of order.* By way of confirmation of this theory,
we would mention a paradoxical finding: many electrocardiograms in patients with severe heart disease reveal disappearance of the chaotic fluctuations, as if disease were a state of stability [Goldberger *et al.*, 1990]. The
nervous system, too, may show a loss of variability and the onset of pathological periodicity in disorders such as epilepsy, Parkinson's disease, and
manic-depression syndrome.

Walter J. Freeman, professor of neurobiology at the University of California, Berkeley, reports: "Our studies have led us as well to the discovery
in the brain of chaos, complex behavior that seems random but actually
has some hidden order. The chaos is evident in the tendency of vast collec-
tions of neurons to shift abruptly and simultaneously from one complex
activity pattern to another in response to the smallest of inputs. This changeability is a prime characteristic of many chaotic systems. It is not harmful
in the brain. In fact, we propose it is the very property that makes perception possible. We also speculate that chaos underlies the ability of the brain
to respond flexibly to the outside world and to generate novel activity patterns, including those that are experienced as fresh ideas" [Freeman, 1991.
p. 34].

In the immune system, too, chaos may play a very important role, especially because this system continually needs to generate new forms of receptors to cope with all the possible antigens that the outside world and
the inside of the body may present. *Fantasy*, then, is a fundamental property of the immune system, without which the body would lack the necessary adaptabilty to a world in a constant state of change and the ability to
defend itself against potential aggressors. Chaos and fractals are essential
in the dynamics of idiotypical networks, as modern immunology is increasingly demonstrating.

In the hematopoietic system there are cells, called stem cells, which can give rise to all the possible cell lines of the blood (erythrocytes, granulo-cytes, lymphocytes, megakaryocytes, monocytes-macrophages). What makes the cell "decide" the evolutionary path it is going to take? There are two interpretations: according to the deterministic conception, the cells obey external signals such as hormones and growth factors; according to the stochastic conception, the choice is made at random. Probably, both theories contain elements of truth: it would appear, in fact, that the stem cell differentiates itself at random, but that, after this choice, it expresses receptors for growth factors, with the result that it is the latter which make the cell proliferate (otherwise it would remain differentiated but useless, in that it would yield no progeny) [Golde, 1991].

It is very likely that in the near future studies on fractals and on chaos will be applied to physiology and pathology to an increasing extent. In fact, if chaotic dynamics is a *normal* aspect of physiological processes, in-vestigating this may furnish more complete predictive information for char-acterizing dysfunctions due to old age, pharmacological or toxic substances, and other pathogenetic processes.

An example of how to control chaos in a living system has been provided by elegant experiments performed on an *in vitro* neural network prepared from a hippocampal slice of rat brain [Schiff *et al.*, 1994]. In this brain area, focal neuronal activity is represented by discharge burst with typical cha-otic behavior (unstable periodicity), that can be monitored by computer-ized recording under suitable experimental conditions. Intermittent electric pulses delivered at appropriate time intervals ("periodic pacing") to the bath where the slice is kept can increase and regularize the periodicity of such neuronal population bursting. Moreover, periodic behavior in cer-tain preparations can be *anti*controlled in order to induce chaos. The au-thors claim that this model could be applied to the control of *in vivo* epileptic spike foci, which share similar characteristics of unstable periodicity.

The existence of chaos and particularly of the possibility of at least study-ing some of its rules carries much more far-reaching implications than one might think. In this connection, it is worth quoting the conclusive part of a study on chaos by a group of American researchers: "Chaos brings a new challenge to the reductionist view that a system can be understood by break-ing it down and studying each piece. This view has been prevalent in sci-ence in part because there are so many systems for which the behavior of the whole is indeed the sum of its parts. Chaos demonstrates, however, that a system can have complicated behavior that emerges as a consequence of simple, nonlinear interaction of only a few components.

The problem is becoming acute in a wide range of scientific disciplines, from describing microscopic physics to modeling macroscopic behavior of biological organisms. The ability to obtain detailed knowledge of a system's structure has undergone a tremendous advance in recent years, but the ability to integrate this knowledge has been stymied by the lack of a proper conceptual framework within which to describe a qualitative behavior. For example, even with a complete map of the nervous system of a simple organism, such as the nematode studied by Sidney Brenner of the University of Cambridge, the organism's behavior cannot be deduced. Similarly, the hope that physics could be complete with an understanding of fundamental physical forces and constituents is unfounded. The interaction of components on one scale can lead to complex global behavior on a larger scale that in general cannot be deduced from knowledge of the individual components.

Chaos is often seen in terms of the limitations it implies, such as lack of predictability. Nature may, however, employ chaos constructively. Through amplification of small fluctuations it can provide natural systems with access to novelty. A prey escaping a predator's attack could use chaotic flight control as an element of surprise to evade capture. Biological evolution demands genetic variability; chaos provides a means of structuring random changes, thereby providing the possibility of putting variability under evolutionary control.

Even the process of intellectual progress relies on the injection of new ideas and on new ways of connecting old ideas. Innate creativity may have an underlying chaotic process that selectively amplifies small fluctuations and molds them into macroscopic coherent mental states that are experienced as thoughts. In some cases the thoughts may be decisions, or what are perceived to be the exercise of will. In this light, chaos provides a mechanism that allows for free will within a world governed by deterministic laws" [Crutchfield *et al.*, 1986, pp. 48-49].

We have sought here to expound, in broad outline at least, the main concepts embodied in the complexity paradigm because they constitute the basis for a proper understanding of homeopathy. The relationship between the discussion on chaos and fractals, on the one hand, and homeopathy, on the other, is neither immediate nor simple. We will return to this subject and discuss it in some detail in Chapters 6 and 7 after presenting the general frame of reference for the hypothesis as to the mode (or modes) of action of homeopathic remedies. Without this frame of reference, any kind of speculation at this point would seem vague and largely unfounded.

5.8

General discussion on complexity

There can be no doubt that living phenomena belong to the category of complex phenomena. Even a single bacterium contains such a large amount of constituent elements interacting with one another in a coordinated manner that there can be no objection to defining it as a *complex system*. On the contrary, the phenomena involved in the physics of nonliving systems (such as gravity and the motion of the pendulum), the various pure chemical substances (in the form of solid, liquid or gaseous matter), and the geometrical forms are usually regarded as fundamentally simple systems, which are at any rate amenable to exact description and whose behavior can be predicted. In recent decades, however, new physical research instruments and new theories applied to classical mechanics show that the dividing line between "simple" and "complex" is much narrower than was once supposed. Even simple systems can present complex behavior in certain conditions. For this reason there has been a whole crop of studies by physicists and mathematicians providing us today with a fairly objective view of complexity and its main properties, which is also undoubtedly of importance in biology and medicine.

Introducing the concepts of complexity and chaos into the fields of biology and medicine is tantamount to introducing a new way of thinking because it is not merely a matter of understanding that things are not as simple as one might have hoped (i.e. that they are highly complicated), but a matter of acquiring a number of categories of thought whereby it is possible to "find one's way" around the world of complexity with a certain measure of familiarity. To put it another way, understanding the peculiar properties of complex systems may help us to avoid being overwhelmed by the infinite variety and the degree of complication of the individual mechanisms involved. This, it goes without saying, is not important only for the homeopathic approach, but it allows us to view that approach within the framework of a paradigm which is now gaining ground and establishing itself in many fields of science.

Nicolis and Prigogine declare: "Our physical universe is no longer symbolized by the regular, periodic motion of the planets which underlies classical mechanics. It is rather a universe of instability and fluctuations, which underlie the incredible wealth of forms and structures we see in the world around us. We therefore need new concepts and new instruments to describe a nature in which evolution and pluralism have become the basic watchwords" [Nicolis and Prigogine, 1991, p. XI].

5.8.1 Birth of a complex behavior

In an attempt to illustrate the concept of complexity from a purely physical standpoint, we have to refer to the properties of those dynamic systems which are in a state of continual change or exchange with other systems. One form of complexity, or rather of complex behavior, may emerge from a dynamic system in equilibrium, when it is subjected to a *flow* of energy (termed by some authors a *constraint*) which reaches a critical threshold (also called *symmetry break*).

For example (Figure 19), let us consider an open system which presents two states A and A' which are theoretically in a state of equilibrium and reversible (A and A' may be state of health and state of disease, or, more simply, a physiological or cellular parameter with values oscillating from a minimum A to a maximum A'. The system is open in the sense that it receives an input (x) of matter, energy, and information from the environment (other systems) and produces an output (x') of matter, energy, and information to the environment. Prigogine defines this system as a *"dissipative"* system, whereas Reckeweg speaks of a *"flow system."*

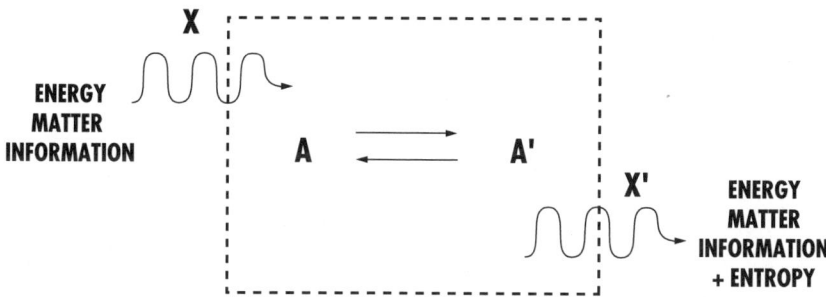

FIGURE 19 Schematic representation of an open system.

The status of A and A' in any given time period will be conditioned by the *constraint* consisting in the change in x and x' in that period. Thus a system of this kind will hardly be stable, but will undergo continual changes.

Unlike the system considered, isolated systems, in which no exchange with the environment is allowed, tend in an irreversible manner towards a final state of equilibrium, in which there is no longer any diversity, asymmetry, or change. In this case, *equilibrium* does not coincide with *order*, but with disorder of all the elements of the system.

This behavior of matter is expressed by the famous second law of thermodynamics:

$$dS/dt \ 0$$

whereby the change in entropy dS over the time period dt is equal to or greater than zero, which is as if to say there is an inevitable tendency towards disorder. In technical terms, *entropy* is a measure of the degree to which the energy in a closed thermodynamic system or process has ceased to be available for some type of work or modification.

On the other hand, open systems are subject to continual modifications; here the entropy is kept under control. In a certain sense, open systems, and among these particularly living systems, evade the second law of thermodynamics, precisely because of the dissipation of entropy in the environment. Internally, these systems undergo the increase in entropy, in the sense that their internal entropy d_iS is 0, but they also depend on an exchange of entropy with the outside environment. If we call this exchange d_eS, we obtain a reformulation of the law whereby:

$$dS/dt = d_iS/dt + d_eS/dt$$

Whereas physical law imposes d_iS 0, there is no law imposing the sign of d_eS, in that the flow of entropy of a system can be positive or negative according to the system considered. It is thus possible that, in some particular system, d_eS may become negative enough to exceed the value of d_iS, with the result that the system presents:

$$dS/dt < 0$$

which is a situation where the disorder decreases and the degree of organization increases. Basically, this would be the fundamental mechanism whereby disorder is diminished in the course of evolution. From the environment the system takes or receives energy, matter, and information; the open system supplies the environment with energy, matter, and information in another form. Within the system, entropy decreases, whereas the total entropy of the universe continues to increase, thus saving the general validity of the second law.

The real situation of physical and biological systems, however, cannot be encompassed within schematic frameworks of this kind, since it would appear that, even within the system itself, large-scale spatial interactions of the various elements may somehow "spontaneously" elude disorder and generate orderly forms and complex behavior patterns [Nicolis and Prigogine, 1991]. More thorough analysis of these issues goes beyond the scope of this book, the intention here being merely to provide an overview of certain as yet unsolved problems in the field of complexity.

An effective example of what is meant by complexity in a physical system might be the field of thermal convection phenomena. If we take a receptacle, fill it with water, and then leave it in isolation ("closed" system), after a short time the turbulence of the liquid which occurred during filling will subside and disappear, the air bubbles will rise to the surface and we will have a homogenous liquid in which all the parts are identical, homogeneous, and at the same temperature. The water molecules move in a state of maximum disorder (Figure 20 **A**).

The tendency of the system towards equilibrium is fairly strong: if a perturbation is applied, for example by stirring (kinetic energy) or dipping a finger into the water (thermal energy), after a short time the water will settle down again and disperse the thermal energy: not a trace of the perturbation will remain. If, however, we subject this system to a *flow* of energy (constraint), for example by applying stable heat which comes from below the receptacle and is dispersed above it (assuming that the side walls have no effect), two different situations can be observed: up to a certain point the system transfers energy from the warmer water (below) to the colder water (above) according to "simple" thermal convection, i.e. a new equilibrium will be created, with molecules moving in a disorderly fashion, faster in the

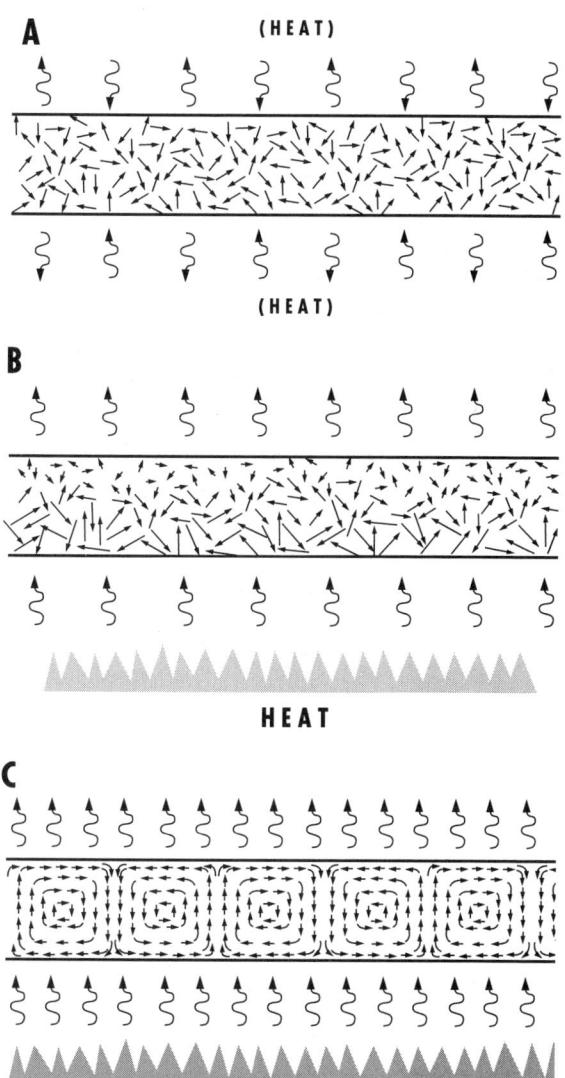

FIGURE 20 Formation of Bénard convection cells. The vectorial movements of water molecules are depicted schematically in a receptacle enclosed between upper and lower partitions, sufficiently far apart for the side walls to have no effect. For the sake of simplicity, only the section of the receptacle is represented. **A:** situation of equilibrium; **B:** new equilibrium, caused by flow of thermal energy; **C:** disruption of the equilibrium, with onset of complex behavior (Bénard convection cells).

lower layers and more slowly in the upper layers (Figure 20 **B**). In this new equilibrium, too, however, the molecules move in disorderly fashion, at higher or lower speed according to the temperature. At a certain point, called the critical point, massive, collective movements of the molecules begin to occur in the liquid. The continuity of the thermal gradient from top to bottom is interrupted and rising (warmer water) and descending (colder water) currents are generated, forming the so-called Bénard convection cells (Figure 20 **C**).

At this point, the water is no longer in the state of disorder which predominated previously; a certain type of order appears in the system, as if the molecules had received their marching orders and had started to move in rank and file, obedient to some form of *coordination* from on high. It is as if each molecule of the fluid "knew" its own position and the movement of the neighboring molecules and took due account of this in its contribution to the overall pattern. The result of these broad-ranging interactions is that the motion is not caused only by kinetic energy and by random impacts between molecules, but also by the collectivity. To this we should add the fact that the new rules not only influence the molecules *within* a convection cell, but also the behavior of adjacent cells: in fact, two adjacent cells present motion in opposite rotation directions.

If we continue to supply energy to this ideal receptacle, above a certain critical value the order is disrupted and so-called turbulence phenomena appear (collective, but chaotic movements) whereupon the motion reverts to being almost completely disorderly. Obviously, the maximum molecular disorder is reached in the gaseous state.

The example we have given, despite its schematic simplification, embraces the main elements of complexity: the birth of the *organization* or *structure* of a system, despite the existence of strong tendencies towards the growth of entropy. This order in the system considered consists in the appearance of *broad-ranging* interactions between many water molecules (it has been estimated that a Bénard convection cell contains roughly 10^{20}). This has been achieved by subjecting the open system to a flow of energy.

How complex and still not entirely understood the behavior of water is can also be deduced from another phenomenon, namely its crystallization. In the phase transition from liquid to ice during the drop in temperature, volume expansion takes place (unlike what happens in the vast majority of other liquids), but, more importantly, in suitable conditions, the occurrence of orderly figures such as snowflake crystals is possible. In the snowflake, the crystal lattice produced by the intermolecular hydrogen bonds has little to do with the development of the snowflake branches in such a great variety of forms, in that the sizes of the latter are of an incomparably greater order of magnitude than the molecular diameters. What happens, then, is a complex behavior of the water vapor in the phase in which it is subjected to nonequilibrium during the drop in temperature. This complex behavior is capable of generating orderly, organized forms on a much greater scale than the molecular crystal lattice.

Many systems have been described as being capable of generating order in complex systems subjected to given constraints: the order may be spatial (waves, spatial structures such as rings or spirals) or temporal (oscillations). There are even chemical reactions which are capable of self-organization in nonequilibrium states in the course of time. The prototype of these reactions is the one described by Belusov-Zabotinskij: in this reaction, the reagents (we will ignore the details) generate a colored product which, however, is not always constant, nor always on the increase, but continues to disappear in the course of time, thus giving rise to talk of a *chemical clock*.

If orderly systems are formed in space (e.g. circles, target-type structures, spirals) this means that each element is affected in its position and speed by the others in the system: it takes its "orders" or information from the adjoining element and behaves accordingly. This results in phenomena of cooperation and coherence, so that the elements arrange themselves in orderly structures. If orderly structures are formed in time (e.g. chemical oscillators, biorhythms, pulsations) this means that the state of the system in any given instant "depends" on the previous one and "conditions" the next one in the series. In complex systems, this is not equivalent to a certain type of inertia of motion according to the classic laws of physics because these orderly structures in time may present, and indeed usually do present, a nonlinear trend. There is transmission of information processed in a complex manner in time, and thus a form of memory.

In brief, it has been claimed that it is the very appearance of *spatiotemporal structures*, due to *broad-ranging* interactions among the elements of a system, that constitutes the most typical feature of complexity [Nicolis and Prigogine, 1991]. It is in this that complex behavior consists in the true sense of the term, and not merely, as one might be tempted to believe, in the continual increase in the factors involved. In other words, complexity contains not only a quantitative factor related to the number of elements involved, but also a qualitative factor associated with the appearance of "structure," or "form."

In cells, *structures* have absolutely indispensable functions: we need only mention the cell membranes, which divide the cells into compartments and separate the cell itself from the surrounding environment. Via the membranes a marked *dysequilibrium* of substances and electrical charges is maintained, which is necessary for a whole series of functions, such as the production of energy (mitochondria), the production and transmission of signals (neurons), and the activation of movement (muscles).

Biologists are accustomed to regarding these types of order as the rule in cell structures (membranes, filamentous proteins, circadian rhythms, cell cycle, and many others), but recently chemists and physicists, too, have devoted their attention to phenomena of this type which occur in nonliving nature. This is important because if the ability to generate order is also found outside the biological setting, this means that we are in the presence of a type of behavior basic to nature itself and thus in a certain sense ancestral or atavistic.

Order, information, and complexity are aspects of one and the same problem, which would appear to be of increasing importance in fields ranging from biology to physics, to the study of evolution and of social and economic systems. The contribution deriving from a physico-mathematical approach to the problem of complexity is much greater than might at first sight be imagined: while it is true that a living system with its thousands of different subcomponents will never resemble a chemical system with two or only a few components and can never be described by a mathematical formula, on the other hand it is equally true that the study of the complexity of "simple" systems may enable us to discover a number of "basic rules" of behavior which are repeated in substantially identical form in systems at different levels of evolutionary development.

In other words, the complexity of biological systems (and their pathological aspects) may be tackled and better understood by reference to a pattern common to all complex systems, i.e. to a model developed in physicochemical reference systems. Knowing the behavior of a system on a small scale may help us to identify some of the properties of a vaster and more complex system. Such a procedure exploits the knowledge accumulated in the study of fractal geometries, which shows us that there is kind of *self-similarity* in many aspects of nature, whereby the fundamental rules (even as expressed in mathematical formulae) remain similar on changing the scale of operations. In the detail, we rediscover the image of the vaster context in which that detail occupies a place (see Chapter 5, Section 7).

5.8.2 Résumé of the properties of complex systems

Without wishing, obviously, to dismiss here in few words such a broad-ranging and difficult topic, we can summarize the particular characteristics, properties, or modes of functioning of complex systems as emerging today in many disciplines:

a) *A complex system presents properties which amount to more than simply the sum of its component parts*. From the interrelations between subsystems new functions are generated, such as, for example the electrical membrane potentials in the field of physiology, or the control of blood pressure at vascular system level, or thought and emotions at central nervous system level. The new functions cannot be deduced from an analysis of the subcomponents, though they are conditioned and determined by them.

b) *In a complex system not all behavior patterns are theoretically predictable and experimentally reproducible*. For example, in the Bénard convection cell system described above, we can predict and reproduce the phenomenon of the appearance of convection motions at temperature values beyond a certain threshold, but we cannot predict what will be the direction (e.g. clockwise or counterclockwise rotation) of the motion of the water of a cell in a given space in the receptacle. This latter parameter is selected by the system at random, probably in response to imperceptible fluctuations of the random motions of the molecules at the critical moment when the orderly flow tends to begin. Thus, the behavior of a complex system is the fruit of cooperation between determinism and chance. The immune system, too, is characterized by this property: the lymphocytes continually generate new receptors with random sequences, and then the information which enters in the form of an antigen selects the corresponding clones and induces them to proliferate, thanks to the intervention of many other components of the system itself (receptors, immunological memory, other lymphocytes, cytokines).

c) *A system which obeys the laws of complexity does not always behave in a linear manner, i.e. the effects are not always proportional to the doses of a given factor which modifies the equilibrium*. Theoretically, the consequences of this factor may be extremely variable. For example, it may happen that a perturbation is "absorbed" without leaving a trace, i.e. it causes the modification of a parameter, immediately followed by a return to the initial state (negative feedback).

It is also possible that the reaction of the system may be such that there are oscillations of the parameters, even in the opposite direction to that of the initial perturbation (what in pharmacology may be defined as a rebound effect). On the other hand, another possibility is that minimal changes in initial conditions or minimal perturbations may activate autocatalytic cycles ("positive" feedback), or interlinked amplification cascade systems, with major consequences (see the butterfly effect).

The field of meteorology, in fact, is one of those in which the problem of complexity and chaos has been grasped and tackled in a highly systematic way owing to the notorious difficulty encountered in forecasting the weather. Amplification systems, however, are present at all levels in the equipment of a complex system receiving external stimuli. "*Pronounced dependency on initial conditions*" is a fundamental property of complex systems, accounting for the occurrence of chaotic dynamic patterns, unpredictability and nonlinearity of responses [Ruelle, 1992].

d) *Complex systems exhibit another singular property—bistability.* Given the same external and internal conditions (temperature, chemical concentrations, mathematical parameters), the system may assume different states. The choice between one state and another possible state often depends on the *past history* of the system itself. For instance, when we consider a liquid "perfect," the melting point and freezing point coincide, but when we consider aggregates of molecules which are midway between liquid and solid (microaggregates), the two points may differ very considerably: on heating a solid composed of microaggregates, it will melt at a certain temperature; on cooling the solution, the microaggregates remain in the liquid phase up to lower temperatures than those they had when they were in the solid phase prior to melting. At one and the same temperature, the molecules may be in the solid or liquid phase according to their previous state: if they come from a liquid phase they tend to remain liquid; if they come from a solid phase, they tend to remain solid.

These models are regarded as being very useful for more thorough study of phase transition processes, which, as is well known, are also of decisive importance in living systems (cf. the continual polymerization and depolymerization phenomena of cellular macromolecules).

e) *A complex system is regulated by communication modes suited to the degree of complexity.* For example, communication between two molecules (fairly simple system) consists in electrostatic attraction or repulsion; communication between several groups of molecules (complex system) consists in ondulatory dynamics and spatiotemporal variations (oscillations of particular signal molecules); communication between organs and systems is entrusted to further complex systems which use both chemical (hormones) and physical (action potentials) means of communication. Lastly, communication between different individuals is entrusted to other means such as words, writing, looks, and broadcasting by cable or over the air. This means that if we want to "enter the communications network" (with a view to understanding and eventually influencing it) we have to use the same method or methods of communication as the system we are interested in. This fact has been clearly appreciated by psychiatrists who, though armed with a vast array of highly effective molecules such as neurotransmitters and transmission inhibitors, know perfectly well that this molecular approach may condition, but not solve a psychiatric problem, the root of which lies in an affective, relational or behavioral disorder.

The comparison, however, can be extended to other fields of medicine because the more we study them, the more these other systems, too, prove to be composed of interactive networks between cells and multicellular centers which, in qualitative terms, resemble the neural networks. If a system is regulated by modes of communication consisting in synergisms between several molecules acting at low doses, to enter this network in an effective way theoretically you would need to use the same method: low-dose modulators exploiting synergisms and antagonisms. If, on the other hand, we use modulators of only one molecular type and at high doses, we obtain effects, admittedly, and even effects in the desired direction, but not in complete harmony with the system itself, the result of which therefore will be a high incidence of unwanted side effects.

f) *Systems far from equilibrium are susceptible not only to dramatic changes but also to having to conserve a spatiotemporal memory of such changes.* Memory in this context means the possibility of an *irreversible change*. Unlike what happens in a system in a state of reversible equilibrium on changing the external or internal parameters (see Figure 19), in a complex system a situation can be reached in which there is a *symmetry breaking*, or irreversible change. Minor localized attempts to deviate from the equilibrium are not necessarily made to fail by the instantaneous development of some form of counteraction, but may be accepted or even amplified by the system, thus becoming sources of innovation and diversification. In mathematical terms, this phenomenon is also called bifurcation. While it is true that random fluctuations and perturbations can usually be damped, beyond certain values, or in the presence of appropriate environmental conditions, these effects are not annulled, but with the system acting as an amplifier, a reaction is triggered which removes the system from the reference state. We thus have the setting up of a new state of the system, which can no longer be restored to the previous state. This phenomenon has proved very important, amongst other things, in the evolution of cells: the spatial symmetry breaking occurring, for example, when the membranes started to separate what was inside the cell from what lay outside the cell marked an irreversible leap forward in the organization of living systems, since it was precisely through these partitions that a gain in information and complexity was achieved, favoring the existence of a new state compared to the previous one.

Complexity, then, is associated with memory, or rather with the storage of information: a previous event may influence other subsequent events.

Information exhibits a special propensity for being transmitted, and thus is particularly capable of generating consequential effects on the receiving system, but also of being stored, and of persisting as a memory of subsequent events. The evolution both of the macrocosm and of each individual (embryogenesis, followed by development and growth) is a progressive increase in the storage and handling of information.

g) *In the behavior of complex systems the quality of the information is far more important than the quantity, or the energy consumed to provide it.* The biological system, in particular, has developed and has integrated within itself the systems of production and use of energy, utilizing various well coordinated metabolic pathways and the rapid availability of phosphorylated intermediates. The functional reserve of these systems is considerable (except in highly pathological cases of cell damage or anoxia), so that normally the functional oscillations and the behavior patterns of cellular or organic biological systems do not depend on addition or subtraction of energy, but on control mechanisms at the information level. Information of such a nature as to be received and processed efficiently by receptors and signal transduction systems is capable of activating energy metabolism and of evoking functional and mechanical response cascades which may be incomparably greater than the initial stimulus in terms of amount of energy and information produced.

The more complex and "flexible" a system is, the scantier may be the amounts of energy capable of altering its behavior. We need only mention, for instance, the brain, which is in all probability the most complex system existing in nature. It can be "mobilized"—and, as a result, so can the entire body—by nonmolecular stimulations, which in a certain sense may be devoid of energy or matter. Biochemical, metabolic, electrical, receptor, and even anatomical systems (in the sense of the physical structure of the neurons) can be activated and modulated not only by chemical or pharmacological substances and electrical stimulations, but also, in an optimally efficient and specific manner, by sounds, visual images, words, ideas, and thoughts. What matters, in this case, is not the quantity or intensity of the stimulus, but its "meaning" in terms of information.

h) *When it comes to describing and understanding complex systems it may be very useful and perhaps indispensable to use archetypes and analogies.* This approach has been strongly emphasized by Nicolis and Prigogine [Nicolis and Prigogine, 1991]. What is meant by analogy is that similarity between two distinct systems which may serve to understand one of them better on the basis of knowledge already gained about the other. Analogy can therefore be used to construct more advanced models compared to those in current use and to make forecasts about unknown systems starting from known systems (usually physicochemical or mathematical) which act as *archetypes*, i.e. as reference systems.

The above-mentioned authors state the case: "The physicochemical systems which give rise to transition phenomena, to broad-ranging order, or to far-from-equilibrium symmetry breaking may serve as archetypes for understanding other types of systems which exhibit a complex behavior, for which the laws of evolution of the variables involved are not known at any comparable level of detail. (...) The analysis proceeds in two steps. Firstly, certain analogies are traced between the observations and the behavior of physicochemical "reference" systems. This defines the type of model which is likely to be the most appropriate representation of the system concerned. Then, an attempt is made to go beyond the stage of plain analogy, to pinpoint, *within the framework of the model adopted*, the specificity of each problem and to incorporate it in the description. Lastly, the predictions of the analysis are compared against experience with past behavior and, assuming an agreement is reached on quality, these predictions are used to foresee future tendencies. If all goes well, the natural outcome of the process should be an ability to come up with concrete, practical suggestions as to how to *dominate complexity*" (authors' italics) [Nicolis and Prigogine, 1991, p. 251].

As we have seen earlier (Chapter 5, Section 7), fractal geometry appears to be the most suitable for describing the forms and properties of many natural systems. The existence of self-similarity on changing the scale, a typical property of fractals, in a certain sense justifies the analogy procedure: an image or behavior pattern is observed in the part which resembles the whole to which that selfsame part "belongs." The part then is significant, and contains information and properties which allow analogies to made with the entire system and with other parts of that system. In a nutshell, the analogy highlights that "hidden order" which exists in complex systems, consisting in scale invariance and thus in the presence of elements of similarity between apparently very different systems (see also Chapter 5, Section 7).

The following chapters will serve to illustrate how the complexity paradigm helps us to get the basic features and principles of homeopathic medicine into proper perspective.

6 *Homeostasis, Complexity and Homeopathy: The Law of Similars*

The relationship between the concepts expounded in the foregoing chapter and the homeopathic medicine may not be directly self-evident, but is very profound and far-reaching: homeopathy presents itself as an approach which expresses a distinct preference for the "subtle" as opposed to the macroscopic, for homeostatic regulation as opposed to intervening drastically on some single factor modified by the disease, the equilibrium of the body as opposed to the organ; in a certain sense the preference is for information as opposed to more material aspects. The very law of similars itself, the cornerstone of homeopathic theory, is founded upon analogical-empirical rather than upon logical-inductive reasoning.

Homeopathy can only be understood within the context of the paradigm of complexity. In this chapter we are going to attempt to analyze the relationship between complexity and homeopathy without, however, laying any claim to solving all the questions raised by homeopathy, but confining ourselves, for the time being, to discussing the law of similars as defined by Hahnemann and the effect of small doses of pharmacologically active substances. In other words, in an attempt to shed light on such an intricate issue, we have decided to leave aside for the moment the problem of infinitesimal doses, which will be dealt with later (Chapter 7).

Here, homeopathy will be treated as *a therapeutic approach which uses compounds at low doses administered according to a rationale which differs from that characteristic of allopathy*. The justification for such a procedure is to be found in the very history of homeopathy, where the pivotal concept for both the founder and the various schools over the years has always been *the law of similars rather than the problem of dilutions*, and in its present-day practice, where we see that a substantial proportion of the drugs sold as "homeopathic" remedies effectively contain ponderal doses of substances of mineral, vegetable or animal origin. All the preparations containing dilutions lower than 20x or 10c belong to this category.

Using this type of approach, the possible mechanism of action of homeopathic remedies can be addressed without necessarily having to take as gospel truth the famous concept of the "memory of water," which understandably may be at variance with the tenets of current biomedical reasoning.

In a nutshell, then, the basic hypothesis considered here is as follows: *a homeopathic drug works by providing information commensurate with the complexity of the organism with which it interacts.* This hypothesis is illustrated in detail and step by step here below.

The possible mechanism of action of a homeopathic remedy is to be sought within the sphere of the regulation of complex homeostatic systems. It is therefore necessary to refer to what we have already said about the characteristics of the functioning of homeostatic systems (Chapter 5, Section 4). By way of an initial approximation we shall attempt to consider the essential phenomena of the variations in homeostasis and the regulatory impact of homeopathic intervention. Thereafter, the model will be enriched with variants and its possible applications will be discussed.

6.1

Mode of action of homeopathic drugs

Given a homeostatic system such as the one described in Figure 8 (Chapter 5, Section 4), we will consider how it is modified when a perturbation of a pathological type comes into play which shifts the equilibrium excessively towards A' (Figure 21). The variable A may thus be regarded as the normal condition and A' as the pathological condition, in the sense of an excessive oscillation of the parameter considered. Another possibility is that A' is a pathological event in the sense of the presence of biochemical alterations coming from the outside, i.e. A' is of exogenous origin, such as a foreign antigen or a toxic molecule: the subsequent chain of events does not change. At this point A' produces an enhanced signal a' which then brings about very marked activation of the regulatory system. We have seen that, following an increase in the signal a', the specific receptor system is *primed*, i.e., to simplify things, it exposes a greater number of receptors for a' (see the homologous priming phenomenon mentioned above in Chapter 5, Sections 2.1 and 6.2).

The primed regulatory system increases its activity by producing more of the signal r, which, in turn, will force the effector mechanisms ($A' \rightarrow A$) towards the normal condition A. In this initial phase of the disease, the body reacts logically and efficiently in the direction of equilibrium and healing. For instance, if a' is a molecule "judged" to be abnormal in terms of quality or quantity by the "immune" regulatory system, the system will produce more receptors for a' (in this example, antibodies and T lymphocyte receptors) and more r signals (interleukins, cytokines, interferons) which in turn prompt the effector system (phagocytes or complement) to restore normal homeostasis by eliminating the excess of A' and re-establishing the condition A (healing).

In this initial stage of the disease, which might be regarded as perfectly "physiological," other phenomena worthy of note occur: the first of these

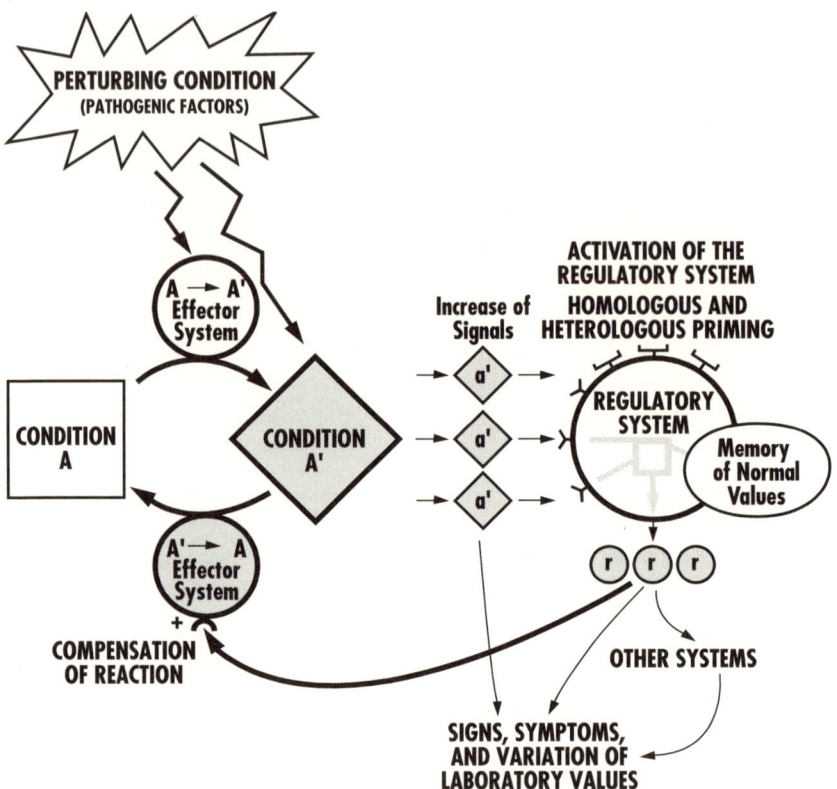

FIGURE 21 Diagram of the modifications induced by an external perturbation in a homeostatic system. The starting situation ("controlled dysequilibrium") is that described in Figure 8. The perturbing condition is posited as being that which acts upon the effector system $A \longrightarrow A'$ or directly upon A', leading to an excessive increase in that parameter. With an increase in the signal a', the regulatory system is activated and reacts by attempting to restore the lost equilibrium. For the receptor dynamics illustrated in this model, see also the text.

is the onset of symptoms. The signals regulating the homeostatic systems are generally endowed with substantial redundancy and pleiotropicity, in the sense that they are capable of activating multiple systems in various ways. Thus, a' will manifest itself by producing some symptom or other depending upon the systems it activates. It has already been said (Chapter 5, Section 1) that *symptoms are usually linked to the activation of endogenous systems rather than to the direct effect of the etiological agent*. The symptoms thus stem from "side" effects produced by a' activating the specific homeostatic systems. In the diagram presented in Figure 21, not only do symptoms appear caused by a', but also symptoms caused by other signals (r), produced by the regulatory system. Referring once again to the previous example, an increase in a' and r may cause symptoms stemming from activation of the immune system, linked to the "side" effects of antibodies, complement, or cytokines (fever, leukocytosis, fatigue, sleep, and other manifestations).

With reference to classic homeopathic theory, as outlined in paragraph 63 of the *Organon* (see Chapter 2, Section 3), it may be said that the effects of signal a' (Figure 21) correspond to the "primary action," whereas those of signal r correspond to what Hahnemann called the "secondary action" of the remedy, which is believed to be of a "life-preserving nature."

A second event worthy of note, contemplated in Figure 21, is the onset of a new sensitivity related to exposure of new receptors by the regulatory system for substances other than a'. This event, too, belongs to the category of "priming" events (heterologous priming) and, in general, to all those modifications of receptor sensitivity and homeostatic system compensatory activity, related to pathological conditions and dealt with in some detail above (see, particularly, Chapter 5, Section 6.3 and Figure 15). The homeostatic systems involved in reactive regulation are thus altered not only specifically by the etiological agent, but also according to a broader spectrum of specificities. This, too, has been clearly demonstrated in many conditions: the interferons produced as a result of a viral or bacterial infection induce a greater resistance to other viruses, other bacteria and even tumor cells; a treatment with barbiturates induces an increase in the activity of microsomal systems in the liver which may serve to offset the effects of other drugs and toxic substances with greater efficacy; when leukocytes come into contact with endotoxins they are also sensitized for other bacterial products such as formylpeptides; when the main hepatic detoxification system (cytochrome P450) is activated by the chronic intake of toxic substances its ability to metabolize other substances is enhanced. There is thus a certain degree of broadening of the spectrum of specific sensitivities in a regulatory system activated during a disease.

After this initial reactive phase, if the perturbation of the homeostasis continues, the regulatory system may undergo a major change in status: it adapts to the altered conditions, progressively suppressing the sensitivity for the persistent, abnormally increased signal (Figure 22). This adaptation enables the system somehow to "survive" with the disease, which otherwise would require an excessive expenditure of energy (continual activation of both the $A \longrightarrow A'$ and $A' \longrightarrow A$ mechanisms) and excessive problems in terms of symptomatology. From the molecular point of view, the cells reduce the receptors for a' to the point where they disappear altogether, or they reduce their affinity, or they produce a decrease in communication with the effector systems (in our case, the production of r). By and large, this phenomenon is specific at receptor level: that is to say, it is the *occupied* receptors which disappear, whereas the others remain or even increase in number. In other words, the desensitization tends to be agonist-specific (though, obviously, exceptions and variants are possible in terms of combinations of groups of different receptors, cell states of overall exhaustion of all activities, etc.).

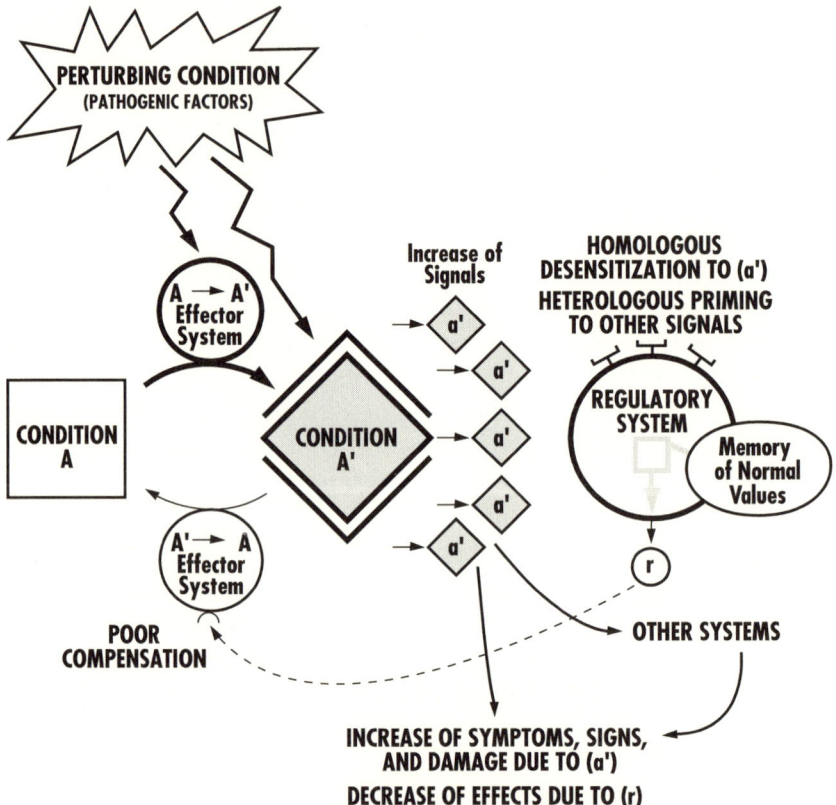

FIGURE 22 Disorder in a homeostatic system due to persistence of the perturbation. It is postulated that the perturbing condition is severe and long-lasting, such as to produce a strong, constant increase in the signal *a'* despite the efforts of the regulatory system. In these conditions, the regulatory system may adapt by reducing the sensitivity to *a'* with major consequences for the evolution of the disease process.

By reference to this basic model, which by the very nature of things is necessarily highly simplified, we are in a position to postulate the mode of action of the homeopathic remedy (Figure 23). It *activates the regulatory system via receptors other than those for* a', *but which produce the same effect, namely that of restoring production of the signal* r *and thus of bringing about activation of the compensatory mechanism A' —> A*. The homeopathic drug is therefore thought to act in lieu of *a'*, to which the system is no longer sensitive as a result of adaptation.

On what do we base such a hypothesis? It rests on the fact that the homeopathic drug necessarily has to interact with the regulatory system concerned, because it has been identified precisely on the basis of its *ability to*

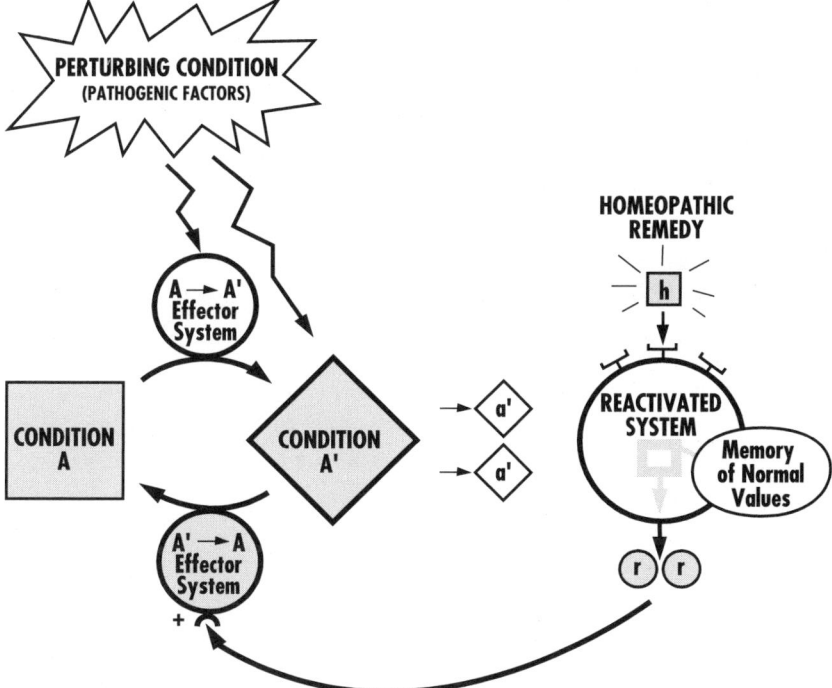

FIGURE 23 Schematic and highly simplified representation of the possible way by which a drug with a "homeopathic" mode of action (h) may reactivate the regulatory system and the homeostatic circuit.

cause symptoms similar to the disease, i.e. symptoms similar to those caused by the mediator a' via activation of the regulatory system. It is clear that, if it is true that most of the symptoms in a pathological condition are due to activation of homeostatic reaction systems, it should be possible somehow to "reproduce" the activation of these same homeostatic systems by administering a compound which "reproduces" the symptoms of the disease. Theoretically, in the healthy, nonperturbed system, symptoms of the disease may be produced by the administration of *a'* and *r*, or of a substance which activates the regulatory system via receptors other than those for *a'*. In the diseased system, *a'* is already present in large amounts and effectively causes the symptoms, but, if the mechanism of receptor adaptation comes into play, we may find ourselves in a situation whereby the regulatory systems become "paralyzed," prove inefficient, and are themselves unbalanced. Since, however, the regulatory system conserves other sensitivities in the disease state, and indeed probably accentuates them, if other sensitivities are brought into play through other signals, the system can be reactivated. *By subjecting the regulatory system to a signal "similar" to a' (in the sense that it causes similar symptoms), the response r is elicited and thus a return to normal homeostasis.*

The *similarity* is therefore between the symptoms caused by the activation of reactive mechanisms by the disease process in the patient and the symptoms caused by activation of the same reactive mechanisms in a healthy subject by a biologically significant external agent (in this case, the homeopathic drug).

The hypothesis put forward here is based essentially on the following points:

a) In the dynamic progression of a disease process, *specific homeostatic regulatory systems may break down or be blocked* following excessive stimulation or as a result of the interference of other pathological factors (metabolic and nutritional problems, toxic factors, heterologous desensitization, neurohormonal disorders, water-electrolyte imbalances, or simply as a side effect of high-dose drug therapies).

b) As long as the disease process does not lead to excessively profound and irreversible impairment of the regulation systems, *this blockade can be by-passed using different receptor sensitivities* (for exogenous or endogenous substances) which the perturbed systems themselves conserve or even accentuate.

c) The identification of suitable substances for reactivating the homeostatic systems *specifically* blocked in a given disease process is hard to achieve *with precision* in any single patient by using the conventional scientific approach, on account of the complexity, variety and multiplicity of the systems involved and because of the dynamic and changeable nature of diseases.

d) The homeopathic approach, particularly through the use of analogy (law of similars) *makes it possible to get nearer to identifying substances capable of interacting specifically with the homeostatic systems involved* in the disease process in each individual case.

At this juncture we feel obliged to quote Hahnemann, who was the first to gain a real insight into this therapeutic approach (forgiving him, of course, for indulging in hyperbole): "The curative power of medicines, therefore, depends on their symptoms (*), similar to the disease but superior to it in strength, so that each individual case of disease is most surely, radically, rapidly and permanently annihilated and removed only by a medicine capable of producing (in the human system) in the most similar and complete manner the totality of its symptoms, which at the same time are stronger than the disease. As this natural law of cure manifests itself in every pure experiment (**) and every true observation in the world, the fact is consequently established; it matters little what may be the scientific explanation of how it takes place; and I do not attach much importance to the attempts made to explain it. But the following view seems to commend itself as the most probable one, as it is founded on premises derived from experience. (...) As every disease (not entirely surgical) consists only in a special, morbid, dynamic alteration of our vital energy (of the principle of life) manifested in sensation and motion, so in every homeopathic cure this principle of life dynamically altered by natural disease is seized through the administration of a medicinal potency selected exactly according to symptom-similarity by a somewhat stronger, similar artificial disease-manifestation" (*Organon*, paragraphs 27, 28 and 29).

The purpose of this presentation here is to provide a model which explains the effect of homeopathic drugs in terms of molecular and cellular biology. This theory is based on an extremely simplified—perhaps over-simplified—model, but this is necessary in order to pinpoint the central concept, around which a whole series of other problems can be identified, which will be dealt with here below.

The theories and models outlined in the foregoing section do not lay any claim to being the only explanation of the action of a homeopathic drug, but are merely a first sketchy attempt at a hypothesis, which is undoubtedly due to be supplemented with new insights and new concepts in the future. The theory offers a frame of reference within which various aspects need to be clarified and a number of corollaries, extensions and variants need to be discussed.

6.2

Discussion of the model presented

(*) That is, those which the medicines are capable of causing in healthy human subjects.

(**) What Hahnemann means by "pure experiment" is one conducted by trying out the remedies in healthy subjects and in patients.

6.2.1 *Aggravation*

From the diagram in Figure 23 we see that the administration of the homeopathic drug may cause symptoms related to reactivation of the regulatory system. Though the doses are low, reactivation therapy is, however, capable of producing effects which in some way match the disease, or which may appear as an acute exacerbation of the symptoms. In point of fact, activation of the regulatory system entails the production not merely of signals directly aimed at restoring homeostasis, but also of signals which are transmitted to systems which produce symptoms. This is a well known fact in homeopathy, so much so, indeed, that it has been termed "homeopathic aggravation." It is the price that has to be paid for the removal of the adaptation system.

It is also conceivable that, if the present disease is the outcome of a succession of pathological events, the regression of the last event may be accompanied by the recurrence of previously disappeared symptoms. In this sense, homeopathic therapy leads the patient to experience in reverse order the history of the particular disease or even of his or her pathological history in general, according to a process which may bear some resemblance to psychoanalytical therapy. A similar concept has also been proposed by other investigators [Laplantine, 1986].

6.2.2 **Further degrees of complexity**

The diagram in Figure 23 (Chapter 6, Section 1) needs to be amplified in view of the fact that homeostatic systems are integrated with one another in complex networks. This interplay underlies one of the main insights of the homeopathic approach. It is clear, in fact, that, in the presence of a practically inextricable network of intertwined homeostatic systems, it is not possible, in any single case, to know sufficient details of the state of each such system to be able to apply effective pharmacological remedies. For example, in the course of an infectious disease, we may know that the thermoregulatory center is altered and institute therapy aimed in such a way as to restore its normal equilibrium (e.g. antipyretic therapy), but at the same time we have no means of knowing the status of the thirst and hunger centers, the macrophagic activity of the spleen, the hepatic synthesis of various mediators such as complement and antiproteases, the influence of the patient's psychological state on regulation of blood pressure or the patency of the airways, the relationship between the various lymphocyte subpopulations, the levels of growth factors in the blood, and thyroid and adrenocortical function, to mention but a few. Even if we were in a position to know these details through appropriate analyses, there is no guaranteeing that we would then be able to implement therapies coordinating all the various imbalances in order to help the patient's body to restore biological order. In most cases, then, there is no alternative but to resort to therapies combating the etiological factors or the symptoms. The regulatory systems, in fact, are too complex for us to be able to act at this level (which, however, is the very heart of the dynamics of a disease process).

This then is what the progress made by homeopathy is all about: realizing that such a degree of complexity exists in the informational disorder associated with the disease and discovering the main way of getting round the problem, namely the empirical-experimental method based on the law of similars. In point of fact, in this way *we have two sets of complex, integrated information*: the set regarding the drug and the one about the patient. It is true that little is known about *which* molecular and cellular alterations take place and particularly about the intimate relationships between them (their "*internal essential nature*," as Hahnemann puts it), but such alterations and such degrees of complexity somehow express themselves as symptoms, which can be observed and documented. On comparing the patient's symptoms and those of the drug, two complex images are brought face to face, the expression of two reactive "patterns," which, if they match, must necessarily refer to the same or similar regulatory systems in the "internal sphere" of the body.

The drug thus "uses" the same systems (which we can even admit we do not know) as the disease. This is a typically *analogical* way of proceeding (what the doctor is basically seeking in the repertorization of the symptoms is an analogy between the patient and the drug), but, on the basis of what we have said, it would also appear to be a logical way of proceeding. The homeopathic approach does not mean that reason gives up the ghost in the face of inextricable complexity, but adopts a realistic attitude towards it. The complexity is accepted as a basic fact of life, but, by knowing a number of general rules (nonlinearity, feedback, integration, analogy), we can make up for our ignorance of the details.

The action of the homeopathic remedy presents itself as highly specific in terms of information. This specificity is based in the first place on the nature of the drug in itself, i.e. on the *low dose* (as a rule, the lower the dose of a drug, the more likely it is to be specific because it acts on the very few highly sensitive targets) and on its *active ingredients*, which are usually multiple and combined in various ways (cf. the vastness of the homeopathic pharmacopoeia, especially of vegetable and animal origin, and the subtlety of the distinctions between apparently very similar drugs such as plants belonging to the same family, to mention but a single example).

The specificity, however, is based not only on the nature of the drug because seemingly very simple drugs are used in homeopathy (mineral salts, metals), but is guaranteed above all by the particular symptom-based individualization procedure. This procedure enables the right remedy to be identified for the largest number of symptoms present and thus for the largest number of homeostatic systems impaired.

The homeopathic drug acts better, the more complex the system and the more subject it is to subtle regulatory dynamics. The use of such a drug as an enzyme inhibitor is unthinkable, and those investigators who have attempted such experiments have reported negative [Petit *et al.*, 1989] or poor and uncertain [Harisch and Kretschmer, 1988] results. The experiments described in Chapter 4 indicate that research is revealing that it is easier (or rather, less difficult) to achieve positive results with homeopathic dilutions when the experimental systems consist in animals or isolated organs rather than in cells or enzymes.

Homeopathy has a pharmacopoeia comprising a whole host of substances stemming from the animal, vegetable or mineral realms. Most of these substances (again, quite apart from the question of high dilutions) are extracts from raw materials, and not purified or synthetic molecules. This adds a further degree of complexity with regard both to the interpretation of their effects and to research in this field. On the other hand, according to the basic "logic" of homeopathy, this could hardly be otherwise. If it is true that diseases present complex dynamics, no action to restore equilibrium can be implemented without adopting a complex approach. In the optimal therapy, many different receptors have to be reached simultaneously in a dynamic, specifically targeted manner, some of which will be activators and others regulators, both in the psychic and physiological spheres. The homeopathic pharmacopoeia offers a vast choice of remedies with differing characteristics. The only clue, or at any rate, by far the most important clue to negotiating this maze of complexity is the similarity of patient and drug symptoms.

It is quite astonishing to find that the animal body presents multiform receptors capable of receiving information from any number of elements present in other animal organisms, in flowers, in the roots of plants, and in a variety of minerals. Often these elements are poisons if used at high doses, which indicates their very substantial reactivity with biological systems.

What is the sense of this "matching" of information from sources within and outside the body, which effectively proves damaging or therapeutic according to the doses? The reasons for this are to be found in the evolution of living creatures: poisons came onto the scene as the products of plants and animals that used them to advantage for defensive and offensive purposes; to achieve these aims they had in some way to "mimic" substances present inside the target organism, otherwise there would have been no specific interaction and thus none of the biological damage intended. Accordingly, poisons and toxins, precisely because they are what they are, are "similars" of certain structures, receptors, enzymes, or signal molecules already present in the body, probably as mediators of physiological functions.

On the other hand, in terms of evolution, we can readily understand why the complexity of the remedy (by this we mean a medicine which comes to hand or is discovered in nature) has evolved along with the complexity of the organism to be treated: living creatures have learnt, often to their cost, but in an increasingly expert manner, to "recognize" what is useful in the environment for therapeutic purposes. Those forms of life with a broader, more versatile and more flexible set of receptor apparati (the receptor is the mirror of the signal) have adapted better to changing environmental conditions. According to this view of things, those forms of life which, when subjected to endogenous or exogenous stress and thus affected by a great variety of diseases, developed receptor apparati capable of recognizing specific substances (foodstuffs, plants, oligoelements, vitamins, *inter alia*) or other signals (light, heat, magnetic fields) present in the environment and useful for restoring normal homeostasis, have had a major evolutionary advantage.

In a word, it could be claimed that the law of similars, as applied in the field of complexity considered here in this section, and particularly with reference to what was said in Chapter 5 with regard to chaotic networks, is tantamount to an attempt to *increase the connectivity* of homeostatic regulatory systems, by introducing into the systems themselves *targeted information* which is of an *adequate degree of complexity and subtlety*, precisely because it has been identified on the basis of a vast array of information stemming from the symptoms. According to the reasoning which has led us here, increasing the *flow of information* which passes into the complex dynamic systems may serve as a guide for restoring their disrupted or dysregulated relationships and thus for redirecting them towards their original functions. In a word, the homeopathic stimulus is aimed to put a specific *form* of order (*in-"formation"*) into chaos.

In Appendix 1 (pages 392 and the following pages) we will further discuss the significance of various types of symptoms in order to connect biological changes and the evolution of disease.

6.2.3 Individualization

The conceptual frame of reference outlined here enables us to grasp one of the cornerstones of the homeopathic approach, namely the fact that one and the same disease can present different, peculiar symptoms in different subjects and may require different treatments. To this aspect, i.e. the individualization of the prescription, homeopaths have always accorded paramount importance.

The same disease may result from alterations of a great variety of homeostatic systems, with subtle differences for the individual patient, depending upon his or her genetic make-up, age, previous medical history, type of diet, and other intercurrent endogenous factors. The "typical" symptoms of a disease, that is to say the "diagnostic" or "pathognomonic" pointers, according to the conventional view, are the same in all subjects suffering from the disease (e.g., the high temperature of influenza, the headache of migraine, the jaundice of choledocholithiasis). These symptoms are of little significance in homeopathic individualization, where they are called "*local*" or "*common*" symptoms, whereas much greater importance is ascribed to those symptoms which differ from one individual to another with the same disease. These latter symptoms are called "*peculiar*" symptoms.

For instance, two subjects with influenza may both have a high temperature, but one may sweat and not the other; one may be in a state of prostration and the other agitated (*Belladonna* and *Aconitum*, respectively). Perspiration and prostration are peculiar symptoms and guide the homeopathic physician in his choice of remedy.

The importance accorded to the peculiar symptoms, within the framework of the theory expounded above, is justified on the basis of the fact that they reflect both the patient's *physiological homeostasis*, regardless of the disease, and the mode of reacting, *the way the body chooses to face up* to the disruption of homeostasis currently under way. It should be recalled that all homeostatic systems are interconnected, with the result that the modulation of one cannot fail to have an impact on the others. In the example we have given, it would seem clear that the imbalance of other homeostatic systems (thermoregulation, general cenesthesia) "conditions" the influenza. It is only by "conditioning" these systems pharmacologically that the particular subject can be helped by a homeopathic treatment.

The *disease*, from the homeopathic standpoint, is not identified either with what the patient complains of or with what he or she is conventionally accustomed to considering as such, but rather it embraces a broad spectrum of interrelated pathophysiological changes. It is common experience for homeopathic practitioners to observe that, in patients who present with organ diseases or diseases located at skin level, the therapy induces improvements in the psychological sphere, or in other diseases which have been present for some time and which the patient had not regarded as treatable. This happens because, by targeting the treatment at the patient's peculiar symptoms, one is operating at a much deeper level than that apparently involved on the basis of the symptoms currently experienced.

6.2.4 Importance of small doses

To reactivate the regulatory system impaired by the disease process, *small doses* of a substance acting at receptor level may suffice. The impaired system, indeed, may be hypersensitive, having a greater number of receptors and a heightened sensitivity at postreceptor (transduction) level. This fact accounts for something which was illustrated by Hahnemann and confirmed by the various schools of homeopathy: to cause the symptoms of the disease in healthy subjects you need higher doses of the remedy than those required for patient remission. On the other hand, considerations of this type also hold good for various nonhomeopathic drugs; aspirin, for instance, lowers the patient's temperature only when it is pathologically high; it does not lower it if it is normal; the thermoregulatory system becomes sensitive to aspirin only if it is operating abnormally.

The fact that the homeopathic remedy may act at low doses is also important because in this way we avoid:

a) The remedy used having toxic effects, seeing that many substances used in homeopathy are fully fledged poisons in their own right when used at high doses.

b) The actual receptors for the drug on the regulation system becoming saturated and thus losing their efficacy for the reasons explained above apropos of receptor dynamics (Chapter 5, Section 6.3).

Within the context of complexity, the issue of doses makes even more sense and appears even more interesting than would appear to be the case merely in the light of receptor dynamics in the classic sense. The sensitivity to small doses of drug is not explained solely in terms of the increase in numbers of receptors, as might appear from a simplified view of the phenomenon, as proposed in the diagrams in Figures 21-23. If it is true that homeostatic systems are governed by the "laws" of complexity, where chaotic dynamics may easily arise and where order (information) and tendency to disorder (entropy) coexist in a state of controlled dysequilibrium, then also their pharmacological manipulation is subject to laws of nonlinearity. When a homeostatic system oscillates between order and disorder, between positive purposefulness and self-damage, or between the option of attacking the disease and that of saving a state of tranquillity, it is in a situation of great "precariousness" and "uncertainty" as regards the possible solutions adopted. This is the point which in mathematics is termed the "bifurcation point" or "symmetry break" point [Nicolis and Prigogine, 1991].

The borderline between what is considered defense and what is considered offense represents a watershed along which the body finds itself "undecided" in critical phases. At this point even the slightest piece of "exogenous" information, if properly directed and thoroughly understood, may be the crucial factor for the system in tipping the scales in favor of one or the other of two opposite attitudes (in our case, to simplify things, adaptation or reaction, receptor expression or their down-regulation, immunity or tolerance, coagulation or fibrinolysis, etc.). It might be postulated that to produce a regulatory effect the drug doses necessary will be all the lower, the more delicate and subtle the choice the system is called upon to make. In other words, in a system which can take on various different configurations or operate at different levels of activity, the intensity of the exogenous stimulus prompting the choice will be lower, the greater is the degree of "freedom" of the system itself.

What is meant here by "freedom" is the possibility of taking on different alternative configurations. In the behavior of complex systems, this may correspond to the possibility of shifting between different attractors, or between attractors of different degree of chaoticity. At one extreme there is maximum freedom, as in the case of a system oscillating through spontaneous and chaotic fluctuations, while at the opposite extreme we have a wholly deterministic system subject to precise controls and periodic behavior. As we have seen, biological systems and the human body as their maximum expression carry both characteristics (order and chaos) within themselves and therefore can be regulated both by "drastic" measures (high-dose drugs, enzyme inhibitors, surgical interventions, ionizing and excitatory radiation, to mention but a few) and by "subtle" measures (homeopathy, acupuncture, psychological and cultural factors, low-frequency electromagnetic fields, and many others).

According to this hypothesis, it would be utterly out of the question for a homeopathic remedy to act at atomic level or on simple molecules. If we want to split the nucleus of an atom (a relatively simple and highly—though not entirely—deterministic system), we must use an extremely large amount of energy, furnished only by special particle accelerators, and it cannot be done using any chemical substance, however powerful and concentrated it may be. If we want to split a cell, we have to use fairly hefty radiation, though the rays emitted by any run-of-the-mill cathode ray tube will suffice, and the splitting can also be done by acids, alkalis, or toxins at adequate concentrations. If we want to kill a man, this can be done with minimum doses of poison affecting only a minimal part of the body, e.g. the cardiac conduction system, or the respiratory center. A man can also be killed—and it happens—by a shattering piece of news (minimum energy in physical terms, maximum informational significance).

In conclusion, then, we would say that *the more complex a system is, the less energy is needed to alter its behavior and structure*. We shall come back to this point when dealing with high-dilution homeopathy (Chapter 7, Section 5.2).

6.2.5 Inhibitory or antagonistic effects

An important aspect which, for the sake of simplicity, has not been previously discussed, but which must be part and parcel of the model, has to do with the possible inhibitory effect of the drug at low doses. Clearly, what we are talking about here is the effect of biologically active substances on homeostatic control systems and therefore the context is the one we have already extensively illustrated regarding the complexity of receptor dynamics (see Chapter 5).

The binding of a molecule to its receptor produce an effect which schematically may be of the stimulatory or inhibitory type, according to which transducers are activated by the receptor and according to the possible interaction of the molecule with other molecules (forms of synergism and antagonism). Within the frame of reference we are dealing with here, then, we should not neglect the possibility that a homeopathic drug may act not so much as an *activator* of the homeostatic system (action contemplated by the model in Figure 23), but rather as a *regulator* of the homeostatic system.

This point is very important because, if things were only as outlined in Figure 23, the action of a homeopathic-type measure would make sense only when the regulatory system is completely dys-regulated, in the case in point by the receptor adaptation which leads to the lack of, or to an inadequate counterreaction to the disease. If things were exclusively in these terms, it would be impossible to understand how a homeopathic drug would be able to act in the early stages of diseases, when the regulatory system is still very efficient and, indeed, in a state of hypersensitivity or hyperactivation. In these early stages, the responsiveness of the regulatory system is intact, and it would make no sense to give the system a further stimulus, "similar" to the endogenous physiological one. This might only aggravate the disease and the symptoms, introducing an additional pathogenetic factor.

By contrast, the homeopathic and homotoxicological experience refers to therapeutic effects obtained also in the initial stages of the diseases, effects which may be regarded essentially as a reduction of symptom (see Chapter 3). Obviously, we are not talking here about suppression of the type caused by allopathic drugs, particularly if used at high doses as enzyme inhibitors, but this reduction of symptoms is nonetheless a form of suppression. When the regulatory system functions optimally, it is this system itself which leads to restoration of the homeostatic balance (healing), and the doctor's action can be no more than an attempt to reduce the subjective symptoms and any complications due to excessive expression of the endogenous reaction (including the occurrence of the blocking of the regulatory system itself).

What conceivable form can the regulatory action of a homeopathic drug take? Theoretically, such action can come about via two main mechanisms:

a) Binding or interference with receptors for endogenous activating mediators. It has been said that, in healthy subjects, a homeopathic drug causes symptoms similar to those it is capable of curing in sick individuals. To explain this apparent paradox we may postulate that the drug in question is molecularly "similar" to the endogenous mediator (a' in Figures 8, 22 and 23) so that, if administered to a healthy subject, it pursues the same line of action as the mediator: causing symptoms similar to the disease and activating the regulatory system.

In sick individuals, on the other hand, *where the endogenous mediator is already present* in large amounts, the presence of a "similar" might express itself as an inhibition of the effect of *a'* through some form of *competition or interference at receptor level*, in a manner cognate to the well known mechanism of drug antagonism in conventional pharmacology. For this to happen, it is not necessary for the drug to be present in high doses because, if it is a "similar," it may show a much greater degree of affinity than the endogenous mediator in interfering with the receptors.

b) *Binding to receptors coupled to inhibitory systems*. Another possibility of moderating the unwanted action of the regulatory system is by activating receptor systems which, once occupied, exert an inhibitory or repressive effect on the cell, on the tissue, or on the global functioning of an organ. Many receptors of this type exist (e.g. the opioid receptors in the nervous system, the adenosine A_2 receptors in blood cells, and the H_2 receptors on mast cells). If a homeopathic medicine interacted with such receptors, activating them, we might expect effects such as an immediate reduction of the extent of the symptoms or other disorders.

At this point, it might well be objected that action mechanisms of this type cannot be called homeopathic, inasmuch as they are receptor manipulation phenomena used in many well established allopathic therapies (ergotamine, beta-blockers, calcium antagonists, and so on). This objection is tenable only within the framework of a schematic preconception that there is some kind of insurmountable iron curtain rigidly separating homeopathy and allopathy. We have already expressed the opinion that many modern therapies are steadily approaching homeopathic principles, in the sense that the precise targets of drugs are being increasingly specified, molecules increasingly similar to naturally occurring substances are being used, and synergisms are being exploited with, as a result, the maximum possible reduction of doses.

6.2.6 Relationships with other therapies

Homeopathic therapy is thus a therapy of reactivation or regulation, unlike other forms of therapy which act on different levels of the pathological process (Figure 24). Most of the therapies currently employed are based either on intervention before (against the etiological factors) or after the fact (against the symptoms). Another type of intervention is replacement therapy, which is necessary when a decisive pathogenetic element in the disease is the lack of some factor, such as a hormone, vitamin, or body organ (transplants). In addition, there are also receptor therapies (cf. cimetidine, antihistamines, etc.) which are based essentially on blockade of the response of the reactive system. The homeopathic approach is quite singular, in that it rests on the endogenous systems.

According to the diagram in Figure 24, there are well established therapeutic procedures in modern medicine which (interferons, cytokines) act in a homeopathic-like way. The same is true for specific immunosuppression. However, here too, we find certain differences. In fact, while in this case the therapy is very specific (precisely targeting the receptors of the allergen), the effect is based more on the suppression of sensitivities than on the exploitation of alternative sensitivities. Actually, the question is subtler because there is evidence that the induction of tolerance in the immune system is not merely an effect of receptor suppression (this might apply to high-dose tolerance), but also an *active response* involving activation of suppressor lymphocytes. In this sense, then, specific immunotherapy might embody a number of elements resembling the action of the homeopathic drug in activating the regulatory system. It is likely that a closer examination of current practice will show that many other drugs used today work on the basis of a mechanism which is at least partly homeopathic.

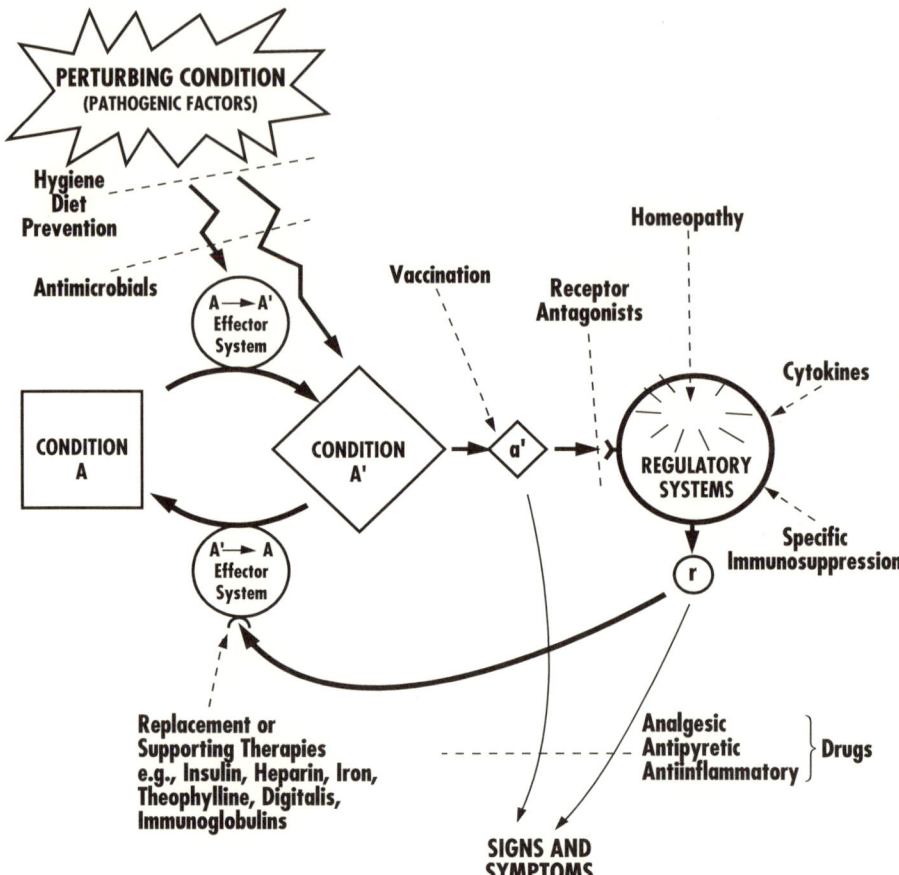

FIGURE 24 Possible levels at which various types of medical and pharmacological intervention act upon the homeostatic system.

Even a number of treatments of nonpharmacological type may act as activators of the regulatory system: for instance, hyperbaric oxygen treatment is used in the therapy of refractory skin ulcers. It is likely that such therapy does not work merely because it supplies oxygen to the tissues (this happens only during the brief period of treatment), but because, by virtue of the production of oxygen free radicals, it rekindles the inflammatory process serving the epithelial and connective tissue repair mechanism. Physical therapies such as marconitherapy or magnetotherapy (used in conventional medicine, particularly in orthopedics, cf. Chapter 7, Section 2) may act in a similar way. Finally, the relief of musculoskeletal pain by subcutaneous injection of distilled water should be mentioned: this effect, also called "counter-irritation" or "hyperstimulation" analgesia, is due to the mechanism of "diffuse noxious inhibitory control" (DNIC), referring to a widespread inhibition of the input from nociceptive afferents to dorsal horn cells [Byrn *et al.*, 1994].

In principle, homeopathic therapy is not at odds with other forms of therapy, and, indeed, may actually integrate the latter. This is a crucially important point, which has played a pivotal role in the history of homeopathy as a form of alternative medicine. It may perhaps be understandable that Hahnemann, in his day and age, when medicine had practically nothing scientific about it, should advocate his approach as the only rational and effective one (see, for instance, the notes on paragraphs 22 and 25 of the *Organon*, in which he defines allopathy as an "irresponsible murderous game with the life of the patient"). Today, however, such an attitude obviously appears anachronistic, in that, from the therapeutic standpoint, it would be desirable to be able to use all such measures as contribute towards restoring human health. For example, it is quite clear that reactivation of the regulatory system fittingly accompanies removal of the etiological factors (environmental prevention, diet, abolition of intake of toxic, allergogenic and carcinogenic substances).

Thus, one can see no reason why homeopathy cannot be combined with antibiotics in cases of bacterial disease. In this latter eventuality, the only objection which could be raised (apart from the problems raised by antibiotics already known to allopathy) is that, if we administer antibiotics when it is not strictly necessary, the regulatory system is not given the chance to function naturally and thus to sensitize itself with a view to an enhanced later response.

Somewhat trickier is the issue of the relationship between homeopathy and drugs acting via symptom suppression. In theory, a combination of the two should not be contraindicated, except, obviously, in the case where suppressor drugs are used at doses that block the functioning of the very system at which the homeopathic drug is aimed. The problem is that, effectively speaking, most of the symptoms are produced by the regulatory systems (see Figures 2 and 21) and that most of the drugs that suppress symptoms (e.g. analgesics, antiinflammatory drugs, spasmolytic agents, bronchodilators) are not very specific in biochemical and biological terms. Consequently, interference with the regulatory action of the homeopathic drug is highly likely.

Another drawback has to do with the fact that suppression of symptoms, though desirable from the patient's subjective point of view, may cause problems in terms of homeopathic *methodology*, because it makes it very difficult for the doctor to get his bearings in the choice of remedy. This is therefore a problem of a methodological type which—who knows?—may conceivably be solved by homeopathy, once the concept has taken root that *some* symptoms (for example, pain) can be removed, while others remain and can be used for homeopathic repertorization.

Lastly, as regards the relationship between homeopathy and other forms of therapy, one fairly banal, but by no means negligible fact is worth stressing. The availability of immediately effective drugs (e.g. antibiotics for infections, antipyretic agents for high temperatures, antihistamines for allergies, sedatives for anxiety, bronchodilators for asthma) tends, almost inevitably, to condition the doctor's activity, diminishing the importance of investigating the causes and of hygienic and preventive measures. Regardless of his or her good intentions, the doctor, under the weight of a heavy workload and pressing patient demands, will be inclined to resolve the symptoms with drugs of immediate efficacy rather than worrying about the underlying causes. Problems of the same ilk are invariably associated with human activities as a result of technological developments: innate faculties and capabilities atrophy owing to disuse.

The homeopathic approach, far from being an alternative to the use of effective drugs when needed, may be of help in tackling this problem because the method entails a shift in the focus of attention from the disease to the patient. For example, it is known that there are people who are prone to frequent infectious episodes, particularly of the upper airways as a result of chills, changes in climate, stress, contact with infected people in particular social settings (schools, barracks, hospitals). It is also well known that, in most cases, no precise biochemical or genetic cause can be pinpointed for such an increase in susceptibility to infection. In these cases, it is clear that the immediate cause of the infection is microbial, but also that the "terrain"—in the case in point, a certain degree of immunodeficiency—plays a decisive role. The use of antibiotics, though resolving the condition if the disease is bacterial, makes it "superfluous" in practical terms to ask oneself why the subject presents such an abnormal risk of infection. Thus, there is a risk of solving the immediate problem well, while leaving the long-term problem unsolved or relegating it to the sphere of possible spontaneous healing. Devoting attention to the "terrain" in these cases would be a more logical and more effectively preventive approach.

6.2.7 Limits of homeopathy

One logical consequence of an analysis of the models presented is also a clearer delimitation of the possible fields of application of homeopathic treatment, this being a subject which is rarely considered, precisely because of the lack of a theoretical frame of reference. Of course, the homeopathic approach, like any other form of medical therapy, presents itself as the only possible approach in certain cases, as an optional treatment in others, and as useless or perhaps even damaging in others still. Though admitting that, being a "global" approach (see below), some kind of effect will always be obtained, our model rules out the possibility that homeopathy can *resolve* the condition in cases such as the following:

a) In diseases in which the genetic component is preponderant, or rather, in the genetic component (meaning a permanent variance of the genetic code) which is present, to a greater or lesser extent, in many diseases.

b) Diseases in which there is an excessively accentuated or irreversible organic type defect, such as, for instance, cases of advanced arteriosclerosis, infarct-associated necrosis, slipped disk, etc.

c) When the etiological factor remains and strongly prevails over the reactive systems: in these cases, though the regulatory system is reactivated, the disease cannot be cured owing to persistence of an excessively intense $A \longrightarrow A'$ perturbation (see Figure 22).

d) When the regulatory system is impaired in such a way as to present no receptors and produce no signals: it might be supposed, for instance, that the efficiency of the various reaction systems declines in the elderly (homeopathy, in fact, is said to be more effective in children) or in subjects taking toxic substances or narcotics.

The logical consequence of this is that homeopathic therapy, based essentially on analysis of the symptoms and on the use of small doses of remedies, cannot be recommended, when there is a well-founded suspicion that we have to do with one of the above-mentioned conditions. To give just one example, precordial pain of sudden onset with characteristics suggestive of angina or infarct precludes an exclusively homeopathic approach and calls for an electrocardiogram and blood-chemistry tests at the very least to substantiate the diagnosis. Concepts of this sort appear only too self-evident today, and the need to integrate homeopathic practice and conventional medicine, tailoring the therapy to the diagnosis, is acknowledged also by modern homeopaths [see, for example, Tetau, 1989].

As far as tumor therapy is concerned, this is an intermediate case. The law of similars, at least in its "classic" form, proves hard to apply in cases in which gross localized anatomical alterations, such as in neoplastic growths, are overlooked by the homeostatic system in general and themselves become the main pathogenetic mechanism of the disease. Moreover, in this type of disease, as we have seen earlier, there is a genetic pathological component (mutation or translocation or insertion of oncogenes) which does not fall within the province of the disorderly functioning of homeostatic systems, but rather figures among those lesions which are practically irreversible on the molecular plane. It is impossible to see how small doses of any drug whatsoever can act on the genetic plane in an extensive cell population. Nevertheless, an approach based on principles analogous to the law of similars and aimed at activating the body's endogenous defences is not only feasible, but also positively desirable. In view of its importance and complexity, this issue will be dealt with in a later section (Chapter 6, Section 5).

Another objective limit to the possibility of effectively applying the homeopathic method may be the practical difficulty encountered in analyzing all the symptoms the patient complains of and attributing the right degree of importance to the various symptoms. In this case, this is not merely a theoretical problem, but also a question of applicability. While it is true to say that homeopathic theory holds that the same drug that causes the symptoms of the disease should be used, in actual fact *diseases are dynamic processes and symptoms often change with great rapidity*. Even the regulatory systems themselves can find themselves in a good response phase or in the phase of pathological adaptation (see Figures 22 and 23, respectively). In the same disease, drugs which are potentially active in one phase may be different from those which are active in another phase. At this stage, the new picture, theoretically, should call for another drug.

In conclusion, then, the activity of the homeopathic practitioner proves highly demanding on account of the continual changes in the clinical picture as a result of the developing course of the disease and the effect of drugs. For this reason, homeopathy, however plausible and useful it may seem in theoretical terms, is hard to apply in practice, requires a great deal of study, very substantial experience and a fair measure of inspired guesswork, and presents all the well-known problems of standardization and reproducibility in the clinical research field.

6.3

The law of similars at a pharmacological and pathophysiological level

6.3.1 Considerations on the scientific validity of homeopathy

When tackling the problem of defining the pathological process in relation to the complexity of homeostatic systems, we admitted that the intimate nature of disease is essentially unknowable and, consequently, that the empirical approach adopted by homeopathy in search of remedies for the diseases themselves is essentially legitimate.

This, however, should not lead us to believe that it is pointless to seek an explanation for the action of a homeopathic drug on the basis of its specific pharmacological properties targeting determined pathophysiological mechanisms. Given a remedy identified empirically on the basis of the global approach advocated by homeopathy (that is to say, the complex of symptoms produced by the remedy), it is always possible to work backwards, from synthesis to analysis, seeking to break down the problem of the mechanism of action by considering, on the one hand, the active ingredients of the homeopathic drug and, on the other, specific informational and regulatory disorders of the likely target systems in the body.

Many homeopathic remedies were initially proposed and studied against a total lack of knowledge as to the possible active ingredients which the extracts and initial dilutions contained and, what is more, against a total lack of knowledge as to the possible molecular, cellular and pathophysiological disorders that such remedies were supposed to cure. Today, the situation is quite different and, on the basis of current scientific knowledge, we are in a position to make many connections which previously were unthinkable. One important concept emerges from these connections: at least some of the actions exerted by homeopathic drugs on organs and systems can be explained on the basis of their active ingredients. In this section, we intend to offer a number of examples of such concepts, without desiring to deal in any way systematically with a topic of such vast scope.

The law of similars, as formulated initially by Hahnemann, was based on the similarity of symptoms, and the reasoning outlined in the foregoing section is aimed at demonstrating its substantial validity. However, precisely from what we have said it emerges that the need to resort to the analysis of symptoms is related essentially to ignorance of the intimate pathophysiological mechanisms involved in the disease. This ignorance will never be definitively overcome, owing to the complex nature of the pathological phenomena in most cases, particularly as referring to the complete analysis of the *individual patient*. According, however, to the reasoning behind the models outlined here, it is to be assumed that, if the mechanism or mechanisms of the disease were known, to achieve effective regulatory intervention it would not be necessary—indeed it would not be enough—to resort to analysis of the symptoms, inasmuch as a knowledge of the relevant biochemical, laboratory, molecular and cellular parameters and of their causes is more scientifically reliable and precise.

Assuming that a similar body of knowledge was achieved in an individual case, at this point Hahnemann's symptom-based approach would be integrated in a thoroughly and unequivocally scientific form of homeopathy. This is precisely what is happening in the field of immunotherapy, with the use of the so-called *biological response modifiers (BRM)*, vaccinations and desensitizing therapies, and even in homotoxicology itself. A factor is used which activates the function of the homeostatic system at a fairly well-known molecular level. It is thus readily predictable that *the principles of homeopathy, though not recognized as such, will increasingly pervade scientific medicine, paralleling the increase in scientific knowledge regarding endogenous regulatory systems.*

This should not prompt homeopathy supporters to fear the total "absorption" of classic homeopathy in scientific medicine because many aspects of diseases, in those areas where complexity predominates, will by the very nature of things elude description in molecular terms. In this sense, it is also likely that homeopathy may be a kind of outpost, or pilot experience, for medical research. Homeopathy, in fact, increasingly provides an enormous reservoir of empirical observations, clinical cases, and theoretical speculation built up over what now amounts to two centuries. This experimental and clinical knowledge might open up and suggest to a careful observer new lines of study of those complex regulatory mechanisms which we are gradually coming to understand in their dynamic aspects.

Also within the framework of the homeopathic world, we encounter tendencies to rationalize the law of similars according to the viewpoints of contemporary science, finding applications for it at cellular and molecular level [cf., for example, Boiron and Belon, 1990]. Thus, for instance, the *isotherapeutic* approach has been developed, whereby the etiological agent is used in a homeopathic preparation: dilutions of pollen to treat hay fever, dilutions of *Herpesvirus* to treat herpes infections, dilutions of *Candida* to treat candidiasis (needless to say, these are sterilized preparations) and similar therapies. It has also been seen that animals intoxicated with arsenic have been treated with dilutions of arsenic [Cazin *et al.*, 1987], which indicates that the similarity was sought and found at the level of the etiological agent. At another level, the similarity may be found in organs or cells: we need only consider the protective effects of phosphorus on liver damage, or the effects of phytolacca on lymphocytes and of histamine on basophils, described in Chapter 4.

There are those who propose, at least as a working hypothesis, the "homeopathic" use of allopathic drugs [Dawley, 1988]. The rationale behind this, at any rate from the homeopathic point of view, lies in the fact that precise, detailed toxicological studies have been conducted for the majority of the modern drugs in use today, i.e., in practice, their overdose effects are known. These effects could be compared to a homeopathic "proving." Thus, according to homeopathic reasoning, it should be possible to obtain therapeutic results using diluted, dynamized preparations of the allopathic drugs in two situations:

a) In patients with symptoms similar to those notoriously caused by the drug in healthy subjects.

b) In patients presenting such symptoms as adverse effects of the drug administered at high doses. In practice, this is a modern version of isopathy, or at any rate an approach that should be pursued with all due attention, also in the light of the widespread occurrence of iatrogenic diseases.

The scientific soundness of homeopathy, or at least of some of its aspects, stems from the possibility that many issues can be tackled according to the tenets of current pharmacology and can be subjected to experimental and analytical review. Whereas, on the one hand, this type of therapy, as a global, integrated approach to disease, will always present areas that are essentially unknowable and unsoundable, on the other hand, it is also true to say that many specific problems can be rationalized and clarified.

References to specific drugs and substances mentioned in the following sections can be found also in other works [Goodman Gilman *et al.*, 1980; Guermonprez, 1985; Evans, 1989; Brigo, 1990; Kent, 1990].

6.3.2 The history of nitroglycerine, a homeo-allopathic drug

To illustrate the relationship, that is evident also in the course of the history of medicine, between homeopathy and conventional pharmacology, it is interesting to note the history of nitroglycerine, which was originally studied as a potentially therapeutic agent by a homeopathic practitioner, C. Hering [Goodman Gilman *et al.*, 1980; Fye, 1986].

Hering tried the substance on himself and on his friends (synthesized not long before that for completely different purposes) over the decade from 1840 to 1850. This was the period which witnessed the birth of the great materia medicas, in whom the results of experiments on an infinite number of mineral, vegetable and animal substances were accumulated and assembled. Hering revealed that the main effects of the ingestion of nitroglycerine (which the homeopaths called *glonoine*) were headache, tachycardia and sense of precordial oppression, in addition to a very unpalatable taste. However, he did not ascribe any great importance to the cardiovascular symptoms and did not include nitroglycerine among the remedies for chest pain, leaving it mainly as a remedy for headache [Hering, 1849]. Perhaps this "oversight" was due to the fact that angina pectoris was a fairly rare disease or, at least, was rarely recognized as such at the time [Fye, 1986]. These early studies, however, are the basis for many other subsequent experiments conducted both by homeopathic and nonhomeopathic doctors, leading in 1879 to the discovery of the efficacy of nitroglycerine in angina pectoris.

This example shows that in-depth analysis of the mechanism of action of homeopathic drugs may bring homeopathy itself closer to conventional scientific medicine, whereas the latter may draw upon the empirical discoveries of homeopathy.

Other examples illustrating the fact that the two approaches are not basically in contrast can be derived from a consideration of what may be regarded as the *active ingredients* of homeopathic preparations in the classic pharmacological sense of the term. As we shall see from the following examples, examination of these active ingredients demonstrates that there is a *biochemical logic* in the use of these remedies, which, at the very least, hints at the reasons why certain drugs have certain effects on precise targets (this phenomenon is also named *biological tropism*).

6.3.3 Belladonna, Hyoscyamus and Stramonium

These are three plants of the *Solanaceae* order containing alkaloids with parasympatholytic activity: atropine, present mainly in *Atropa belladonna* and scopolamine mainly in *Hyoscyamus niger* and in *Datura stramonium*. They are extensively used in the homeopathic pharmacopoeia. According to the law of similars, these plants should be expected to be effective in syndromes with *parasympathetic blockade symptoms*, and, according to their pharmacological composition, the three remedies should present several similarities. Both of these assumptions are adequately corroborated.

According to classic pharmacology and toxicology [Meyers *et al.*, 1981; Goodman Gilman *et al.*, 1992], the effects of atropine drugs can be summarized as follows:

a) *Effects on the vegetative nervous system (VNS)*: mydriasis, dry mouth, tachycardia, postural hypotension, urinary retention and difficulty with micturition, and constipation. All these effects (except for constipation) are listed in the "pathogeneses" (list of symptoms caused in healthy human subjects) of homeopathic materia medicas. Mydriasis, dry mouth, tachycardia with a hard solid pulse and difficult micturition are characteristically present for all three plants.

b) *Effects on the central nervous system (CNS)*: drowsiness and depression, then delirium, hallucinations, sensory hyperexcitability and, with massive doses, convulsions and respiratory depression. In homeopathy, the three plants are indicated in various sleep disorders including *drowsiness* (sometimes accompanied, paradoxically, by inability to drop off to sleep), sleep too deep for arousal or agitated sleep with nightmares.

What distinguishes these three *Solanaceae*, however, in the homeopathic pathogeneses is *delirium* which is a furious, violent manifestation in all three: the patient tends to hit out, bite and tear; it is accompanied by visual hallucinations of men, ghosts, animals, and monsters. *Hyoscyamus* differs from the other two in the verbal excitement with shouting, singing, imaginary disputes or continuous incomprehensible muttering, and in the exhibitionism it produces.

Hyperesthesia is characteristic only of *Belladonna*, while impaired perception is frequent with *Hyoscyamus*. Another important coincidence of effects in toxicology and homeopathic pathogenesis is represented by the *convulsions*, which are present with subtle differences in the pathogeneses of all three *Solanaceae*. *Belladonna* acts better in the feverish convulsions of infancy. *Hyoscyamus* acts on those accompanied by automatic movements of scratching or plucking (carphology), which, moreover, are often triggered by swallowing (eating or drinking). *Stramonium* causes violent contractions of one or more muscle groups, particularly the muscles of the nape of the neck, in those experiencing its effects. As far as *respiratory depression* is concerned, the homeopathic action is more controversial, considering that *Belladonna* and *Hyoscyamus* can cause both a slowing and an acceleration of breathing, whereas *Stramonium* has no effect. Atropine and scopolamine are also known to have stimulating effects on the respiratory centers.

c) *Effects on extravascular smooth muscle*: whereas, for the CNS and VNS, the coincidence of effects in toxicology and homeopathic pathogenesis is almost total, there is a difference in the effects of homeopathic dilutions of these solanaceous plants on extravascular smooth muscle, where the coincidence can be observed not with the overdose (toxicology) symptoms, but with the ponderal therapeutic use of atropines.

These latter drugs are used in traditional therapy as spasmolytics, e.g. in hepatic and renal colic or in spasms of the gastrointestinal tract. Such indications coincide perfectly with those of *Belladonna* in its homeopathic dilution. *Hyoscyamus*, on the other hand, is used by homeopaths in spasms affecting the eyes (nystagmus) or the eyelids (blepharospasm) or bronchial muscle (spasmodic cough). In healthy subjects, *Stramonium* causes, and therefore cures, violent tics of the face and body as well as a spasmodic constriction of the muscles of the pharynx and esophagus which impedes swallowing. At the present time it is difficult to comment on such behavior on the basis of the law of similars (which would involve inversion of the effect) and of our pharmacological knowledge. However, the action of atropine on Oddi's sphincter is also unexpected: the latter contracts as a result of the action of the sympathetic fibers, while the parasympathetic fibers relax the sphincter; this, despite the fact that atropine inhibits sphincter spasm. One plausible explanation of these apparent discrepancies is to be found only if we consider the fine regulatory mechanisms at receptor and post-receptor level (presence of multiple types of receptor for the same substance, active or inactive state of the receptors, agonist and antagonist effects of the homeopathic remedy), which are topics we have already touched upon at some length in other sections (Chapter 5, Section 4, Chapter 6, Sections 1 and 2).

d) *Effects on perspiration and thermal regulation*: according to classic pharmacology, the atropines can cause suppression of perspiration, with consequent hyperthermia and redness of the skin, particularly in children. It comes as no surprise that, in homeopathy, *Belladonna* and *Stramonium* and, less often, *Hyoscyamus* are used in childhood for the treatment of fever of rapid onset accompanied by signs of parasympathetic inefficiency, mydriasis, dry mouth, and facial flushing and congestion, regardless of bacterial or viral etiology. It should be noted, however, that the feverish conditions of *Belladonna* present red, dry skin only initially, later followed by a characteristic and copious perspiration.

6.3.4 Chemical groups present in plants with a spasmolytic effect: polyenes and coumarins

An example of the possible rationale underlying the use of homeopathic remedies is provided by the study of the active ingredients present in a series of plants used with spasmolytic and analgesic indications, though the relationship with conventional pharmacology is less clear than in the previous example. Among these plants, the most representative is *Matricaria chamomilla (wild chamomile)*, the common chamomile, which, in homeopathy, has a spasmolytic, analgesic, antiinflammatory and sedative action. The classic disorders in which it is indicated are unbearable pain, neonatal and infantile flatulent colic with foul-smelling diarrhea, intolerable dysmenorrhea, certain types of fever and otitis, and a number of convulsive syndromes. Bringing it down to three words, we are talking about inflammation, spasms, and hyperesthesia.

In the case of chamomile, the entire flowering plant is used, from which the mother tincture is obtained according to the international standard procedures [Brigo, 1990]. The most interesting constituents are: an essential oil containing chamazulene, a proazulene (matrizin); a polyene dicycloether; a number of polyphenols; coumarins and flavonoids.

Particularly worthy of note is the combination of *coumarins* (products containing a C=O carbonyl group) and *polyene derivatives* (with several C-triple bond-C acetylene groups). This combination is found not only in chamomile, but also in other plants used by homeopaths in convulsive syndromes: *Cicuta virosa* (water hemlock) contains coumarins (umbelliferone and scopoletol) and polyacetylene derivatives (cicutol and cicutoxin); *Oenanthe crocata* contains numerous polyacetylene derivatives and a carbonylated derivative, a ketone, latifolone or crocatone; *Artemisia vulgaris* (mugwort) contains a polyacetylene derivative with a ketone function, artemisia ketone. This type of combination thus appears to be a constant feature of many plants with an anticonvulsive effect. It should be noted that the homeopathic use of such plants seems to be directly related to their very similar chemical composition, despite belonging to very different families from the botanical point of view. *Cicuta* and *Oenanthe* are *Umbelliferae*, while *Chamomilla* and *Artemisia* are *Compositae*.

The polyene derivatives are to be found in two groups of plants:

a) Those with a homeopathic action in the convulsive syndromes: *Cicuta virosa* (spasms in hypertension, epilepsy), *Oenanthe crocata* (epilepsy), *Aethusa cynapium* (convulsions of newborns unable to tolerate mother's milk and suffering from gastroenteritis), *Artemisia vulgaris* (menstrual or peripuberal epilepsy), or, in any event, in various diseases with spasms: *Chamomilla* (in certain convulsions), *Conium maculatum* (tremors, esophageal spasms), and *Grindelia* (dyspnea, bronchoconstriction).

b) Those with a homeopathic action on the inflammatory process and on hemostasis: *Chamomilla matricaria*, *Arnica montana* (traumatisms, ecchymoses, toxic-infectious syndromes), *Bellis perennis* (traumas, ecchymoses, hematomas), *Echinacea angustifolia* (suppuration, abscesses), and *Erigeron canadiensis* (traumatic hemorrhages, ecchymoses).

Lastly, we should mention those plants with carbonyl function derivatives other than coumarins: *Strichnos nux vomica*, *Strichnos ignatii* (strychnine and brucine, indole alkaloids), *Moschus moschiferus* (muskone, an aromatic ketone), *Anamirta cocculus* (picrotoxinin, a highly oxygenated sesquiterpene with several ketone groups), *Crocus sativus* (an essential oil with carbonyl derivatives from safranal and isophorone), *Castoreum* (acetophenone, a ketone), *Ambra grisea* (dihydro-g-ionone, a volatile compound with a ketone function), *Valeriana officinalis* (pyrryl-a-methylketone and the dipyridylmethylketone, an alkaloid called the "main" alkaloid), *Oenanthe crocata* (crocatone, a polycyclic ketone), *Actea racemosa* (carbonyl of the ester function of actein), *Artemisia cina* (santonin, a sesquiterpene lactone), *Gambogia* or *Garcinia hanburyi* (numerous compounds with a carbonyl function including benzophenone), *Cephaelis ipecacuanha* (carbonyls of ipecoside, an azotized heteroside). Also the mollusc Sepia officinalis contains a black pigment with double carbonyl groups (sepia-melanin). All these compounds, when diluted and dynamized and then administered to healthy human subjects in the so-called homeopathic pathogeneses, produce symptoms related to spasms of smooth or striated muscle fibers (in very different areas of the body), and in many of these the presence of such symptoms is essential for the prescription of the remedy (e.g. *Nux vomica* or *Ignatia* or *Moschus*), while in others it is secondary (e.g. *Sepia*). A fair number of these (*Ignatia*, *Moschus*, *Castoreum*, *Ambra grisea*, *Actea racemosa* and *Valeriana*) are indicated for subjects with a hysterical temperament who manifest changeability of humor, loquacity, paradoxical behavior, and frequent fainting.

The fact that several plants share similar components such as the carbonyl and acetylene groups and that it is these components which at least partly explain the pharmacological effect strongly suggests the existence of a non-casual biochemical and pharmacological basis for the effects of homeopathic drugs.

6.3.5 Ipecac or Cephaelis ipecacuanha

This plant is a *Rubiacea* native to Brazil and Central America, but which is also cultivated in India and Malaysia. The part of it used is the dry root which contains 4–5% of minerals, 30–40% of starch, an allergizing glycoprotein, a tannin (ipecacuanic acid), 1.1% of ipecoside (an azotized heteroside with an isoquinoline ring) and 2–3% of isoquinoline alkaloids, the most important of which are emetine, cephaeline and psychotrine.

Ipecacuanha syrup is used in therapy as an emetic, particularly on account of its *emetine* content, which toxicologically causes:

a) Gastrointestinal symptoms, such as diarrhea, nausea, vomiting and cramping abdominal pains, due to its direct action on the intestinal musculature.

b) Neuromuscular symptoms, such as weakness, pain and stiffness of the skeletal muscles, particularly those of the neck and the extremities.

c) Cardiovascular symptoms including hypotension, tachycardia, dyspnea and ECG abnormalities.

This justifies the homeopathic use of *Ipecac* in diarrhea syndromes, especially if accompanied by nausea, and also in the most disparate syndromes where nausea of central and not gastrointestinal origin is experienced. It may be noted here, in support of the rationale underlying the use of homeopathic remedies by analogy with the pharmacological knowledge, that the specific indication for *Ipecac* is not nausea of gastrointestinal origin, which is characterized by a dirty tongue and is improved by vomiting, but only that where the tongue is clean and moist, salivation is copious and the attacks of nausea are not improved by vomiting. This observation was made by homeopaths back in the last century, long before such nausea could be defined as *central* and, above all, long before it was known that there is a chemoceptor trigger zone in the medulla oblungata and that emetine acts precisely at this level. Furthermore, emetine hydrochloride in a homeopathic dilution is generally preferred to the dry root *in toto* if the diarrhea and nausea are accompanied by hypotension and tachycardia, which are toxic manifestations of emetine and not of the extract of the dry root *in toto*.

Another rational comparison of the use of ipecacuanha in the conventional vs. the homeopathic pharmacological traditions can be done at the level of the respiratory tract. In fact, this vegetable drug is undoubtedly active as an expectorant, but its use has been substantially limited by the presence of the appreciable side effects mentioned above (nausea and vomiting); it was present in a number of antitussigenic preparations and was used at times by asthma sufferers who were unable to tolerate other drugs. The homeopathic use of this plant is fairly similar, and is prescribed in respiratory tract diseases with cough, dyspnea, bronchospasm and bronchial hypersecretion; yet, to stress once again the global action of homeopathic drugs, it is particularly indicated if the bouts of coughing are accompanied by nausea or if nausea and diarrhea figure frequently in the patient's medical history.

Summarizing the tropism of *Ipecacuanha* and referring back to the previous chapter, it can be said that *Ipecac* has a distinct spastic tendency in its effects on both the gastrointestinal and respiratory tracts. From the biochemical point of view, this is probably due to the presence of several carbonyl groups in the ipecoside.

6.3.6 Anthraquinone derivatives and diarrhea syndromes

Another example confirming the link between the constituent vegetable active ingredients and the actions of the homeopathic remedies obtained from these plants is provided by the plants used as laxatives both in the popular tradition and in modern pharmacology. These are a liliaceous plant, *Aloe ferox*, a leguminous shrub, *Cassia angustifolia*, or senna, and two *Polygonaceae*, *Rheum officinalis* or rhubarb and *Rumex crispus*. These plants all contain anthraquinone derivatives (aloin and rhamnosides of aloin) the laxative action of which is well known; in homeopathy, the action of these plants on the large bowel is confirmed, though obviously with inversion of the effect. In fact, all these plants are characterized by action on diarrhea syndromes, especially *Aloe*.

6.3.7 Coffea

Originating in the highlands of Abyssinia, the coffee plant was introduced into numerous tropical regions of Asia, America and Australasia. In homeopathy green coffee is used, that is to say the coffee bean stripped of its coverings, as it presents itself prior to torrefaction, which produces the aroma. For this reason the remedy is called *Coffea cruda*. In the green coffee bean some 3–4% of minerals can be measured, mainly calcium phosphate and sulphate; citric, malic and oxalic organic acids; carbohydrates and glycosides (over 50% of dry weight); lipids (from 10 to 15%); abundant acid phenols (from 5 to 10%), the most important of which is chlorogenic or 3-caffeoylquinic acid; scopoletol; azotized compounds including serotonin amides and particularly caffeine (from 0.6 to 3%).

Of all these compounds the most interesting and intensively studied is undoubtedly *caffeine*. Caffeine, like theophylline and theobromine, is a purine-based methylated xanthine derivative. Its best known pharmacological action is stimulation of the CNS: in experimental conditions it induces an increase in ability to sustain intellectual effort, a reduction in reaction time and a better association of ideas. However, after ingestion of 1 g (15 mg/kg) or more of caffeine, corresponding to plasma concentrations of more than 30 µg/ml, insomnia, restlessness, excitation and hyperesthesia occur. Another effect of caffeine on the CNS is stimulation of the bulbar respiratory centers, probably because it raises sensitivity to CO_2 stimulation; this action, however, is encountered much more often when respiratory function has been depressed by certain drugs, such as opioids. One last effect on the CNS is nausea and vomiting.

The cardiovascular system is also subject to the action of caffeine. Doses greater than 400 mg, i.e. approximately 5 cups of coffee, increase the sinus rhythm, the formation of ectopic impulses and the cardiac contraction force.

Lastly, caffeine is capable of stimulating both acid and pepsin gastric secretion and the secretion of catecholamines.

To explain the therapeutic effects of methylxanthines, reference is frequently made to their ability to inhibit the phosphodiesterases for cyclic nucleotides. Pharmacological studies, however, clearly show that the therapeutic concentrations do not coincide with those necessary to bring about an increase in cyclic AMP. On the other hand, methylxanthines act as competitive antagonists on the adenosine receptors at concentrations which fall very comfortably within the therapeutic range. Adenosine is actively involved in numerous local regulatory mechanisms, especially at CNS syn-apsis level; for example, adenosine inhibits the release of neurotransmit-ters from the presynaptic structures and reduces the neuron discharge rate; in addition, it induces dilation of the coronary and cerebral blood vessels and slows down the activity of cardiac pacemaker cells.

In homeopathy, *Coffea* is used in three main conditions:

a) The most frequent is *insomnia*, and particularly that due to cerebral excitation with continual hyperideation; the subjects for whom it is usually prescribed are agitated, excitable and inclined towards euphoria. In the materia medicas they are described as "full of ideas and quick to act." Thus, the homeopathic therapeutic use appears to coincide with the toxic effect of caffeine on the CNS at ponderal doses.

b) A second indication is *hypersensitivity to pain* and of all the senses, particularly the sense of hearing, in view of the fact that any pain is aggra-vated by noise. Some authors claim, however, that this sensitivity is due not so much to caffeine as to the chlorogenic acid contained in green cof-fee [Guermonprez, 1985].

c) The third indication is a condition of *hypersympathicotonia* which also embraces tachycardia and tachyarrhythmias. This latter indication of *Coffea* in homeopathic dilution may also be compared with the action of caffeine at pharmacological doses on the myocardium.

6.3.8 Active ingredients and inverse effect

The indications outlined above are only a few examples of how, taking homeopathic empiricism as our starting point, a line of study akin to mod-ern pharmaceutical reasoning can be pursued. Of course, a broader-rang-ing effort of analysis and experimentation would be necessary to provide systematic documentation of the soundness of these concepts.

Table 6 schematically summarizes the possible relationship existing be-tween active ingredients in the preparation, the "homeopathic" effect and the biological and biochemical action of the active ingredients themselves.

The result is a significant demonstration of how, once we admit the possibility of inverse effects, the homeopathic effect can be viewed in terms of an action pharmacologically targeted at one or more physiological sys-tems: the biological effect of the active ingredient is "similar" to the ho-meopathic indications of the remedy itself. Considering the fact that many homeopathic remedies were identified and applied empirically long be-fore their targets at pathophysiological level could be understood, the re-lationships illustrated here provide surprising "a posteriori" evidence of the soundness of the homeopathic empirical tradition. It goes without saying, of course, that the examples given here constitute only a small, indicative part of a field which is extremely vast and highly complex, inasmuch as homeopathic remedies often contain a multiplicity of active ingredients. The inverse and paradoxical effects of many drugs have been discussed also by others [Teixeira, 1999; Eskinazi, 1999].

TABLE 6 **Relationships between a number of active ingredients of homeopathic remedies and their possible pharmacological effects**

Drug	Homeopathic indications	Active ingredient	Biological effects
Apis	Edema Pomphi Itching	Melittin	Activates mast cells
Phytolacca	Lymphadenitis Pharyngitis	Mitogenic pokeweed	Activates lymphocytes
Nux vomica	Spasms Hyperesthesia	Strychnine	Blocks post-synaptic inhibition
Ipecac	Nausea Vomiting	Emetine	Activates spinal chemoreceptors
Silica	Chronic inflammation	Silica	Activates macrophages
Opium	Drowsiness Euphoria Constipation	Morphine	Mimics endorphins and enkephalins
Belladonna	Mydriasis Dry mouth Agitation	Atropine	Blocks muscarinic and cholinergic receptors
Iodum	Tachycardia Anxiety Hot flushes	Iodine (via thyroid hormones?)	Activates metabolism
Coffea	Insomnia Hypersensitivity Sympathicotonia	Caffeine	Increases cAMP Adenosine antagonist

6.4

Considerations on auto-hemotherapy

In our account of the variants of homeopathy (Chapter 2), mention was made of autohemotherapy as a particular form of isotherapy performed with the patient's own blood. It consists in withdrawing a certain amount of the patient's blood, treating the blood with ozone or homeopathic drugs, and re-administering it to the patient, usually by the intramuscular route [Kief, 1988; Kirsch, 1989; Kief, 1991]. Other authors make high homeopathic dilutions (30c or 200c) of patient's blood in distilled water and give it *per os* [Richardson-Boedler, 1994]. Since in this section we do not deal with high dilutions but are interested in the application of the *similia* principle in this particular sector, the topic is discussed considering the use of whole blood or of blood used at low dilutions, i.e. containing putative active principles in molecular form.

As can be seen, the procedure is technically simple, but what is not clear is its efficacy, its mode of action, its indications and its contraindications. We cannot review here all the problems, some of which serious, which make this modality a subject of much debate and indeed a questionable practice. The procedure is interesting because it may provide a valid example of an "interface" between homeopathy and problems within the domain of modern immunology. Autohemotherapy is based on the homeopathic principle: administering to the patient something which contains active ingredients of the disease, in this case autologous blood.

Here we shall consider a number of hypotheses as to the possible mechanism underlying the therapeutic procedure termed autohemotherapy, particularly when this is applied to the treatment of allergies. The mechanism of action of autohemotherapy may be interpreted in the light of the most recent advances in knowledge regarding immunological homeostatic systems, most notably in the context of the idiotype network theory.

Up until the mid 'sixties the reactions of the immune system were viewed in terms of the ability to recognize and eliminate, through the antibody (B lymphocytes) or cellular (T lymphocytes) response, non-self antigens, largely originating outside the individual, or antigens deriving from abnormal modifications of endogenous substances. Following the discovery of anti-antibody antibodies, it was appreciated that the interplay between antigens, antibodies and cells of the immune system is a far more complex matter.

Credit is due above all to N. K. Jerne, the 1984 Nobel Prize-winner for Medicine, for constructing a model (the *idiotype network*) to explain these interactions. According to this theory, which is universally accepted today [Jerne, 1974; Blaser and Weck, 1982; Golub, 1984; Male *et al.*, 1988; Perelson, 1989], the antibodies, as proteins, are themselves antigens and thus an antibody (antibody-1, or "Ab1"), directed specifically against a certain foreign antigen (in our case, for instance, an allergen) presents a particular structure (*idiotype*) in its variable part called Fab (Fragment antigen binding), and this idiotype may evoke the formation of specific antibodies (*antiidiotype*, or "Ab2") (Figure 25).

These antiidiotype antibodies in turn evoke the formation of anti-antiidiotype antibodies, or "Ab3." Ab1, Ab2, and Ab3 are produced in different (decreasing) amounts in the course of a normal immune response. We do not know what the effective degree of "ramification" of the system is, but it would not appear to go beyond Ab3 or Ab4 [Male *et al.*, 1988].

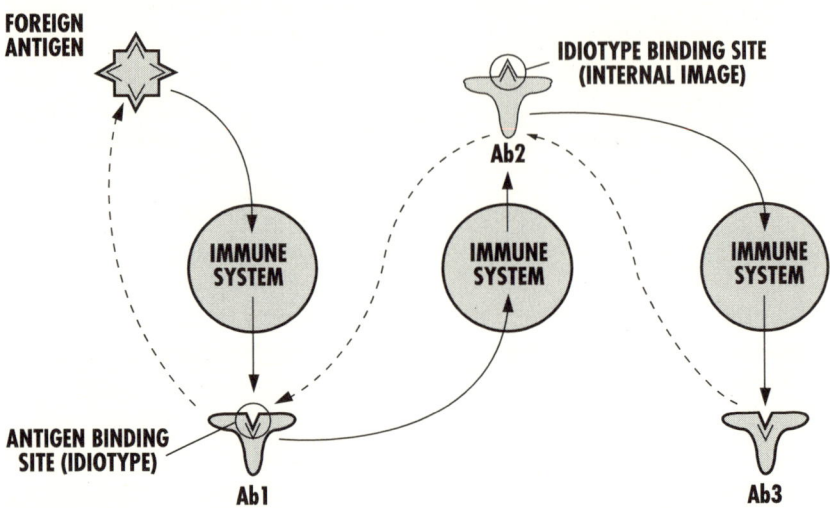

FIGURE 25 Schematic representation of the formation of antibodies to a foreign antigen (Ab1) and of antiidiotype antibodies (Ab2 and Ab3). Solid lines = stimulation of the system or production of antibodies; dashed lines = blockade of the antigen or idiotype regulation. For the sake of simplicity, the antibody is represented as univalent (i.e. binding an antigen with only one region).

On this basis, various mathematical models have been developed in order to be able to make quantitative predictions regarding the behavior of lymphocyte clones during the immune response [Perelson, 1989]. On analyzing immune dynamics (e.g. the trend of the production of a certain antibody) by these means, it has been seen that it always presents oscillations in which the concentrations of idiotype and antiidiotype antibodies fluctuate inversely with peaks recurring roughly every 80 days. If. however, a number of parameters of the system-model are changed, even only slightly (such as, for example, the rate of formation of new B cells in the spinal cord), the fluctuations become irregular or even aperiodic (chaotic). An interesting point is that such substantially irregular oscillations have also been found in experimental immunizations in the rat [for a review see Perelson, 1989].

Since the antiidiotypes recognize and bind to Ab1, they have a physicochemical structure "*similar*" to the allergen (which also binds to Ab1) and represent, so to speak, the "*internal image*" of it produced by the body (see Figure 25).

The fact that the antiidiotype (Ab2) is in many respects similar to the original antigen has already been exploited by immunologists to produce vaccines which are used when the administration of the original antigen is inadvisable for reasons of safety (e.g. particularly dangerous viruses). In this case, the patient who receives an antibody resembling the pathological antigen will produce anti-antiidiotype antibodies (Ab3) which will be similar to Ab1 and thus will furnish a certain degree of protection against the antigen we are seeking to induce immunity to. Another possible application, still, however, at the experimental stage, is the use of antiidiotype antibodies in autoimmune diseases [see, for example, Verschuuren *et al.*, 1991].

This whole series of interactions does not have the pathological significance of the known anti-antibody antibodies present in autoimmune diseases, but appears to perform important regulatory functions. In fact, the binding of an antibody to the idiotype of another antibody may have a number of major consequences, namely:

a) The neutralization of the possibility of binding the "natural" antigen (or allergen), by masking the recognition site.

b) Elimination of the aggregate antibody complex by the phagocyte system.

c) Blockade of the receptors for the antigen on B lymphocytes, these being receptors which notoriously present the same idiotype as the antibody that the cell will produce; thus blast cell formation, cloning and maturation of the B plasmacell line specific for that antibody are also blocked.

d) It cannot be ruled out that a strong antiidiotype response may even lead to the elimination of the lymphocyte clones through cytolysis or apoptosis, with the result that a state of permanent desensitization might be expected.

Though the theory was originally proposed in terms of interactions between antibodies and B cells, it now also embraces T cells, which present antigen-specific receptors on their surfaces. T-lymphocyte receptors also present a variable part which therefore expresses a particular idiotype, which can be recognized and may interact with an antiidiotype receptor on the T cells or with an antiidiotype antibody. Inclusion of the T cells makes the interpretation of the possible physiological functions of the system enormously more complex. There are, in fact, various types of T lymphocytes, the main ones being those of the *helper* type (which increase the immune response) and those of the *suppressor* type (which inhibit it). There is evidence that idiotype-specific cells of both helper and suppressor type can be formed.

The interactions at idiotype network level, both of B and T cells, are very important in the regulation of processes controlling both the quantity and quality of the immune response. Malfunctioning of the idiotype network forms part of the mechanisms causing the onset of autoimmunity: since a certain amount of autoimmune reaction is also present in the healthy body, it is the idiotype networks (and more specifically their "*connectivity*") that govern the transition from innocent to aggressive autoimmunity [Kumar and Sercarz, 1991; Cohen, 1991; Varela and Coutinho, 1991].

Other experiments, conducted in the mouse [Kelsoe *et al.*, 1981; Blaser and Weck, 1982] have shown that injection of idiotype has modulatory effects on the immune system depending upon the dose injected. For example, 10 µg of antibody suppress the production of anti-antibody, whereas 10-100 ng stimulate it. It has also been seen that it is easier to obtain suppression in young animals than in adults [Male *et al.*, 1988].

The induction of T cell mediated suppression can be explained by the fact that the idiotype injected binds with T suppressor cell receptors and stimulates them, inducing the proliferation of a clone of antiidiotype T lymphocytes. These cells then interact with and suppress B cells expressing the idiotype, blocking the production of antibodies. There is experimental evidence that B cells, antibodies and T cells have receptors with similar or identical idiotypes [Blaser and Weck, 1982]. It should be noted that, for the T-B interaction (in which cells of the macrophage series also participate) to be able to take place, recognition of the HLA group is also necessary. In other words, these mechanisms operate only between cells belonging to the same HLA group.

What we have said here above refers to studies conducted on the normal IgG immune response. Evidence is available that the idiotype network also plays a role in the regulation of the IgE response, which is the most important (though not the only one) in the pathogenesis of allergic manifestations. In synthetic and necessarily simplified terms, the main pathogenetic factor in allergy, or type I immediate sensitivity, is excessive production of IgE antibodies in subjects who are particularly sensitive to given allergens. These antibodies then bind with their constant fragment (Fc) on the membrane of the circulating basophils and mast cells in the connective tissue, mainly subepithelial. When the allergic (sensitized) subject again comes into contact with the allergen, this binds to the Fab part of the cellular IgE and triggers the release of histamine and of other inflammation-promoting substances. According to the area where the reaction is maximal, there will be various manifestations such as urticaria, rhinitis, conjunctivitis, edema of the glottis, asthma, and diarrhea, and even anaphylactic shock if the reaction is generalized.

According to some researchers [Katz *et al.*, 1979], the formation of IgE is minimal in normal subjects and kept at low levels by a disactivation mechanism consisting in T suppressor cells and their soluble factors. Depression or malfunctioning of this disactivation mechanism might trigger sensitization whereas the stimulation of IgE-T suppressors might restore the state of health. Neuroendocrine mechanisms are also certainly involved in allergic reactions, if we consider, for example, that cortisone has a potent depressant effect on lymphocyte responses and that some nerve endings in connective tissue can release neuropeptides (substance P) which are capable in themselves of stimulating the mast cells to secrete histamine.

Going back for a moment to autohemotherapy, it can therefore be postulated that this procedure could enable us to intervene in the delicate equilibrium regulating the IgE response and thus the allergy. By introducing the patient's own blood by the intramuscular or subcutaneous route, critical factors are introduced into the network, which are vectors of specific information: antibodies, immune complexes and lymphocytes (especially T lymphocytes, which are the ones most commonly present in the bloodstream) bearing particular idiotypes. Aided by the inflammatory reaction caused by the blood in an extravascular site and, possibly, by the large amount of lipid material supplied by the erythrocyte membranes (that could work as an adjuvant), these factors may stimulate the production of antibodies (IgG or IgM) capable of neutralizing IgE, or may stimulate the production of idiotype-specific T lymphocytes capable of suppressing their corresponding IgE-producing B cell counterparts.

The administration route is of considerable importance. In fact, one possible objection to the hypothesis propounded here might be based on the fact that in autohemotherapy what is administered is the patient's own blood and thus something which is obviously already present throughout the immune system and tolerated as "self." This would therefore fail to explain an anti-idiotype response greater than the physiological one. One answer to this objection, hypothetically, may be that via the intramuscular or subcutaneous administration route the idiotype-specific factors (B or T receptors or antibodies) are expected to reach the immune system (lymph nodes) across the cortical sinus, which is the most appropriate route for it to be recognized, processed by the phagocytes and presented to the lymphocytes. As already discussed previously (Chapter 5, Section 6.1), by changing the introduction route of the antigen opposite effects can be achieved in the immune response.

Equally important may be a partial chemical modification of the antibody (or of the lymphocyte receptor) [see Sehon, 1982]. This modification, which transforms the "identical" into the "similar," might come about during the inflammatory response (intervention of proteases, formation of carrier-hapten processes, protein and proteolipid aggregates) as a result of the very presence of blood in an extravascular site. The transformation of the "identical" into the "similar" may be a mechanism for bypassing immune tolerance and inducing the anti-idiotype response.

In the context of this type of reasoning, an explanation may be found for the fact that, according to certain authors [Kirsch, 1989], on treating blood with ozone prior to reintroducing it into the body, earlier and more effective therapeutic responses are obtained. Ozone, a potent oxidizing agent, would make the idiotype (or the adjacent parts of the protein structure) slightly different from the naturally occurring idiotype, thus stimulating a much more intense response. In animal models of autoimmune diseases (experimental allergic encephalomyelitis) it has been seen that modification of no more than a single amino acid in the protein inducing the autoimmunity (myelin basic protein) transforms it into an agent capable of preventing the autoimmunity itself [Smilek *et al.*, 1991].

The regulation of the formation of antibodies involves both helper and suppressor effects, and an alteration in the equilibrium between them may be triggered by an antiidiotype response. In this connection, it is significant that the formation of IgE is particularly susceptible to suppression by the antiidiotype. In some cases, concomitant suppression of the IgE response and activation of the response of other antibody classes have even been observed. This is important because the specific suppression of the entire immune system may be deleterious for defense against a pathogenetic antigen and its elimination [Blaser and Weck, 1982].

Among the possible mechanisms involved in autohemotherapy we would probably also be well advised to consider the "aspecific" reactions, namely those reactions which are not directly related to immunity to a certain substance. In a patient's blood, in addition to the antibodies and activated lymphocytes, there are many other components potentially endowed with biological significance. For example, cytokines, interleukin soluble receptors, and cytokine antagonists, are all highly active substances, even in small doses. It is plausible that, in every disease and at every stage of the disease, particular "constellations" of various compounds of this type are created for regulatory purposes. In other words, there is also a *cytokine network*. At this point, the use of blood of this type may prove very efficacious in regulating nonspecific responses. The inhibition of the degranulation of basophils *in vitro* by blood dilutions may be due to such effects [Sainte Laudy *et al.*, 1986].

Despite the fact that the foregoing considerations may conjure up suggestive intervention possibilities, we must make it quite clear that, owing to the complexity of the immune system, it is to date impossible to construct a model which enables us to establish with certainty what happens as a result of the introduction of autologous blood according to the auto-hemotherapy procedure. It is by no means easy to predict the response in the individual patient or even to know whether this procedure, which undoubtedly constitutes a "perturbation" of a delicate equilibrium embracing many components, may entail a risk of aggravating the patient's immunological status.

In a critical review of the problem, one point which can hardly fail to capture our interest is the fact that the clinical evidence is in favor of auto-hemotherapy, in that it shows a significant number of cures or improvements in allergic patients. What is more, no serious side effects have been reported, if we exclude the occurrence of fever syndromes. Since, however, the literature on this subject is fragmentary and for the most part not retrievable by consulting current texts of immunology, further and more detailed research is necessary. Particularly in the treatment of severe diseases of the immune system such as AIDS, where the use of auto-hemotherapy has also been proposed and experimented with (apparently unsuccessfully) [Garber et al., 1991], it is absolutely mandatory to proceed with all due caution using reliable assessment procedures for evaluating the efficacy and harmlessness of such techniques. It has been recently reported [Schirmer et al., 2000] that intramuscular injection of autologous blood in combination with *Formica rufa* D6 failed to improve the clinical course of ankilosing spondylitis. In conclusion, then, it would be desirable to clarify the biological basis of a method which might, if properly known and conducted under strict surveillance, constitutes a valid approach in the management of various disorders of the immune system and of inflammation. Essentially, two main avenues of research could be explored:

a) Conducting large-scale strictly controlled clinical trials to establish the validity of the procedure and its adverse side effects, if any. In these clinical trials the investigators should take into account not only the subjective symptomatological aspect, but also the instrumental aspect (e.g. spirometric determinations in forms of asthma) and, above all, the laboratory aspect (antibody assays, assays of lymphocytes belonging to the various subclasses, all the relevant allergy tests).

b) Intensifying research into the biological basis of autohemotherapy, investigating, for example, whether the effect depends on administration of antibodies, or of lymphocytes, or other blood components (cytokines, immune complexes). Furthermore, animal models could be developed (particularly in mice) which are much easier to manipulate in experimental terms. Most of the studies on the idiotype network have, in fact, been conducted in mice, so much so indeed that many aspects of this theory in human subjects are purely hypothetical.

In this section we shall tackle the problem of possible new therapeutic approaches to tumors, not with the intention of providing indications for therapeutic practice (this would be both beyond the bounds of the aims of this book and beyond the sphere of competence of its authors), but with the intention of illustrating how complex the problem is and the possible contribution of the homeopathic approach in this field, at least from the theoretical point of view.

The giant strides made by oncology in recent years in the fields of surgery, radiotherapy and chemotherapy are there for all to see. Malignancies which until not so very long ago carried a thoroughly negative prognosis are now treatable and even curable today. At the same time, the necessary awareness and means of intervention have also increased as a basis for an effective prophylactic effort. Much, however, still remains to be done and to be understood before we can claim to be satisfied with the therapeutic measures available to medicine in the struggle against these diseases.

On the basis of our analysis of the situation in Chapter 5, Section 3, where we reviewed the basic elements of our knowledge of molecular pathology in cancer, we might be tempted to ask ourselves whether the dispelling of the darkness shrouding the pathogenesis of cancer allows us to project new and more effective therapeutic measures. Realistically, we are still a very long way from seriously capitalizing on such knowledge from the therapeutic point of view, though certain tendencies and lines of research now appear highly promising.

6.5.1 Problems related to possible therapeutic measures

The existence of various phases linked to epigenetic events (see the concept of neoplastic "*promotion*" illustrated in Chapter 5, Section 3.3) and to the intervention of exogenous and endogenous factors which control and promote tumor growth (see the concept of neoplastic "*progression*") partly modifies the notion of a tumour as a chance event, subject to the laws of probability and ultimately unmodifiable in its dynamics, unless through some form of destructive attack (surgery, chemotherapy).

The basic question is the following one: *if it is true that neoplastic disease is subject to a progressive dynamic trend, might there also be a regressive dynamic trend?* The recent studies on this issue enable us to give a partly affirmative answer, at least from the theoretical standpoint and on the basis of experiments in cell cultures. It would appear, in fact, that tumor growth is not inevitably progressive, not entirely uncontrollable, and not necessarily irreversible. Little can be done to modify the transformed gene (oncogene), but a great deal could be done to block its deleterious effects. Hope lies therefore in being able to act effectively at epigenetic level, as argued, for instance, by L. Sachs: "*The genetic abnormalities that give rise to malignancy can be bypassed and their effects annulled by inducing the differentiation that blocks multiplication*" [Sachs, 1989].

A number of theoretical possibilities of inducing tumor regression using means other than conventional radio- and chemotherapy or surgical approaches are the following:

a) *Immunotherapy*, consisting in potentiating the defenses of the host organism by administering immunotoxins (antibodies to the tumor, acting as vehicles for toxins), interferons and cytokines, or cells treated with interleukin 2 (LAK), or other natural or artificial immunostimulating agents such as bacterial extracts or polysaccharides (research here is breaking extensive new ground) [Uchida, 1993].

b) *Blockade of oncogene expression*, by means of the addition of appropriate agents such as interferons (α-interferon seems particularly important, above all because its efficacy in certain tumors has been demonstrated [Gutterman, 1994]) or antagonists of the tumor promoters, such as, for example, bryostatin, genistein or corticosteroids.

c) *Blockade of the protein production of oncogenes*, by means of the administration of antisense oligonucleotides specific for the oncogene or oncogenes involved, which would interfere with the mRNA and thus with protein synthesis in the tumor cells.

d) *Induction of cell differentiation*, by means of specific tissue-specific factors, hormones, vitamins (e.g. vitamin A, or vitamin D3), sodium butyrate, and other agents which would bring the cells to more mature stages, with consequent arrest of proliferation.

e) *Induction of expression of anti-oncogenes* (very important, but for the time being purely theoretical, since little is known about their products and their modes of regulation).

Among all these possibilities corticosteroids have been in use for some time now in the treatment of leukemia, but more recently there has also been the use of vitamin A (retinoic acid) and, particularly, that of cytokines (such as interleukins, interferons, and tumor necrosis factor), because these agents have pleiotropic effects, acting both on the host and on the tumor. It would appear important to base the intervention not so much on a single cytokine as on a combination of two or more cytokines so as to be able to exploit their synergistic effects and thus reduce the doses and home in on the target or targets. From tests in cell cultures it would also appear that the combination of a cytokine (such as tumor necrosis factor) and a chemotherapeutic agent (such as adriamycin) makes it possible to use very low doses of both to overcome the resistance of the tumor cells to the treatment [Bonavida et al., 1991; Taylor Safrit et al., 1993]. In view of their importance, these lines of research are actively pursued with promising results.

The problems that hinder a simplified approach to the modulation of the neoplastic growth are multiple, and this is all the more true, if we consider the possible clinical applications. We can do no more here than merely touch upon a number of open questions:

a) Therapy with cytokines or with LAK cells has often been characterized by serious side effects and, moreover, appears effective only in a minority (albeit by no means negligible) of the tumors in which it has been tried.

b) The differentiation factors and the cytokines themselves may be mitogenic factors in some cancers, thus accelerating tumor progression.

c) The proliferation-inhibiting factors can hardly be expected to possess such a degree of specificity as to be able to inhibit only the tumor, and thus they may have immunosuppressive side effects (e.g. corticosteroids).

d) The antisense oligonucleotides (which theoretically would have the enormous advantage of selectivity) work in cell cultures, but only at doses that could hardly be used in vivo, where they would also be rapidly degraded.

e) In general it is difficult to predict the actual doses that reach the target cells, especially in the case of molecules with a poor tissue diffusion capability or which are not easily picked up by the receptors.

f) One last problem has to do with the fact that the trials with the new drugs must first be conducted in animals, despite the fact that, in this field, animal models are not always predictive of the outcome in human subjects.

What we have said thus far may suggest, by and large, that a disease as complex as cancer necessarily calls for a subtle, sophisticated, complex diagnostic and therapeutic approach, taking good care to individualize the treatment. Alongside the traditional strategy of "attack" (surgical, pharmacological or radiotherapeutic), which, as is well known, is capable today of resolving many cases of cancer, we may postulate that the identification of the various and multiple factors contributing towards cancer development may enable us to take efficacious remedial action for inducing regression, or at least for slowing down tumor progression.

Faced with all the various possible levels of dys-regulation in the system as a whole, we can hardly suppose that the reductionist approach will prove resolvent, whereby, knowing the molecular mechanism involved, we can then intervene with a specific drug, just as we can hardly suppose (and history demonstrates it) that pure empiricism will prove resolvent, whereby on the strength of continual trial and error a recipe will be found for curing cancer. It is, however, experience, scientifically based and methodically controlled, that will have the last word regarding the usefulness of a treatment. Faced with a problem of enormous complexity, modern biomedical science and the empirical approach, which often comes up with new and unexpected aspects of reality, can meet on common ground and integrate one another, each providing its own specific contribution.

6.5.2 The law of similars in oncology

In this context, what role can homeopathic medicine play? First and foremost, we should stress the serious danger posed by those methodological approaches which expressly claim to be an alternative to conventional medicine—aiming at its exclusion—on the basis of purely empirical or intuitive reference markers. Such approaches, which are perhaps less open to criticism in other fields of medicine where the patient's life is not at stake, take no account of the biological reality or of the advances in scientific knowledge of cancer and therefore cannot fail to be inadequate in terms of results. It goes without saying that, in those cases where healing by allopathic means is reasonably possible, homeopathy can play no more than a secondary role. In the current state of our knowledge and experience, homeopathy cannot be considered as an antitumor therapy, in the sense of being able to attack the tumor directly. In this field, there are no important, convincing studies, but there are theoretical objections regarding the efficacy of homeopathic remedies in resolving diseases involving the genetic component of the cell (cf. Chapter 6, Section 2.7).

In tumors, particularly when diagnosed at an advanced stage, the molecular, cellular and systemic alterations are so advanced and serious that the "similarity" between the symptoms of the remedy and those of the patient, as expressed in the classic version of the law, proves hard to detect and is barely applicable. In other words, since the identification of suitable remedies is supposed to be based on experiments with such remedies in healthy subjects, where they are supposed to cause symptoms similar to those of the disease, it is unthinkable that such experiments can be conducted in such a way as to cause tumors in healthy people. To this one might object that it is, in any event, possible to implement homeopathic therapy not aimed directly at the tumor, but at the overall complex of the subject's neuroimmunoendocrine characteristics, in an attempt to restore their homeostatic equilibrium. This is undoubtedly true, but two major outstanding problems remain:

a) How can such characteristics be identified in a situation where the tumor has created such a severe and profound upheaval in the patient's body?

b) How can a treatment aimed at the fine regulation of homeostasis act within the context of such a strongly and progressively degenerating clinical and biochemical picture?

Having said this, it does not mean that we cannot express a number of general considerations on the subject, which is most certainly of considerable topical interest.

If the basic problem is at the informational level (genetic or epigenetic), it ought to be expected that, in theory, a good therapeutic intervention should consist in providing the system with the "right" information in a form that can be received and utilized at the level of the control system that has undergone a loss of homeostasis. In this sense molecules, too, are items of information (good or bad, as the case may be; for example, the viral oncogene is "bad news" for a cell!) and in this sense they are often used in therapy. Once we have excluded the possibility that the weak and complex information provided by homeopathic medicines can have any chance of defeating a tumor in its progressive phase, we have to ask ourselves whether or not the homeopathic approach can have a positive impact *on a number of aspects of the body's struggle against the tumor.*

As regards the contribution that homeopathy, and natural medicine in general, might perhaps be able to make in the field of modern oncology, one aspect which in the first place appears to be of particular interest is the study of a number of drugs of vegetable origin such as the extract of *Viscum album*, which first came to light in the empirical tradition and today have clearly and surprisingly (if we think of the way they were discovered) been shown in scientific studies to contain active ingredients of both immunostimulant and cytotoxic type against cancer cells [Koopman *et al.*, 1990; Gabius *et al.*, 1992a; Gabius *et al.*, 1992b; Kuttan and Kuttan, 1992].

The methodological approach of homeopathy and homotoxicology, however, is not only important for its ability to supply empirically identified natural remedies, but is worthy of note above all because it tends to provide an overall picture of the patient in his or her entirety and particular pathophysiological individuality, the essential programmatic and methodological characteristics being the painstaking, systematic effort to gather the greatest possible amount of information about the patient's state and history, together with the basic guiding concept that to be effective a treatment must aim first of all at treating the "host" or "terrain," i.e. at treating the patient before treating the disease.

In this connection, it is worth recalling that homotoxicological theory [Reckeweg, 1981] defines cancer as a dynamic process which is in a certain sense progressive vis-à-vis inflammation, when the latter has not been completely resolved (see also Chapter 2, Section 6). From the therapeutic point of view, homotoxicology has introduced the concept of *"regressive vicariation,"* according to which stimulating the process of expulsion of "homotoxins" ("excretion phase") and inflammation ("reaction phase") with various biological means may constitute a way of preventing or combating the transition to degenerative or neoplastic phases of disease.

These concepts, though generic, appear to be consistent with modern cytokine therapies which, while being much more controllable and scientifically sound, are based essentially on the same biological principle: activating inflammation and immunity for the purposes of utilizing these systems to the full to attack the tumor. Using purified cytokines or mixtures of them, as is done today in a number of antitumor protocols is not *substantially* very different from the administration of the old B.C.G. (bacillus Calmette-Guérin, an attenuated strain of the Koch bacillus) or of the homeopathic nosodes (which are essentially extracts of tissues with pathological processes in progress and thus containing mixtures of cytokines in addition to the etiological agent). Cytokines, in fact, are normally produced *endogenously* whenever the inflammatory reaction is activated.

From a theoretical standpoint, cytokine therapy is, in a certain sense, akin to the homeopathic approach. These molecules, in fact, are produced in the cancer patient and are responsible for a fair amount of the symptoms: we may recall, for example, the effects of the tumor necrosis factor, which causes lack of appetite, weight loss to the point of cachexia, fever, shock and a whole series of biochemical disorders. In small doses, the same molecule serves to activate the leukocyte antitumor defenses.

An even more marked degree of analogy with the homeopathic approach can be found in treatments aimed at providing specific immunotherapy for cancer. In this field there have been many attempts in the past, and interest in this line of research has been rekindled thanks to new ideas and new experiments [see, for example, Chen *et al.*, 1992; Boon, 1993; Fathman, 1993; Dranoff *et al.*, 1993; Dalgleish, 1994; Gong *et al.*, 1997; Kugler *et al.*, 2000]. Though this is not the place for a systematic analysis of such a vast and varied problem, some brief mention at least of the basic principle of this specific immunotherapy is worthwhile. What the various proposals have in common is the use of the cancer cells themselves, suitably treated in order to "unmask" their antigens so as to specifically stimulate the defenses against the tumor. A very interesting way of achieving this "unmasking" would appear to be to insert into the tumor cells by genetic engineering additional signals for the lymphocytes, which, in this way, may be able to "understand" that the tumor cells are extraneous to the body and thus give the go-ahead for rejection of the tumor. In other words, an attempt is made to "present" the tumor cells to the immune system, which previously failed to recognize the tumor, the purpose being to activate the reaction of the immune system.

The above-mentioned approach is a very sophisticated use of a "similar" in order to enter into the subtle information network of that complex homeostatic system known as immunity. The law of similars is transferred from the sphere of similarity between symptoms to that between cellular and molecular mechanisms. This is not entirely in keeping with classic homeopathic reasoning, which, for the reasons already discussed, programmatically seeks to focus upon the entirety and the complexity of the human being. The fact, however, that it does not fully comply with the law of similars does not mean that it conflicts with it. Rather, we might start thinking—without departing from the province of theoretical indications—in terms of intervention at various levels:

a) Fighting the tumor mass according to the conventional "allopathic" approach (surgery, chemo- and radiotherapy).

b) Regulatory measures on the biological plane and nonspecific immunotherapy (see previous section).

c) Specific immunotherapy using the tumor cells themselves.

d) An attempt to restore overall psycho-neuro-endocrine homeostatic equilibrium by means of psychotherapy and/or the classic homeopathic approach.

The possibility of integration between conventional and complementary approaches to cancer treatment is also suggested by a recent survey in the *British Medical Journal*, which reported that in Britain a sizeable percentage (16%) of patients receiving conventional treatments for cancer also use complementary therapies, the most commonly used being healing, relaxation, visualization exercises, diets, homeopathy, vitamins, and herbalism [Downer *et al.*, 1994]. The study was not an attempt to investigate the efficacy of complementary therapies in these diseases, but rather to look at what proportion of patients used complementary therapies and at their satisfaction with these treatments. Apart from the difficulties caused by diets in some patients (weight loss, unpalatable nature of the diet, time and money spent preparing the food), patient satisfaction with complementary therapies was in general high, even without any hope of an anti-cancer effect. Benefits were mainly psychological, such as an increase in optimism and feeling emotionally stronger. Individual patients also reported physical effects, including less difficulty in breathing, reduced nausea, and increased energy.

As regards the above-mentioned study, it is worth stressing that even if the main outcome of such complementary therapy in cancer was of a psychological nature, it would in any case be an important result in this type of patient.

We can conclude, then, by saying that, despite all the inaccuracies related to the paucity of scientific research conducted in this field (a situation which is improving today), the homeopathic and homotoxicological approaches appear to integrate the modern concepts stemming from experimental oncology. Obviously, we should stress once again that the considerations expressed here remain within the province of theoretical speculation and that the intention is not to champion the actual usefulness of homeopathic and homotoxicological remedies as a primary prescription in oncology. Any such usefulness, to our mind, has still to be demonstrated in practice by means of appropriate clinical trials.

The relationship of cancer therapy and homeopathy (as a complementary approach in addition to conventional treatment) has recently been discussed by others [Montfort, 2000; Schraub, 2000].

7 *The Biophysical Paradigm*

The search for a scientific rationale on which to base a hypothesis regarding the mechanism of action of homeopathy led to examination of the subject of complexity, within the framework of which, essentially, the rational explanation of the "law of similars" and of the possible effects of very small doses of natural compounds and extracts deriving from pathological processes has been inserted. We have already stressed that this is the inspiring concept of homeopathy and makes it relatively easy for homeopathic drugs to play a complementary role in the context of scientifically orthodox pharmacology.

We must now continue further along these lines and address the problem of ultra-low doses (more precisely termed *high dilutions*, or *high potencies* according to classic homeopathic parlance), i.e. those which contain virtually no molecules of the active compound. There can be no doubt that the conceptual leap here is enormous and that the topic we are about to address appears so much out of this world as to make any attempt to suggest that such issues can be investigated scientifically seem no more than mere folly. In the face of such challenging objections, which critics of ours have raised on numerous occasions, since we have no incontrovertible proof (we have seen that the clinical trials and biological tests have yet to yield definitive evidence, and many apparently outstanding results need to be repeated and reproduced), we have no alternative here but to refer to what more authoritative figures than ourselves have had to say apropos of studies in the frontier areas of science.

We are all familiar with the position of the philosopher of science, Karl Popper, one of the best known and most widely accepted modern epistemologists, according to whom scientific method does not consist in demonstrating and affirming certainties, but rather in the continual invalidation of previous theories. In other words, it is a matter of "learning systematically from errors," in the first place by having the courage to commit them, i.e. by propounding new and even daring theories, which one then attempts to confute by means of experiments [Popper, 1969].

A similar concept had already been voiced by Claude Bernard, who might be defined the father of the experimental method in medicine: "Those who have condemned the use of hypotheses and preconceived ideas in the experimental method have made the mistake of mixing up the process of designing the experiment and the ascertainment of the results. It is perfectly true to say that you have to ascertain the results of an experiment with the mind unbiased by hypotheses and preconceived ideas, but absolutely nothing must prevent you from making hypotheses when setting up an experiment and searching for means of information. On the contrary, as we shall see below, imagination must be given free rein; ideas are the source of all reasoning and all invention; it is to ideas that all forms of initiative are due. The imagination should not be suffocated or crushed under the pretext that it may be harmful: it only needs to be controlled and given a decisive cast of truth, and this is something quite different. (...) Even if the hypothesis is not confirmed and has to be abandoned, the facts that it has helped to unearth will remain an integral part of the indestructable body of scientific knowledge" [Bernard, 1973, pp. 33-34].

Later, Bernard goes on to say: "When, in our science, we construct a theory, the only thing we can be certain of is that, by and large, this theory is false in terms of absolute value. Theories are only partial and provisional truths which are used in order to proceed with the research, as we use the landings of a staircase to rest on the way up; they correspond to the present state of our knowledge and therefore are necessarily bound to change with the progress of science, and this process will be all the more rapid, the more backward science itself is in a given field. On the other hand, as we have said, our ideas arise from the study of previously observed facts which are interpreted at some later stage. Now, countless causes of error may creep into our observations, and, despite all our attention and perspicacity, we can never claim to have detected them all because often we do not possess the means, or the means are still far from perfect. Our reasoning, then, if it is to guide us in experimental science, does not oblige us to accept all its consequences. Our mind remains free at all times to accept them or to question them. One should not reject an idea, when it comes into being, simply because it is not consistent with the tenets of some prevailing doctrine. One should rather heed one's feelings and give free rein to one's imagination, on condition that all our ideas only serve as a pretext for other experiments that may provide us with new and fruitful data" [Bernard, 1973, p. 46].

Those who propose to tackle subjects such as the ones we intend to deal with here, at least in terms of ideas and hypotheses, are therefore not operating beyond the pale of the scientific method. Of course, what we report here constitutes a body of facts and theories which still need to be properly systematized, but can certainly offer scope for experimental tests which will eventually confirm or disprove various specific points.

The need to go beyond chemistry and biochemistry, thus entering into the domain of a *biophysical paradigm*, to explain the effects of very high homeopathic dilutions is obvious: if we do not wish to accept *a priori* (as we do not wish to here) either the "null" hypothesis (= it's all an elaborate swindle) or explanations of an extra-scientific type (the action of certain, undefinable "entities" or "energies"), once the lack of molecules beyond the 24x or 12c dilutions has been ascertained mathematically, we are obliged to think in terms of information related to phenomena of a physical nature, such as vibrations of electromagnetic fields or particular spatial structures of the solvent which in some way reproduce the "image" or "information" of the original solute.

In addition to theoretical considerations, the participation of physical mechanisms in the action of high dilutions of homeopathic remedies can also be deduced from the results of several experiments already reported in Chapter 4, demonstrating that:

a) The dilution-dynamization phase is critical and is influenced by the nature of the solvent and by the atmospheric environment in which it takes place.

b) The activity of high dilutions can be destroyed by heat and by electromagnetic waves.

c) The specificity of the effect (biological tropism) also exists in the absence of the original substance.

Though it is premature to draw general laws of action of homeopathic remedies from such indications, all these considerations prompt us to focus our attention on the physicochemical characteristics of the solutions used and on the role played by electromagnetic phenomena in the structuring of liquids and in biological communication.

The possible application of electromagnetism in medicine was envisaged, albeit with a great deal of caution, by Hahnemann himself, who, in paragraph 286 of the *Organon*, stated: "The dynamic force of mineral magnets, electricity and Galvanism act no less powerfully upon our life principle and they are not less homoeopathic than the properly so-called medicines which neutralize disease by taking them through the mouth, or by rubbing them on the skin or by olfaction. There may be diseases, especially diseases of sensibility and irritability, abnormal sensations, and involuntary muscular movements which may be cured by those means. But the more certain way of applying the last two as well as that of the so-called electro-magnetic machine lies still very much in the dark to make homoeopathic use of them. So far both electricity and Galvanism have been used only for palliation to the great damage of the sick. The positive, pure action of both upon the healthy human body have until the present time been but little tested." These comments highlight once again, on the one hand, Hahnemann's perspicacity and insight as a forerunner of modern developments in medicine, and, on the other, the ingrained characteristics of the medical researcher and experimenter.

In summary, to be able to accept that the ultra-diluted homeopathic drug acts via a biophysical mechanism, two basic questions need to be answered:

a) Can a solvent, such as water or water containing various percentages of ethanol, incorporate and maintain some form of order or organization acting as a vehicle for information in the absence of the original solute? In other words: does the notorious "memory of water" exist and, if so, how can it be accounted for?

b) Admitting that order and information can be incorporated and maintained in the highly diluted solutions, how can they interact with biological phenomena? In other words: how does the body interpret and receive these properties of the homeopathic remedy and use them in a regulatory sense?

It must be perfectly clear to all and sundry that it is only by providing convincing answers to these questions that any serious claim can be made for the existence of a scientific basis for high-dilution homeopathy.

In this chapter we shall present many indications, reported in the literature, regarding the peculiar properties of water, which may be of interest with a view to providing an answer to the first of the two above-mentioned queries. In this case, too, of course, we will not be able to develop the topic in systematic, specialistic terms, which would be a task beyond our personal expertise and outside the scope of this book. The study of water is one of the major chapters in physics [Franks, 1982; Franks and Mathias, 1982]. Despite the fact that the knowledge of this extraordinary substance is far from complete, what is known for sure at present *does not rule out* the possibility, at least, that water may act as a store and transmitter of biologically significant information.

7.1

The biophysics of water

7.1.1 Certain characteristics of water

As we have already pointed out, water, despite the simplicity of the molecule, exhibits a typical complex behavior in phase transitions and in the liquid state, when it finds itself in an *"open"* system which exchanges energy with the environment (Chapter 5, Section 8.1). The topic is analyzed here in greater detail, providing notions of a theoretical type and indications of an experimental nature.

Interpretations of the behavior of water in the liquid state are generally formulated in terms of short-range interactions, such as, for instance, the hydrogen bonds and the van der Waals forces, which in some way link together the water molecules in a kind of *network*. Since the hydrogen-oxygen bonds are polar covalent bonds, with the hydrogen positive compared to the oxygen, the attraction between the negative region linked to the oxygen atom and the positive region associated with the hydrogen atom of another molecule leads to a combination of various water molecules, with the result that an irregular network of interlinked tetrahedral forms is created (see Figure 26) [Stillinger, 1980]. Moreover, the water molecule is not linear, but the oxygen atom forms an angle of 104.5° with the two hydrogens. As a consequence, the molecule has a resultant *dipole* moment.

In three dimensions the interlinked tetrahedral structure forms very regular pentagonal and hexagonal figures in ice, though such as to be present also in the liquid, except that they continually vary in a chaotic manner in the latter. Statistically, a network structure with a certain form changes to a different form every 10^{-11} or 10^{-12} seconds. The changes can come about as a result of the fact that the molecule is sufficiently elastic to support minor distortions of the aperture angle.

Each water molecule is capable of forming four hydrogen bonds with the neighboring molecules, in each of which a proton (H^+) is directed towards the electrically negative zone of the oxygen atom. One molecule behaves as a donor of protons to another two, whereas it also becomes an acceptor of protons from another two: the protons are therefore shared by two oxygen atoms and consequently are in continual *movement* or *oscillation* between two atoms.

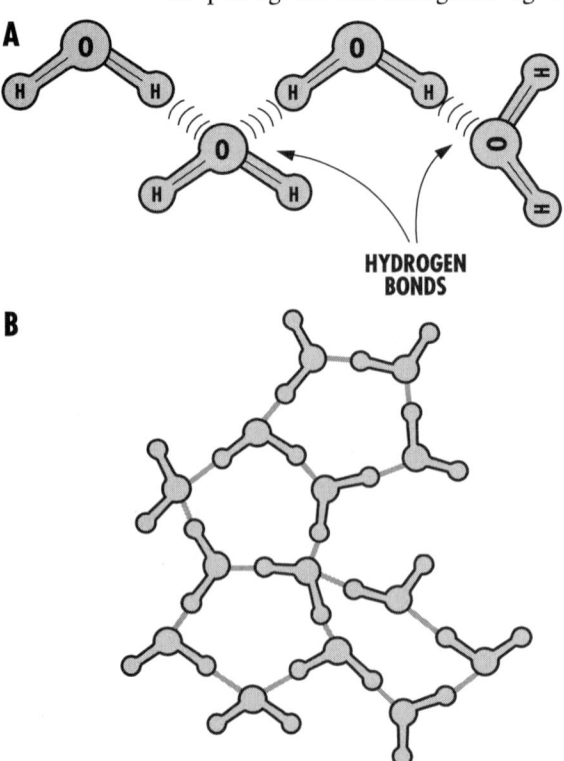

HYDROGEN BONDS

FIGURE 26 A: hydrogen bond between water molecules; **B**: tetrahedral and irregular polygonal structures in liquid water.

These types of interactions have been described as "hooks" which link up the neighboring water molecules and constrain them, when the temperature is below 100 °C, in a more condensed (fluid) physical state compared to water vapor where there are no bonds, but only random collisions between molecules.

The liquid must be defined as a homogeneous yet irregular arrangement of molecules. The structure of the liquid is not crystalline as occurs in the case of ice, and research has also ruled out the possibility that there may be crystalline areas in the liquid [Finney, 1982], though certain investigators talk about a "quasi-crystalline" structure [Stillinger, 1980]. In fact, to say that the arrangement of the molecules is irregular does not mean that the water molecules are in a state of total disorder; the disorder is limited by the particular geometry of the molecules, which tend to form bonds in the form of tetrahedra, and probably by other phenomena related to the dipole moment which will be considered here below.

No anywhere near precise description of the laws governing the arrangement of water molecules and thus of the phase changes of water has yet been produced. Here, for instance, is what the physicist D. Ruelle has to say about it: "Here we have a tricky problem for theoretical physicists: demonstrating that, if we increase or decrease the temperature of the water, there will be phase changes that yield vapor or ice. A tricky problem, alright... but too difficult! We are still a very long way from providing the demonstration required. Effectively speaking, there is not a single type of atom or molecule for which it can be demonstrated that crystallization will occur at low temperatures. These problems are too difficult for us. In actual fact, it is by no means rare in physics to find oneself faced with problems that are too difficult to solve..." [Ruelle, 1992, p. 136].

There are two major unsolved problems: the first has to do with the interaction between neighboring molecules. In the model presented above (chaotically interlinked tetrahedra) we need to assume that the total energy of N molecules depends on the sum of the energies of interaction between each individual pair of molecules, i.e. of each hydrogen bond. Given two molecules that interact in a liquid, it must be assumed that the binding energy is not altered by other neighboring molecules. This assumption would not appear to be applicable to water on the basis of both theoretical and experimental considerations [Finney, 1982]. The existence of influences of other neighboring molecules on the binding of two molecules is certainly not devoid of consequences: multiple cascade interactions are generated which may substantially change the random behavior of the molecules, introducing phenomena of *cooperativity* and *coherence*.

A second major point has to do with what happens when a different molecule is dissolved or immersed in water: the structure will certainly change and break, according to the properties of the new molecule. In addition, at the interface between macromolecules and solvent, an enormous structural reorganization of the water takes place, the latter taking on thoroughly new configurations, even at a considerable distance from the solute molecule. In this case, the cooperative effects are undoubtedly very important. In this connection, various investigators talk about "*vicinal water*" by which they mean water which is near to solid surfaces or macromolecules and is influenced by these. For instance, a protein chain with alternating positive (NH) and negative (CO) chemical groups should polarize the surrounding water, reduce the rotation and translation movements and give rise to the formation of many orderly states of water molecules. These particular modifications of the structure of water extend, according to the various investigators, over distances measuring from 5 to 200 molecular diameters from the surface considered.

This phenomenon does not coincide with the well-known molecular interactions between water and surfaces (e.g. ion-dipole or dipole-dipole interactions), which are of the high-energy, short-range type. Vicinal water, on the other hand, extends much further than the specific surface interactions [Drost-Hansen, 1982]. This may have major implications in the functioning of cells, which are known to be rich in macromolecules, fibers and membranes.

The properties of vicinal water are peculiar: it is denser than normal water and freezes only at temperatures many degrees below zero, and its solvent properties are also altered. It has been suggested that many enzymes, thought to be dissolved in the cytoplasm, are actually weakly associated with the surfaces of fibers or membranes by interaction with vicinal water, with the result that many metabolic processes are thought to occur in conditions of organization on two-dimensional planes rather than in the chaotic motion of free water [Clegg, 1982].

For the purposes of illustrating the possible implications that acceptance of the existence and importance of "vicinal water" would have in the cell, we can refer to the theory expounded and developed primarily by Ling and coworkers [Ling et al., 1973; Ling and Ochsenfeld, 1983; Rowlands, 1988]. Sodium ions are known to have a low concentration within the cell as compared to outside it, whereas the opposite is true of potassium ions. The current theory is that these differences in concentration are maintained by membrane pumps, but, according to Ling, if this were true, there would be an excessive energy consumption just to operate the pumps. Ling thus suggests the hypothesis that the potassium inside the cell is almost entirely bound to proteins, whereas the sodium ions, which have a greater hydration volume, are less soluble in the orderly, polarized vicinal water of the intercellular fluids, compared to the ordinary water present in the extracellular fluids. Thus potassium is thought to be retained and sodium excluded from the cell by means of mechanisms which do not require a constant supply of energy.

The possible implications of vicinal water for cell physiology have also been discussed and documented by Bistolfi within the framework of a biophysical theory of biological communications systems [Bistolfi *et al.*, 1985; Bistolfi, 1989]. Following in the footsteps of Hameroff [Hameroff, 1988], Bistolfi postulates that the water adjacent to the cytoskeleton is highly ordered, i.e. aligned with polar bonds on the surface of the filamentous proteins. This ordered water may be coupled with the coherent dynamics of the proteins (which, as is known, are made by the assembly of a large number of subunits), opposing the thermal dissipation of the protein oscillation energy. In other words, the filamentous proteins may be conductors of vibrational signals and the vicinal water may be a kind of insulating agent favoring conduction.

Recently, evidence has been accumulating in favor of the hypothesis that water molecules participate in proton transfer in various biochemical reactions, including, among others, the photoreceptors [Khorana, 1993]. A series of concatenated water molecules joined together by hydrogen bonds are thought to form a system whereby protons (H^+) "hop" from one oxygen atom to another and travel significant distances. In other words, the water molecules arranged in order are thought to resemble a lead carrying a current of positive charges.

7.1.2 Superradiance

After outlining some of the unsolved problems in the study of the properties of water in the liquid phase, we can now tackle certain issues with a closer bearing on homeopathy. These relate to theoretical models and empirical experience which suggest the existence of a real physical basis for the homeopathic phenomenon.

A group of physicists from the Milan Institute of Nuclear Physics (Emilio Del Giudice, Giuliano Preparata, and coworkers) have for some years now been working on the formulation of a descriptive model of the physics of dense matter and in particular of water in the liquid state, which may make a by no means negligible contribution towards solving the enigma of homeopathic phenomena, or, at least, may serve as support for those who regard some form of biological activity of ultra-diluted solutions as "theoretically not impossible."

We shall attempt here to summarize the essential aspects of the work of this group [Del Giudice *et al.*, 1988a; Del Giudice *et al.*, 1988b; Del Giudice, 1990], ignoring many of the technical details and mathematical formulae to be found in the above-cited studies.

These investigators take as their starting point a critique of the theory of water in the liquid state which contemplates only interaction via the hydrogen bond between one molecule and another. According to their calculations, when the water vapor liquefies, the gas-liquid phase change, which involves something like 10^{23} molecules/liter, is too swift and massive (also bearing in mind that it takes place at 100 °C, under very strong thermal agitation counteracting the electrostatic attraction) to be explained solely by a model based on the existence of the hydrogen bond uniting two neighboring molecules. A more satisfactory model should also include another ingredient, which is lacking in the previous models, namely the *electromagnetic radiation field*, i.e. a long-range messenger which brings order to the vibratory motion of the molecules.

It has been seen that water molecules are electric dipoles. The contribution of this small electromagnetic field to the dynamics of water is negligible in quantitative terms if the interaction between molecules is taken as the sum of intermolecular binary interactions. When, however, a large number of elements (molecules) interact via the electromagnetic field, beyond a certain density whose value depends on the wavelength of the electromagnetic field, the system sets itself in a configuration in which most of the molecules *move coherently, being kept in phase by the field itself.* This phenomenon is termed *superradiance* and consists practically in an oscillation of a large number of water molecules (an estimated 10^{15}) in unison over time in a certain space (corresponding to half the wavelength). Given that the typical wavelength of electromagnetic radiation is 200 μm, the coherence domain would extend approximately 100 μm.

The studies of the Milan group have now gone far beyond the discovery of superradiance, in that another two issues of basic importance for the problem of high-dilution homeopathy are dealt with in their model:

a) The stability of such a phenomenon over time (something similar to a "memory").

b) The interaction between the superradiance regimen and the solute molecules.

According to quantum theory, it is possible that two separate phases coexist in liquid water: one phase subject to the coherence regimen, and another made of molecules that move randomly like a gas, which is a situation also described for superfluid helium and in keeping with experimental observations whereby the hydrogen bonds between the water molecules are much fewer than would be theoretically possible if all the molecules were involved [citations in Del Giudice, 1990]. That proportion of the molecules that vibrate coherently "see" one another as immobile and thus the electrostatic attraction due mainly to the hydrogen bonds is not random as in the gas, but sequentially ordered in packets in which the forces of interaction are enormously greater than in the gaseous phase.

Del Giudice and Preparata's theory is that the groups of molecules that move coherently are maintained in the superradiance regimen both as a result of the actual electromagnetic field produced (which, as we have seen, controls significant distances) and because they are protected by the "shell" of strong hydrogen bonds formed as described. The coherent phase of the water is therefore rather stable and other molecules find it hard to enter. According to Del Giudice, within the coherent phase the entropy is virtually zero, and the thermal and solvation properties of water depend only on the fluid (gas-like) phase.

What we have to ask ourselves now is how such a model can be the basis for the storage of some type of information. This would be possible if the coherent electromagnetic vibration could be influenced, or *modulated*, by outside chemical or physical forces, so as to take on a certain frequency and somehow enter into communication with other chemical, physical or biological systems. This hypothetical property of water is supported by the model according to which it resembles a *free electric dipole laser*. In this type of laser, an ondulatory field induces, in a beam of free electrons, an oscillating electric dipole, transverse to their movement, which is coupled to the electromagnetic radiation and vibrates coherently with the latter [Del Giudice *et al.*, 1988a]. Starting from the finding that water molecules possess a considerable dipole moment, these investigators have provided the theoretical demonstration that they *can interact coherently* with a suitable form of electromagnetic radiation. Given the phenomenon of collective interaction, it is not necessary to postulate a very strong electric field, since even the slight electric perturbation around a macromolecule with a dipole moment, or the field present on the surface of a colloidal aggregate would be enough. Around such "impurities" present in the water, then, a macroscopic domain could be generated, of the order of a few hundred µm, formed by the superradiance of water. Since distances of this order might involve tens or hundreds of cells in a body tissue, the potential importance of such a phenomenon on the biological organization will be immediately appreciated.

To get back to the subject of homeopathy, according to Del Giudice the particular preparation of the homeopathic drug enables us to postulate that the succussion accompanying the dilution produces a regime of turbulence such that for a moment or so the shell of hydrogen bonds of the coherence domains *relaxes*, thus offering an external electric field (such as that generated by the dissolved material) a chance to communicate with the polarization field of the water and assign it its new vibratory frequencies. At the end of the succussion, the shell will re-form, protecting the new frequencies from outside disturbances.

According to this model, the presence of other molecules dissolved in the water (as impurities, mineral salts, or biological molecules) causes no problems for the frequencies thus stabilized, both because the solute is in the fluctuating phase and does not interact with the coherent phase, and because the frequencies of the molecules in solution are much greater than those of the semi-solid dispersion grains and macromolecules with which homeopathic drugs are normally prepared (see trituration process) [Del Giudice, 1990].

It may seem advisable at this point to recall that, given the present state of our knowledge, the theories set forth above still await convincing experimental confirmation demonstrating, for instance, by chemical or physical means, the existence of the superradiance domains postulated. However, we feel we should stress that modern quantum physics does not rule out the possibility that water may possess hitherto unknown properties and that these are somehow compatible with the empirical observations of homeopathy. Those who accuse homeopaths of scientific inconsistency should first familiarize themselves with the physics of water in the liquid phase, so as to be in a position to raise objections (whereby certain theories are in themselves absurd, or certain phenomena impossible) not based merely on so-called "common sense." Judging natural reality on the basis of common sense, or even on the basis of prejudice, has often proved a substantial source of error, and this is all the more true when we enter the various fields of quantum physics.

Though far from clarifying or unequivocally demonstrating the physical basis of homeopathy, physical theories such as the superradiance theory enable us to confute those who, being unaware of the possibilities of water-mediated long-range interactions, consider it theoretically impossible for a molecule to transmit information independently of direct contact with another molecule.

7.1.3 "Activation" of water and colloidal reactions

On dissolving a normal substance, such as an electrolyte or sugar, in water, a system is obtained consisting of molecules or ions dispersed in the aqueous medium, which cannot be separated by filtration and are invisible with optical means, even under the electron microscope. If, however, we suspend a powder of insoluble substances in water, a heterogeneous system is obtained consisting of microscopic solids in a dispersing aqueous phase, such that the various phases are easily separable using filter paper. Somewhere between these two extremes there is a range of sizes of particles suspended in a dispersing medium, such as to make it hard to establish whether it is a homogeneous solution or a heterogeneous suspension. Such systems are called colloids, and the colloidal state must be regarded as a special state of matter, with its own particular properties.

These properties are, for example, the fact that colloids are not retained by common filters; they spread slowly in electrophoretic fields; they can easily pass from the colloidal to the gel state, forming reversible or irreversible clots. In addition, colloids present particular optical properties such as the Tyndall effect (visibility of light rays passing through a colloidal solution) and the absorption in particular bands of the visible spectrum depending not only upon their chemical composition but also upon their physical state (particle size, surface charge, variations according to pH). Colloidal systems consist of particles made up of from 10^3 to 10^9 atoms, with sizes ranging from 1 to 100 nm. There are both inorganic (e.g. colloidal gold, colloidal sulphur, silver bromide) and organic colloids (starch, cellulose, agar-agar, natural rubber, polymerized cell proteins).

The formation of colloidal particles (clusters) occurs from atoms and molecules according to the "rules" of aggregation by diffusion, complicated by the fact that even the particles themselves have a tendency to aggregate. As mentioned previously (Chapter 5, Section 7), these physical processes are neither fully ordered nor completely random, being part of those growth phenomena which can be interpreted in terms of the geometry of fractals and chaos [Sander, 1986].

At a level of magnitude smaller than colloids, but still larger than molecules, are the so-called microaggregates. These consist of a group of atoms or molecules which may range from 4-5 to 100-200, and may form a very large number of structures, all stable, though to different extents [Berry, 1990]. In these microaggregates, the forces of attraction and repulsion between the various atoms or molecules make for the best conformation in terms of potential energy, bearing in mind the obvious fact that protons and electrons attract one another, whereas there are repulsive forces within the pairs of protons and electrons. Normally, the proton-electron interactions are important only within the same atom or molecule, but when various atoms or molecules approach one another beyond a *critical point*, the interactions with neighboring elements become very important. Formation of the aggregate is determined when the energy is minimal, but calculation of the permitted energies on the basis of quantum physics shows that the energy of the aggregate is confined to a series of levels, or steps.

Another interesting property of microaggregates is that they go over from the solid to the liquid phase and vice versa on variations in temperature, but, unlike ordinary matter, the melting point and freezing point do not necessarily coincide, with the result that it can easily come about that both solid and liquid phases of a microaggregate suspension may coexist over a broad range of temperatures.

This situation is reminiscent of the properties of colloids and of the aggregates of organic molecules which oscillate between monomeric and filamentous forms, or between sol and gel. This is an example of the *bistability* phenomenon, typical of complex systems (cf. Chapter 5, Section 8.2).

Microaggregates can change configuration not only as a result of variations in temperature, but also as a result of other energies supplied by electromagnetic vibrations (a microaggregate normally vibrates approximately 10^{10} times per second) [Berry, 1990].

Despite the objective difficulty this field of study presents (it cannot be tackled either by using the investigational means of molecular biology, nor by using those of solid-state physics), its importance also in the sphere of medicine is only just beginning to emerge: we know that many reactions of living cells occur at microaggregate level or in the colloidal phase of many proteins, consisting in rapid monomer to polymer transitions and vice versa. The structure and function of the cytoskeleton are determined to a substantial extent by the microtubules, whose most characteristic - and largely mysterious - property is their *dynamic instability* due to their easy dissolution and reassembly.

The editors of the journal *Current Biology* claim that dynamic instability promises to be one of the most interesting biological processes for biochemists and biophysicists in the near future [Pollard and Goldman, 1992]. Extracellular matter also exhibits behavior patterns typical of colloids: we need only think, for example, of blood clotting phenomena or the thixotropy (conversion of gel to sol) of fluids bathing the articular cavities during movement.

We concern ourselves with colloids here because this particular field of chemistry enables us, on the basis of published experiments, to illustrate an interesting physico-chemical phenomenon which occurs in water treated according to particular procedures. Essentially what interests us is the fact that the formation of colloids is speeded up very considerably by water treated with electromagnetic waves.

The phenomenon of so-called *"activation"* of water was extensively described by Piccardi, Director of the Institute of Physics of the University of Florence, back in the '30s [Piccardi, 1938; Piccardi and Corsi, 1938; Piccardi and Botti, 1939], but it did not cause quite the stir that perhaps it deserved to cause. The revealing reaction is easily reproducible: solutions of gold chloride, formaldehyde and sodium carbonate are mixed in adequate proportions and heated; in the space of a few minutes the color of the colloidal gold formed (blue-violet) can be observed. With numerous variants, this type of reaction is described in text books of colloidal chemistry, amongst other things because these substances today find practical applications in various fields, including electron microscopy.

Piccardi noted that if the water was treated with various agents causing the formation of electromagnetic radiation phenomena (shaken glass bulbs containing mercury, electric arcs, rods of electrically charged ebanite, for example), the water acquired the ability to bring about the formation of colloidal gold (and also of other colloids) at a faster rate. What most astonished Piccardi was that this property *persisted for months* after the treatment. This prompted him to perform countless check tests, all of which he meticulously described, and eventually, as he himself admitted, he was forced to "bow to the evidence." The fact is hardly any less amazing today, but there is no sign that the phenomenon described by Piccardi has led to any further advances in our knowledge of the structure of water. Probably, the time was not ripe and the discovery was seen more as an oddity or freak phenomenon than as a true scientific breakthrough.

It has been shown [Fesenko and Gluvstein, 1995; Fesenko *et al.*, 1995] that preliminary irradiation of a saline physiological solution with electromagnetic waves in the wavelength range of microwaves (without thermic effects) modifies the capacity that this solution has to modulate the opening/closing of membrane ionic channels. This modification of physiological properties of the solution is maintained even after the period of irradiation, in a way that according to these authors suggests the existence of some kind of "memory" of the applied treatment. Interestingly, when ionic channels are already open, the irradiated saline solution has inhibitory effects, while when they are initially closed the solution has stimulating effects on membrane ionic permeability.

A series of trials, with results in keeping with those reported here above, have been described by Markov and coworkers [Markov et al., 1975]. These investigators described a "magnetization" phenomenon in water exposed to a static magnetic field of 450-3500 G for periods of 30 to 120 minutes. The water thus treated is reported to show marked alterations (persisting intact for at least 24 h) of the Raman spectrum and of electrical conductivity, and also a greater degree of germination-stimulating activity of various seeds.

The results reported above serve essentially to support the hypothesis that water possesses particular properties which have yet to receive due consideration and which are evidentiated by its ability to catalyze colloidal reactions. Since these properties are acquired not by the addition of particular substances, but by means of physical treatment, we must deduce that water is endowed with various physical states which are chemically significant, i.e. they act as vehicles for information or energy utilizable by chemical systems. As these physical states are maintained for significantly lengthy time periods, we can by and large speak about a "memory" of water, even though this kind of test tells us little about the type of specificity or selectivity this phenomenon may present. The colloidal gold formation reaction appears to be influenced by a series of possible different treatments of water, and therefore cannot depend on any precise form of electromagnetic radiation. In a certain sense, then, it is a broad-spectrum reaction which is not very specific, but which may, perhaps precisely for this reason, be of great importance all the same for laying the foundations for a properly documented controlled study of the physicochemical properties of water. In the not too distant future we may perhaps find other systems, possibly nearer to the biological colloids, which are more sensitive or more selective for this type of study.

A series of studies by Benveniste's group are significant in this context. These researchers have used the experimental model of the isolated and perfused guinea-pig heart (see Chapter 4, Section 2) to test the transfer of molecular signals via an electronic circuit [Aïssa et al., 1993; Benveniste et al., 1994b]. Closed ampoules of histamine, ovalbumin or LPS, and water (as controls) were placed inside a coil through which an electric current was passed. An amplifier then delivered the current to another coil in which was inserted a closed ampoule of water. The water treated with the current from the coils with histamine, ovalbumin and LPS and perfused through the guinea-pig heart was capable of increasing coronary flow. The water treated with the current from the coil containing water, on the other hand, had only a minimal effect. The differences were highly significant (P < 0.001). A similar phenomenon, consisting in the "frequency-operated transfer of drugs" (TFF) had been previously described by M. Citro, who reported achieving pharmacological effects on cells and animals and even in man, using water exposed to electromagnetic frequencies "modulated" by substances of various types (therapeutic effects in the case of drugs, toxic effects on cell cultures in the case of toxic agents such as atrazine, and inhibition of the metamorphosis of frogs in the case of thyroxine) [Citro, 1992; Citro et al., 1993; Citro et al., 1994]. The phenomenon of electronic transmission of molecular information was further confirmed using a cell activation system by researchers from the Benveniste's group [Thomas et al., 2000; related reports can be found also in the website www.digibio.com].

Another approach to the study of activated water has been developed by G. Arcieri [Arcieri, 1988]. Confining ourselves to essential notes and referring the reader to the cited literature for details, the author maintains that water can be "enriched" with electromagnetic frequencies by means of treatment with physical energies (lasers) or with chemical substances, including samples of biological materials such as the blood of healthy and diseased subjects. The demonstrations of the physicochemical changes induced by these treatments were obtained both with nuclear magnetic resonance spectrometry and with Doppler flow-metry (according to Arcieri, this latter procedure serves to highlight physiological changes induced by activated water).

7.1.4 Water clathrates, isotopicity and similar models

According to some investigators [Smith, 1988; Anagnostatos et al., 1991; Anagnostatos, 1994], the "memory of water" may be based on the formation of aggregates of water molecules in the form of clathrates. What is meant by clathrates, from the Latin "clathrus" (= lattice or grating), are hollow formations which the water molecules are thought to assume with a grid-like arrangement, set around an internal niche or cavity. The possibility of the formation of cavities in liquids is universally accepted. In water, the molecules can align themselves in pentagonal or hexagonal forms thanks to their hydrogen bonds; in turn, in certain conditions (agitation or sonication of the liquid) various polygonal conformations can form complex, internally hollow geometrical figures [Gregory *et al.*, 1997].

On forming the cavities, the surface tension produces a negative pressure inside, which, in the smallest form, takes the form of a dodecahedron (12 pentagons bound together in a geometrically ordered manner), but which may also include nonplanar hexagons. In addition, varieties of chemical bonds other than hydrogen bonds may be involved, such as dipoles between hydrogen and hydroxyl ions [Smith, 1990].

A certain number of molecules of the original compound are thought to be surrounded, once dissolved in water, by a greater number of water molecules which form a kind of shell or niche. Such a niche might possess stability even if the original compound is expelled from the niche itself. Thus, with continual dilutions and succussions, empty clathrates would begin to form inside, which in turn may become the nucleus for the formation of other clathrates, all with the same original pattern [Anagnostatos, 1994].

A considerable variability of forms and combinations would thus be possible in the formation of such micro-cavities. The dodecahedral forms should be capable of binding together in forms similar to helicoidal chains joined by their pentagonal faces. These chains may represent the site of coherent interaction between water and the magnetic field of a current which might cause synchronized "hopping" from one proton (hydrogen atom) to another linking adjacent oxygen atoms [Smith, 1990; Smith, 1994].

Thanks to the ordered, sequential arrangement of the hydrogen bonds, such cavities may be capable of vibrating coherently in resonance with a magnetic field. The frequency of the vibrations would depend upon the shape and length of such structures (in turn dependent upon the original solute), as well as the degree of progressive structuring of the water, as the dilution-dynamization process progresses.

It has been noted [Smith, 1990] that such a model of water makes no provision for the fact that water *emits* radiation or magnetic fields, i.e. that it is an active source of coherence for other systems, but allows only that it may be *a "mirror" of coherence* via weak interactions between external magnetic fields and those generated as a result within the water. This is important, because if there were *emission of energy* by a particular physicochemical structure of water, the latter would be subject to exhaustion in a very short space of time owing to dissipation of energy. If, on the other hand, the interaction occurs as a result of a kind of resonance between a coherence pattern of the solution (caused by the fine structure deriving from the solute) and a frequency pattern of the living organism (deriving from the state, whether normal or pathological, of oscillatory systems), such communication of information by the electromagnetic route does not require the solution itself to emit any radiation or energy.

An analogy could be made with other types of information: a book *contains* information, but does not *emit* it. The information may be fixed on paper for a long time and become significant, in the sense of being able to organize the reader's thoughts, only when it starts to be "in tune" with the reader's receptor and cognitive systems (and here is where the concept of tone, vibration and frequency comes into the picture).

The clathrate model is interesting in that it helps to explain how "aggregates" of water molecules can become the means of transmitting information. It has to be admitted, however, that there is no physical basis to explain the *permanence* of such aggregates in definite forms for sufficiently lengthy periods.

Another interesting theory providing a framework for an explanation of the homeopathic high dilution effects has been proposed by Berezin [Berezin, 1990; Berezin, 1991; Berezin, 1994], based on the physical phenomenon of isotopic diversity (*isotopicity*), i.e. on the well-known fact that most chemical elements are mixtures of several stable isotopes (atoms having a fixed number of protons but a different number of neutrons in their nuclei). Water, for example, is formed mainly by hydrogen (H) and ^{16}oxygen (oxygen isotope ^{16}O), but a small proportion of the molecules are formed by the isotopes deuterium (D) or ^{17}O, or ^{18}O. All these isotopes are stable in solution over time, are present in substantial amounts (^{18}O represents 0.2% of oxygen molecules) and are assumed to be randomly distributed in normal water.

In brief, the essence of the hypothesis is that the distribution of isotopes in water can generate an *"information-carrying pattern,"* due to different possible positional organizations of the different molecules. These patterns, which have been named "isotopic lattice ghosts" [Berezin, 1991], may form when the presence of certain molecules in solution causes some specific readjustment in the positional distribution of isotopes in the vicinity. During the preparation of dilutions according to the homeopathic methodology the "seed" molecules would operate as "symmetry-breaking agents" in a system which is put far from equilibrium by the energy provided by succussion. Symmetry breaking in a physical system results in a decrease in its entropy and is equivalent to the generation of information within this system.

Any theory regarding the homeopathic phenomena should indicate some mechanism whereby the coded information is protected from thermal disordering and is multiplied in serial dilutions in the absence of the original molecule. According to the Berezin's theory, the isotopic configurations could be preserved by *polarization effects*, which energetically stabilize the interactions between the various isotopes. The transmission of the pattern from one configuration to other randomly distributed water molecules should be possible because the imposition of a weak perturbation on a highly degenerate system (i.e. having a variety of possible configurations with the same total energy) often "dictates" the choice of a pattern at which the system eventually arrives, a phenomenon similar to the influence of trace substances on the process of crystallization under specific conditions [Berezin, 1994].

As stated for the above-mentioned clathrate theory, in the case of the isotopicity theory, too, it can be said that even if the suggested model is self-consistent, it still provides no guarantee that it describes actual physical reality. The author of the hypothesis recognizes the need for experimental demonstrations, but at the same time maintains that "the very fact of the existence of an *operational model* for the alleged effect might be a stimulating factor for more focused experimental studies" [Berezin, 1994, p. 138].

7.1.5 NMR, infra-red and Raman-laser spectroscopy

The foregoing sections, devoted to superradiance and clathrates, basically have to do with theories which, however, have yet to be confirmed experimentally. The experiments on the activation of water bear witness to the permanence of particular properties capable of catalyzing colloidal chemical reactions. These experiments, however, like the more biologically oriented experiments in Chapter 4, do not enable us to gain insights into the intimate physical mechanism whereby such properties may be justified. In other words, the answer to the question whether homeopathic remedies possess special physical properties remains very much in the dark.

A tentative approach to solving this problem in terms of experimental physics has been adopted by various investigators by means of analysis of *spectra* (bands of absorption, emission or resonance of electromagnetic waves at different frequencies or intensities) obtained with the Raman-laser, infra-red absorbance (I.R.) and, above all, the nuclear magnetic resonance (NMR) techniques on homeopathic preparations.

NMR is known today mainly for its applications in diagnostic imaging (MRI), but it has been used above all to study atoms and molecules, in that it allows investigation of the behavior of the atomic nucleus when subjected to a magnetic field. Since the nucleus has a dipole moment, the dipole may enter into resonance with sufficiently strong electromagnetic waves, and each type of atom has its own particular resonance frequency. Thus, the NMR spectrum (i.e. the graph plotting the resonance peaks) is directly related to the components of the sample measured and the "geometry" of the molecules. In addition to the spectrum, other parameters considered are resonance relaxation times ($T1$ = longitudinal relaxation time; $T2$ = transverse relaxation time). Relaxation is a complex parameter resulting from the dipolar magnetic interaction between intra- and intermolecular vicinal protons, from the molecular rotation and translation movements, from the exchange of protons and the presence, if any, of paramagnetic substances (certain metals, molecular oxygen, free radicals).

The very first studies in this field were those conducted by Smith and Boericke [Smith and Boericke, 1966; Smith and Boericke, 1968], which showed that the structure of the solvent (ethanol and water) as it appears in the region of the OH and H_2O signals in the NMR spectrum, is modified in serial dilutions. The modification is more marked, if succussion is also performed as compared to dilution alone and, even more remarkably, does not diminish, but rather increases with increasing dilution.

Later, other researchers [Young, 1975; Sachs, 1983; Lasne *et al.*, 1989] were to make similar observations, which were then taken up by Weingartner [Weingartner, 1990; Weingartner, 1992], who clearly demonstrated that the difference between an NMR spectrum of a solvent in which sulphur (Sulphur 23x) has been diluted and a spectrum of the solvent alone relates to the intensity of the H_2O and OH signals, whereas that of the CH_2 and CH_3 signals does not vary (the chemical formula of ethanol is CH_3CH_2OH). In particular, the peaks of a homeopathic dilution of sulphur are significantly lower (probability > 99.9%) and broader compared to the peaks for the solvent alone. Weingartner also reports that this difference is not observed for the Sulphur 13x dilution, in the sense that at this dilution the spectrum cannot be distinguished from that of the solvent. He suggests that the lowering of the peaks observed at NMR is indicative of an accelerated proton exchange. This finding may lend itself to many interpretations, but it would appear to be in keeping with the tendency to attribute an important role to the hydrogen bond in the non-random association of water molecules.

It should be pointed out that hydrogen bonds play a key role not only in the structuring of liquid and solid water, but also in a number of biochemical and biological reactions where information and energy transfer occur. For instance, it is well known that protein secondary structures (alpha-helixes and beta-sheets) are formed by hydrogen bonds between amino acids and that DNA and RNA structures are maintained by intranucleotide hydrogen bonds. Moreover, it has been shown that ligand-receptor interactions may involve proton donation by the receptor and proton acceptance by the ligand [Fay *et al.*, 1993] within the binding pocket, and that the transmission of the light signal into the rhodopsin molecule involves conduction of protons via "chains" of water molecules interlinked by hydrogen bonds (see Section 7.1.1. above) [Khorana, 1993].

Variations in NMR resonance characteristics, and in particular in the relaxation times T1 and T2, in highly diluted solutions of silica have also been measured by another research team in France and published in an official journal of physics [Demangeat *et al.*, 1992]. In brief, it was observed that solutions of silica/lactose, prepared in centesimal dilutions according to homeopathic methodology, presented an increase in T1 and in the T1/T2 ratio as compared to distilled water or to diluted and dynamized solutions of NaCl. These changes were also detectable with silica concentrations of the order of 10^{-17} moles/liter. This experiment is also important because a stimulatory effect of high dilutions of silica had previously been demonstrated on mouse peritoneal macrophages [Davenas *et al.*, 1987; see also Chapter 4, Section 1]. This was therefore the first case in which a difference of a physical nature was rigorously demonstrated between the solvent and the high dilution of a homeopathic remedy whose biological activity was established experimentally.

More recently, NMR spectra of high dilutions/dynamizations of the homeopathic medicine *Nux vomica*, showed significant difference from control solutions (alcohol unagitated) with respect to the spin-lattice relaxation time (T1) of the deuterium nuclei [Sukul *et al.*, 2000; 2001]. The method also allowed the distinction between different potencies of the same drug. However, two other studies attempting to reproduce the findings of specific physical properties of homeopathic soltions by NMR have been unsuccessful [Aabel *et al.*, 2001; Milgrom *et al.*, 2001].

It would also appear that I.R. spectrophotometric analysis enables us to detect physicochemical changes in high dilutions of homeopathic drugs. Heinz's team [data reported by Barros and Pasteur, 1984] appear to have demonstrated the importance of succussion or dynamization in the preparation method by means of the I.R. procedure. In fact:

a) Substances diluted and dynamized to 30x present absorption bands on the I.R. spectrum.

b) These bands are not presented by solutions which are diluted to 30x but not dynamized.

c) A 30x dynamized dilution loses its property of producing absorption bands at I.R. spectroscopy if subjected to boiling.

d) The absorption bands decrease alternately and unevenly: maximum activity corresponds to the 6, 9, 12, 14, 18, 21, 28 and 30 decimal dilutions, and minimum activity to the 7, 10, 13 and 16 decimal dilutions.

Another method which was used for the study of physical changes in homeopathic dilutions is analysis of the Raman laser spectrum. When a laser beam illuminates a substance, a small proportion of the light rays is diffused with a different wavelength to that of the original light. On examining the emission peaks of these diffusion rays (Raman effect) information is obtained about the physical state (viscosity, molecular distortions, dielectric constant) of the liquid analyzed. It has been reported that homeopathic dilutions of various plants (e.g. *Aesculus*, *Bryonia*, and *Rosmarinus*) produced in 70% ethanol modify the Raman-laser spectrum of ethanol, in the sense that they cause a significant lowering of the spectrum peaks at various frequencies [Luu, 1976]. This lowering of the peaks has been observed in the dilutions from 1c to 7c (and in this case is attributed to a mass action, due therefore to the molecules dissolved), but also in the dilutions from 11c to 30c (maximum dilution tested).

In the case of high dilutions, the lowering of the intensity of the Raman-laser effect has been attributed to an electrostatic rearrangement of the molecular environment [Luu, 1976].

There is still no exhaustive explanation of how a transfer of information from the homeopathic remedy to the body can take place, but, if the problem is couched in physical and not merely in chemical terms, it is very likely that any such explanation must necessarily take account of electromagnetic phenomena in living systems.

The study of the effects of electromagnetic fields in the body has come to take on increasing importance and scientific dignity in recent years, while at the same time that aura of mystery which has favored the exploitation of such phenomena by charlatans has steadily declined. It is true, on the other hand, that even in recent times scientists who devote their attention to the study of electromagnetism in medicine and biology, such as Tsong, for example, are still liable to be accused of dabbling in "magic" [Tsong, 1989]. It is indeed singular that such accusations, sometimes accompanied by negative verdicts regarding the subject's mental faculties, have been levied against many scientists operating as pioneers in this field, including a certain Guglielmo Marconi.

The main reasons for the renewed interest in interactions between electromagnetic fields and living systems consist in three types of factors:

a) Evidence has been building up regarding the efficacy of extremely-low-frequency (ELF) pulsed magnetic fields in therapy, and most notably in orthopedics.

b) From the standpoint of public health, there is a heightened awareness of the risks associated with technological development and thus also with exposure to electromagnetic fields generated, for instance, by high-tension electrical power lines, video terminals, diagnostic equipment, household electrical appliances, and other sources.

c) The topic is being tackled increasingly in experimental terms with studies on cell and molecular models, with the result that a number of possible explanations of the biological effects of low-energy magnetic fields are beginning to emerge.

These matters will be briefly illustrated here below, as a contribution to a better understanding of the emerging biophysical paradigm in medicine and thus of the possible relationship between electromagnetic phenomena and homeopathy. In this case, too, we feel we should stress that our discussion of these issues lays no claim to being in any way systematic, but rather constitutes an attempt to compare in outline and put into perspective many different problems which are otherwise regarded as strictly pertaining to other specialist sectors or as being "alternative" medical practices, inasmuch as they are based on phenomena which are largely unclear from the scientific point of view.

For the purposes of making it easier to understand the basic concepts used in bioelectromagnetism and the experimental evidence reported here below, we will briefly explain the terminology and the measurement units used. A diagram illustrating the various types of electromagnetic waves, together with their wavelengths and frequencies is given in Figure 27.

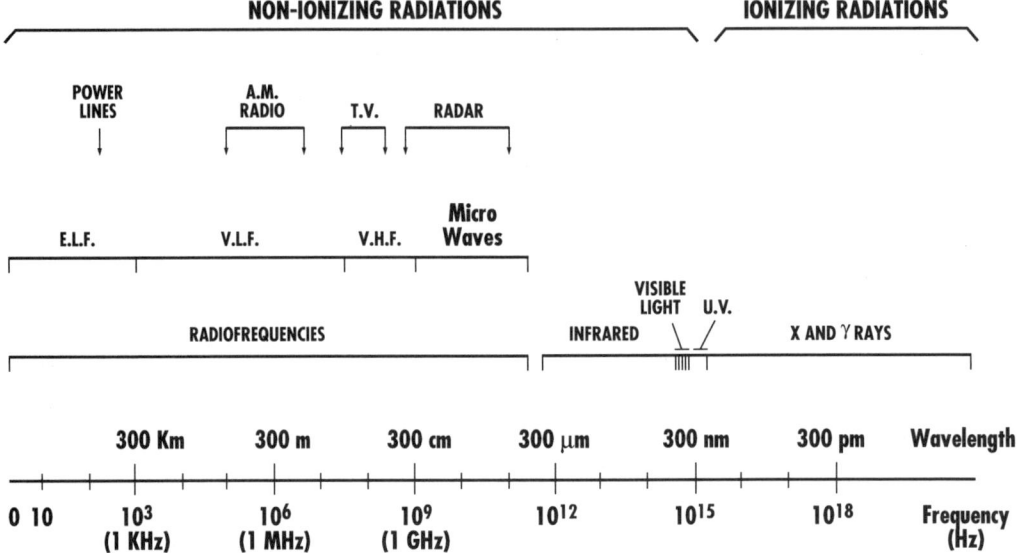

FIGURE 27 Electromagnetic radiations of various wavelengths and frequencies.

The frequency of an electromagnetic field is the number of cycles per second of the electromagnetic wave, or the number of pulsations of the field itself per second and is measured in Hertz (Hz). The wavelength (λ) is the distance between two wave peaks and is measured in meters (or in multiples of submultiples of a meter). Obviously, the higher the frequency, the lower will be the wavelength.

Electromagnetic waves are used, as is known in the case of telecommunications, as *information vectors*. For this purpose a *carrier* wave is used with a frequency selected in a very broad range according to the transmission and reception systems. This carrier wave is specifically *modulated* in relation to the information to be conveyed, i.e. its length and height are subtly altered and can be slightly increased or reduced to a variable extent over time (frequency and amplitude modulation, respectively). In this way, a piece of equipment *tuned* to the carrier wave can perceive the modulation and, after decoding it, the information contained in it.

The *intensity* of the electrical field is provided by the electric potential over a given distance and is expressed in volts/meter (V/m) or millivolts/centimeter (mV/cm). When a biological system is exposed to an electrical field, the mobile charges shift in the direction induced by the field itself, thus forming a *current*, which is measured in amps (A) or in submultiples of an amp. With reference to a certain area of tissue or organ traversed by electrical charges, there will be a certain density (J) of the current itself, which is measured in amps/square meter (A/m^2) or in mA/cm^2.

The electric field and the magnetic field are closely related according to Faraday's law of induction. When a pulsed magnetic field is applied to an electrically conducting material (such as living matter), an electric field is induced perpendicular to the direction (vector) of the magnetic field. This electric field obviously depends on the surface of the area concerned and is proportional in intensity to the frequency of the magnetic field and its intensity.

The intensity of the magnetic field is measured in Gauss (G) or, to use the more modern SI unit, in tesla (T) or submultiples of a tesla (1 T = 10^4 G). To have two terms of comparison, the intensity of the earth's magnetic field is of the order of 0.02 to 0.07 mT (0.2 to 0.7 G), whereas that used in diagnostics by magnetic resonance is of the order of 0.1 to 10 mT (1 to 100 G) [Walleczek, 1992].

7.2.1 Effects on the body

We intend here to examine low-energy, low-frequency radiation, which acts with very different mechanisms compared to ionizing radiation. The latter causes biological effects through ionization (detachment of electrons from the atomic orbits) of the molecules and thus gross alterations such as damage to chromosomes, peroxidation of lipid membranes, and so on. In contrast, the energy of radiation with frequencies from 0 to a few hundred GHz is too low to cause physicochemical changes of this type and at most is able to yield thermal effects (heating, used, amongst other things, in the functioning of microwave ovens).

The effects of non-ionizing electromagnetic fields on the human body may be both of a pathological type and useful for therapeutic purposes. As regards the damaging effects most commonly studied, we have to refer essentially to studies which appear to demonstrate an increase in tumors in exposed subjects [Pool, 1990]. The topic is much debated and the epidemiological data have been confirmed only with regard to a few childhood tumors (leukemias). As regards the uses for therapeutic purposes, the techniques most extensively employed are electromagnetic stimulation of osteogenesis, in cases of pseudoarthrosis and retardation of fracture consolidation [Chiabrera *et al.*, 1984]. This is not the place for a detailed review of the pathological or therapeutic effects of electromagnetic fields, this today being an area of major development, and so we will confine ourselves to outlining the basic molecular and cellular aspects.

There are many natural sources of weak electromagnetic fields: sources outside the body include, for instance, the earth's magnetic field (which is exploited by a number of birds, fish and dolphins for direction-finding), radiation from the stars which emit radiofrequencies, the sun itself (particularly in certain phases of its activity) [Konig, 1989], the waves irradiated by telecommunications and radar systems, and electrical power lines. The sources inside the body are multiple and range from the electrical activity of the nerves and muscles to the electric fields generated by a number of fish and other marine organisms (used for the purposes of recognition in the dark and for defense), to the generation of light by cells such as leukocytes (chemiluminescence).

The electrocardiogram and electroencephalogram are no more than two methods of measuring the endogenous electrical activity of the heart and the nerve centres. Electrical activity is also generated in bone when it is deformed; such activity can be defined as piezoelectric and appears to be important for directing the growth of bone trabeculae along lines of force. In actual fact, one of the first clinical uses of weak magnetic fields was precisely the induction of bone repair [Bassett *et al.*, 1974].

Animal organisms have developed very marked sensitivity to electromagnetic waves. Without going beyond the most obvious field, we need only mention the sensitivity of the eye to light, which makes it capable of perceiving only a few photons.

The experiments by Smith and Monro [Smith *et al.*, 1985; Monro, 1987; Smith, 1988; Smith, 1989; Smith, 1994] illustrate the concept of "sensitivity" to minimal perturbations of electromagnetic fields. These investigators (Smith works in the Department of Electronic and Electrical Engineering of the University of Salford) have reported a series of experiments performed in collaboration with allergologists from the Lister Hospital in London, in which they succeeded in inducing allergic manifestations in patients with immediate hypersensitivity to many substances, simply by bringing them into close contact with sources of electromagnetic radiation. The allergic manifestations could set in rapidly at particular frequency bands ranging, according to the individual patients, from only a few mHz to a large number of MHz. It was not, then, so much the intensity of output of the oscillator (a few V/m) that was important as the frequency and coherence.

It is not only curious that these investigators demonstrated the ability to trigger allergic attacks with electromagnetic waves, but also that the patients sensitive to this type of stimulation themselves produced electromagnetic signals during the allergy attacks, though the latter were provoked chemically. Such emissions could be documented by interference with the recording of magnetic tapes and even, in some cases, by interference with the functioning of electronic equipment such as computers. According to Smith [Smith, 1988], these are electrophysiological phenomena very similar to those known to us from many species of fish.

It has been demonstrated that a number of species of fish are capable of perceiving and responding to electric fields with intensities as low as 0.000001 V/m [Bullock, 1977], which corresponds to the most marked sensitivities found in allergic subjects. Again according to Smith, such sensitivities may enable the fish to locate food at great distances: it has been seen, in fact, that living cells, such as, for instance, yeasts, emit electromagnetic waves in radiofrequencies at levels of approximately 0.1 V/m [Smith, 1988; Pollock and Pohl, 1988]. The same ability, Smith claims, may have served primitive man in his search for food.

In the studies conducted by Smith and Monro, the authors talk about homeopathy and the memory of water. In the course of the allergometric tests in the sample of hyperreactive patients, the researchers realized that allergic reactions triggered by contact with chemical agents could be neutralized by treating the patients with particular frequencies. If the same frequencies were used to treat mineral water, the latter acquired the neutralizing therapeutic properties. If, on the other hand, the water was exposed to frequencies capable of triggering the attack, it acquired the properties of an allergen.

The treatment of the water was done by inserting glass test tubes containing the water in solenoids or thoroids powered by an oscillator. The changes induced in the water, capable of triggering allergic attacks in hypersensitive patients, persisted for 1-2 months. Incidentally, at this point it is interesting to note that the stability of the homeopathic remedy in aqueous solution is traditionally short-lived, of the order of months, whereas Hahnemann himself used water-alcohol solutions precisely because they were much more stable and long-lasting (years).

Quite apart from the fact that only a minority of allergic patients exhibited this extreme sensitivity and were suitable for the execution of such tests, the demonstration of the ability of water to incorporate electromagnetic information and transmit it to individuals reactive to it remains of great interest and significance. This series of experiments should therefore be repeated by independent centers and, if confirmed, may constitute a valid argument in favor of the effective presence of metamolecular information in aqueous fluids.

7.2.2 Molecular and cellular effects

It is well known that electromagnetic radiation can cause substantial changes at molecular level, but the bulk of attention, up until not very long ago, was devoted to the effects of medium-to-high energy radiation, such as X-, gamma- and ultraviolet rays. As mentioned above, investigations into the mechanisms of the biological effects of nonionizing radiation have recently begun (see Figure 27).

Most protein molecules are capable of passing reversibly from one conformational state to another by virtue of various possible combinations of hydrogen bonds, disulfide bridges and hydrophobic forces. These passages occur by means of nonlinear changes, or hopping, to overcome the energy barriers between one state and another. The proteins are thus dynamic, vibrating structures whose components undergo continual oscillatory movements, which take place over a time scale ranging from femtoseconds (10^{-15} s) to several minutes. The most significant vibrations in biological systems are of the order of nanoseconds [Hameroff, 1988]. It is very important to stress the fact that, in biology, many proteins (and also other chemical species such as lipids) are assembled in multimeric or polymeric groups. In these structures, cooperative, or collective, interactions easily occur, with the result that the vibrations may propagate themselves in *coherent* ways and, as such, may take on a biological-informational significance [Frohlich, 1988; Del Giudice *et al.*, 1988b; Bistolfi, 1989].

Electromagnetic waves, even if of low energy and broad wavelength, are known to generate heat, when absorbed by biological matter. The question whether millimetric waves cause effects independent of absorption of heat, i.e. so-called nonthermal effects, has been the subject of lengthy scientific debate. The controversy regarding the existence of cell responses to low-energy waves is due both to the fact that the reproducibility of many experiments has proven difficult, and to theoretical objections that the energy of such weak fields would be less than the energy of the background noise due to the temperature at which the cells are studied (*thermal noise*). If we are to expect an effect of an electromagnetic field applied from the outside, this field will have to cause significantly greater changes than would in any event occur casually in biological systems even in the resting state (e.g. the continual opening and closing of ion channels, oscillations in membrane potentials and in many metabolic activities, etc., all these being processes which are in any event active at a certain temperature). Today, however, the existence of nonthermal effects of weak electro-magnetic fields has been demonstrated in many experimental systems and may now be regarded as generally accepted [Kremer *et al.*, 1988; Aldrich and Easterly, 1987; Magnavita, 1989; Tsong, 1989].

A major contribution to this issue can be found in a critical study published in *Science* [Weaver and Astumian, 1990]. These authors propose physical models according to which the cells are considered as detectors of very weak periodic magnetic fields and where the relationships between the size of the cell and the changes in membrane potential due both to temperature-induced fluctuations and to the application of electromagnetic fields are established. In the simplest version of the model, the calculation estimates at around 10^{-3} volts/cm the intensity of the minimum field to which the membrane macromolecules could be sensitive. However, if the model parameters considered take into account the so-called frequency "windows," i.e. the possibility that certain responses occur only within a restricted frequency band, then the theoretical intensity necessarily proves to be several orders of magnitude lower (10^{-6} volts/cm), thus closely approaching the data from various experiments in cells and animals.

The growth of the nerve processes is guided by weak electric currents [Alberts *et al.*, 1989]. When a nerve process lengthens in culture or even in connective tissue, at its apex a structure called a growth cone is formed, which appears as the expansion center of many long filaments (filopods) which look like continually slow-moving finger-like processes, making ameboid movements: some retract, and others stretch out, as if exploring the terrain. Within the filopods many actin filaments are to be found. The net vectorial shift of the growth cone in one direction is followed by a lengthening of the nerve fiber (at an estimated rate of 1 mm per day). The direction of the movement depends on various local factors, such as, for instance, the orientation of the fibers of the connective tissue matrix, along which the growth preferentially occurs, and even the existence of specific membrane recognition systems between adjacent cells. The cells, however, are also powerfully influenced by electromagnetic fields: the growth cones of neurons in culture are oriented and direct themselves towards a negative electrode in the presence of low-intensity fields (70 mV/cm).

The cells have an ability to receive and integrate light signals, perceiving both their frequency and direction. This has been demonstrated by means of special phase-contrast microscopy equipment with infra-red light [Albrecht-Buehler, 1991]. 3T3 fibroblasts in culture extend the filopods preferentially towards light sources, the most effective being the intermittent ones in the 800-900 nm range with 30-60 impulses per minute. According to the author of these experiments, the cell receptor for the radiation is the centrosome.

There is also evidence that cell proliferative activity is influenced by electromagnetic fields, albeit of very low intensity (0.2-20 mT, 0.02-1.0 mV/cm) [Luben et al., 1982; Conti et al., 1983; Cadossi et al., 1992; Walleczek, 1992].

It is important to note that on the basis of the literature data available to date it is impossible to draw any definite conclusions as to the positive or negative, stimulatory or inhibitory effects of weak electromagnetic fields on cellular or molecular systems and above all as to doses and application modalities [Walleczek, 1992]. In fact, the bioactive electromagnetic signals used vary very considerably in terms of intensity, frequency, duration, and waveform (sinusoidal, square, sawtooth, etc.). Moreover, the effect may also depend on the biological status of the cells exposed [Cossarizza et al., 1989; Walleczek and Liburdy, 1990], indicating that mechanisms of very complex interaction between various different factors are involved.

Many enzymes and receptors appear to be sensitive to stimulations of a physical as well as a chemical type [Adey, 1988; Tsong, 1989; Popp et al., 1989]. The cell membrane, by virtue of its bioelectrical properties, is the site where influences of this type are most likely to be exerted [Kell, 1988], though other possible candidates are the large macromolecules organized in repetitive units, such as the nucleic acids [Popp, 1985], or the proteins of the cytoskeleton, particularly the microtubules [Hameroff, 1988].

The biological basis of the effect of magnetic fields on cells is highly complex and cannot be analyzed exhaustively here. The cell constitutes a typical electrochemical system, with a transmembrane potential difference (negative outside compared to inside) and a very large number of proteins endowed with electric charges of varying sign. According to the fluid mosaic model of the membrane (a model which is still valid, at least in general terms) in an ideal cell at rest, the proteins are distributed evenly over the membrane, but, in the presence of an electric field crossing the membrane, they undergo electrophoretic attraction or repulsion, tending to shift towards the poles which the cell presents in the direction of the electric field. A current of electrons or ions invading a cell flows around it, causing a movement of (electrically charged) proteins in the opposite direction.

The rearrangement of the position of the proteins on the surface of the membrane is not devoid of consequences, in that it favors contact between neighboring proteins and slows down contact between distant proteins [Chiabrera et al., 1984]. Since the functioning of receptors and membrane transduction systems depends on aggregations of proteins or at least on contacts between proteins, the consequences of the electric field for cell activation are easily imaginable. The aggregation phenomenon normally occurs in the case of a chemical signal, because the signal molecule may serve as a bridge between two or more receptors, which are mobile in the plane of the membrane.

Of course, this model is a very substantial simplification of what happens in reality, where the concentrations of calcium, magnesium, sodium, potassium and hydrogen ions come into play, as well as the possible direct effect of the magnetic field on the macromolecules of enzymes, receptors or the cytoskeleton (see below).

In cell biology and biochemistry, it is known that many elements with receptor, structural and enzymatic functions are sensitive to changes in weak electromagnetic fields (see Table 7).

TABLE 7

Molecular systems possibly interacting with electromagnetic fields

Molecules	Reference
Photoreceptors	Alberts *et al.*, 1989
Chlorophyll	Alberts *et al.*, 1989
Receptors with 7 transmembrane domains	Bistolfi, 1989
G-proteins	Adey, 1988
cAMP-dependent protein kinase	Byus *et al.*, 1984
Protein kinase C	Adey, 1988
Lysozyme	Shaya and Smith, 1977
Receptors (aggregation)	Chiabrera, 1984
Chromosomes	Kremer *et al.*, 1988
Protein and lipid biopolymers	Hasted, 1988
Na^+/K^+ ATPase	Liu *et al.*, 1990

Across the double lipid layer of the biological membranes, measuring approximately 40 Å in thickness, an electrical gradient of a few tens or hundreds of mV is established, which means something like 10^5 volts/cm. Theoretically this gradient should constitute an effective electrical barrier against minimal perturbations such as those created by low-frequency electromagnetic fields present in the extracellular membrane. In other words, the natural electrical activity of the membrane would constitute a kind of "background noise" which would prevent the possibility of perceiving minimal variations in potential. Very recent research, however, has shown that electromagnetic fields various orders of magnitude weaker than the transmembrane potential gradient are capable of modulating the actions of hormones, antibodies and neurotransmitters at receptor and transduction system level. This suggests that *highly cooperative processes* are set up, i.e. that repeated minimal variations cooperate to cause major movements. It is an effect similar to that which occurs when a bridge starts to oscillate whenever a body of men cross over it at marching pace, or when a glass breaks as a result of resonance.

The sensitivities observed in these biological processes of electromagnetic modulation are of the order of 10^{-7} volts/cm in the E.L.F. (extreme low frequency) range. Note, for example, that electric phenomena responsible for the EEG create gradients of 10^{-1} to 10^{-2} volts/cm [Adey, 1988]. Moreover, many of these interactions depend more on the frequency than on the intensity of the field, i.e. they occur only in certain *windows of frequency*, which would suggest the existence of *nonlinear* regulation systems far from equilibrium [Adey, 1988; Weaver and Astumian, 1990; Yost and Liburdy, 1992]. Similar sensitivities have been detected in a broad spectrum of tissues and cells, indicating that we are faced with a general biological property characteristic of cells.

The transfer of both chemical and electromagnetic signals from the external surface of the cell across the membrane consists in the transmission of conformational variations and oscillatory motions of proteins which have transmembrane domains (segments of the molecule). It has been claimed that a key role in this transmission is played by portions of proteins that have helical or pleated-sheet-shaped fibrous structures [Bistolfi, 1989]. Such structures are characterized by a substantial degree of order and by arrangement in repetitive sequences, as well as by the existence of hydrogen bonds between the amine residues of adjacent amino acids arranged longitudinally along the fiber. These protein structures are characteristic in their ability to *resound* according to nonlinear modes of vibration as a result of interaction with electromagnetic fields.

The prototype of this type of receptor is rhodopsin, the light receptor in the retina, which consists of 7 α-helixes arranged in orderly fashion transverse to the plane of the membrane on which it is situated. In this type of receptor-transducer, the excitation resulting from absorption of the photon is linked to the pumping of a proton and to the stabilization of a transmembrane potential.

It should be noted, however, that this structure with 7 α-helixes crossing the membrane is also found in an extensive family of glycoproteins involved in cell transmission systems coupled to G-proteins: the β-adrenergic receptors, the muscarinic receptors for acetylcholine, various receptors for neuropeptides, the receptors for chemotactic peptides in the white blood cells and even the mutual recognition systems in yeast cells involved in replicative fusion [Alberts *et al.*, 1989]. It is therefore likely that these characteristic structural features render the transmission systems they are present in susceptible to electromagnetic modulation.

Studies conducted on electromagnetic modulation of collagen production by osteoblasts are consistent with this view. It has been demonstrated, in fact, that parathyroid hormone in osteoblasts binds to external receptors and activates the enzyme adenylate cyclase via the mediation of a G-protein. An electromagnetic field with a 72 Hz frequency and an electrical gradient of 1.3 mV/cm induced 90% inhibition of adenylate cyclase activation without interfering either with the receptor binding or with the enzyme itself. As a result, the inhibitory effect was attributed to blockade of the G-protein [Adey, 1988].

Cyclic AMP (cAMP) is an important element in controlling the function of many enzymes, particularly insofar as an intracellular increase in cAMP constitutes an activatory message for the protein kinases (enzymes which phosphorylate proteins). In precise experimental conditions of frequency and duration of exposure, the cAMP-dependent protein kinase of human lymphocytes has been inhibited by electromagnetic waves (field of 450 MHz modulated in amplitude to 16 Hz). Type C protein kinase, the involvement of which in important cell processes as well as in carcinogenesis is beyond doubt, can also be modulated by electromagnetic waves [data from Byus, cited in Adey, 1988].

The catalytic activity of the enzyme lysozyme is sensitive to electromagnetic waves (radiofrequencies from 0.1 to 150 MHz) [Shaya and Smith, 1977]. In these experiments, solutions of lysozyme were exposed, in the presence of submaximal doses of the competitive inhibitor n-acetyl glucosamine (NAG), to various electromagnetic frequencies supplied by an oscillator by means of a coil wrapped around a polycarbonate container of the enzyme solution. The main effect observed was a modification of the inhibition produced by NAG. Interestingly, specific frequencies (e.g. 40 MHz) increased the effect of the inhibitor, and other frequencies (e.g. 100 MHz) decreased the effect, enhancing the activity to the level of the uninhibited lysozyme, while yet other frequencies (e.g. 150 MHz) had no effect. Inspection of the whole range of frequencies between 0.1 and 150 MHz showed alternating peaks of stimulation and inhibition of the enzyme activity, without any apparent regularity. Subsequent measurements between 30 MHz and 50 MHz showed further fine details in the effects produced. Therefore, the relationship between frequency and activity appears to show a chaotic trend and fractal behavior.

According to Tsong and coworkers [Tsong, 1989; Liu *et al.*, 1990], the conventionally known forms of intercellular communication, such as ligand-receptor interaction, are slow processes operating over short distances, but cells also need rapid forms of communication over long distances, with the result that it has been postulated that the various biochemical reactions, which are in any event necessary, are regulated by forces of a physical nature. Given that oscillating weak electromagnetic fields are capable of stimulating or suppressing many cell functions and that, from the thermodynamic point of view, this is possible only if mechanisms of amplification of the signal exist, it is postulated that the cell membrane is an amplification site.

The experiments carried out be Tsong's team indicate that a weak electric field (20 V/cm) is capable of activating the function of Na^+/K^+-dependent ATPase only if specific frequencies are simultaneously used, corresponding to 1 kHz for the pumping of K^+ and 1 MHz for the pumping of Na^+. These results have led to the formulation of the concept of "electroconformational coupling." This model postulates that an enzymatic protein undergoes conformational changes as a result of a Coulomb interaction with an electric field (or with any other oscillating force field with which the protein can interact). When the frequency of the electric field corresponds to the characteristic kinetics of the conformational transformation reaction, a phenomenological oscillation is induced between different conformations of the enzyme. At the optimal field force, the conformations thus achieved are functional and the oscillations are utilized to perform the activity required, such as, for example, the pumping of Na^+ and K^+.

The organization of DNA in the chromosomes is affected by influences of an electromagnetic nature, as demonstrated in an extensive series of studies by Kremer and his coworkers [Kremer *et al.*, 1988]. These authors used the model provided by giant chromosomes of insects (to be precise, the larvae of *Acricotopus lucidus*), which are easily visible and can be studied under the microscope. It is well known that when information has to be transcribed from DNA to RNA, the chromosomes (compact rods containing thousands of genes packed and stabilized by istonic proteins) have to partially decondense, showing puffs of genetic material issuing from the rod in the relevant segment. This phenomenon is strongly and significantly inhibited - in the sense that the puffs are much smaller - by irradiation of the chromosome with frequencies of around 40 to 80 GHz and outputs of only 6 mW/cm^2. The nonthermal nature of the phenomenon has been demonstrated by many control experiments.

A substantial contribution to the understanding of homeopathy stems from the acupuncture tradition and, particularly, from experience with Voll's electroacupuncture, with the result that some mention of the practice is called for in this book.

Acupuncture today is more accepted, or better tolerated, than homeopathy in the medical world. In fact, though the theoretical basis derives mainly from Chinese medical thinking, the numerous instances of therapeutic success and the incontestable demonstration of the existence of acupuncture points and of a number of physiological correlates have made it easier for this approach to be integrated into western medicine [Di Concetto, 1989]. We are interested here in acupuncture only as regards its relationship to homeopathy, and particularly in view of the fact that certain aspects of the latter can be studied by means of electroacupuncture techniques [Leonhardt, 1982; Fuller Royal, 1990; Fuller Royal and Fuller Royal, 1991; Meletani, 1992]. Voll's electroacupuncture (EAV) constitutes a special synthesis between oriental medical thinking and western technology. Of Chinese acupuncture the "energy" conduction routes are used, such as the meridians and the points lying on them. Of the electronic knowhow and procedures those used are the ones that enable cutaneous resistance to be measured in appropriate voltage and current intensity conditions.

7.3
Electro-
acupuncture

7.3.1 Points and meridians

Before addressing the topic of EAV, we should first make a few brief introductory remarks about traditional acupuncture and the lines along which it has developed. The acupuncture points appear to be windows which give access to information on the state of functioning of specific organs and body systems. The electrical characteristics of the acupuncture points consist in a reduction of cutaneous electrical resistance. The cutaneous electrical resistance at these points is approximately 50,000 ohms, as compared to the rest of the skin, where it is above 200,000 ohms [Fuller Royal and Fuller Royal, 1991]. At the same time, it is known that to these points physical stimuli (needles, electric charges, pressure, laser beams, heat) can be applied, which are transmitted to organs and apparati and act as agents restoring the amount and balance of the "vital force" ("*Ch'i*" according to the Chinese tradition) which has been lost or become deranged (Yin-Yang imbalance).

From the points depart the *meridians* which "link" the body surface to specific organs and to an internal bioenergy network the nature of which is still largely unknown, not coinciding either with the nervous system or with the vascular or lymphatic circuits. It has been demonstrated [see review in Smith, 1988] that on injecting radioactive isotopes at acupuncture points, they travel along the meridians at a rate of 3-5 cm/minute and that the speed is reduced in the case of diseased organs. The propagation rate increases on stimulating the entry point with needles, electric current or light produced by a helium-neon laser. On injecting the isotope into other skin areas not coinciding with the acupuncture point, no appreciable propagation is observed.

Acupuncture meridians and points are known to be distributed nonrandomly on the surface of the body, and in many cases constitute areas with a so-called somatotropic distribution. For instance, in areas such as the tips of the fingers or toes, the ears, the sole of the foot, or the tongue, the points present themselves according to precise maps of organs and systems, arranged with a certain degree of order. Also in this phenomenon the fractal geometry of the body structure and physiology may be thought about: a portion of the body contains a special kind of representation of the whole.

Despite this and other evidence, there is today still no satisfactory scientific theory to account for the effects of acupuncture. Everything we know, however, leads us to believe that underlying the functioning of acupuncture therapies is not simply a nerve reflex (there are no precise anatomical correlations), but a transmission of energy or information of an electromagnetic nature along communications networks of different types.

It has been claimed [Kroy, 1989] that in the philogeny and ontogenesis of living creatures there is a more ancestral cybernetic order than that based on the nervous system or on the humoral system (blood, hormones). This ancestral system is thought to be of an electromagnetic nature, because electromagnetic radiation is the most basic form of information present in nature. Electromagnetic signals have constituted (and still constitute) both the language of communication between atoms and molecules and the means whereby primordial organisms received a series of items of information on the environment (sunlight, other cosmic waves). There can thus be no doubt that living organisms have learnt to use electromagnetism as an information signalling system and thus as a means of communication between cells and tissues. According to the studies by Popp and coworkers [Popp, 1985; Popp et al., 1989], many biological systems are capable of producing, receiving and even of "storing" electromagnetic waves such as light.

The discussion of acupuncture could go on indefinitely. Whatever its mechanism of action, the procedure remains one of the main demonstrations of how biological and therapeutic effects can be achieved (cf., for example, the increase in endorphins, or the activation of the immune system [Chou *et al.*, 1991]) by stimulation of a physical type (mechanical stimulus, weak electric currents, or laser light) and not by drugs.

7.3.2 EAV

As mentioned above, Voll's electroacupuncture is a diagnostic and therapeutic method which combines the basic principles of Chinese acupuncture and the possibilities of modern electronics. This method was introduced by the German physician Reinhold Voll in 1955, and indeed is still known as Voll's electroacupuncture (EAV) [Voll, 1975]. Later it was perfected and elaborated both in theory and in its applications. There are today many variants on the original procedure and many types of instruments capable of carrying out bioelectronic measurements - even of a type distinctly different from those of EAV - so much so indeed as to constitute an extensive area of what is termed *bioelectronic functional diagnostics*.

EAV and bioelectronics in general are widely used in Germany (the Society of Bioelectronic Medicine numbers a thousand or so members), but are becoming increasingly well known in Italy as well, particularly as a result of the work of naturopaths and homeopaths. Unfortunately, the virtually total lack of knowledge (or interest?) in this area in academic circles inevitably means that there is very little scientific research in this field, which, as we shall see, is highly promising.

This is not the place for a detailed review of bioelectronic techniques and procedures, for which the reader is referred to other studies in the literature [Voll, 1975; Leonhardt, 1982; Kenyon, 1983]. Here we shall confine ourselves to schematically outlining the basic principles and applications of EAV, with a particular view to understanding the relationships between EAV and homeopathy.

Thanks to the studies conducted by Voll and others, new measurement points hitherto unknown to classic acupuncture have been identified, and precise clinical correlations have been established between variations in cutaneous resistance and organ diseases; in addition, procedures have been identified for assessing the efficacy of drugs (both homeopathic and allopathic) by using EAV to test their effects. The task of EAV is thus primarily to provide an aid to diagnostics based not on the objective assessment of biochemical or anatomico-pathological alterations, but on the evaluation of the electrophysiological perturbations associated with the diseases. In this sense, there is no conflict between bioelectronic diagnostics and conventional medicine: "The basic opinions of clinical medicine and acupuncture appear at first glance to be opposed, but actually they complement one another to a very considerable extent; whereas the domain of classic medicine is curative medicine, that of EAV is primarily prophylactic. Prevention and cure, prophylaxis and curative medicine, both serve for the patient's well-being and to a greater extent if the two proceed in harmony, hand in hand, and complement one another without gaps" [Leonhardt, 1982, p. 312].

There are measurement points for all the major organs, for the tissue systems, for the bone, articular, vascular, nervous and lymphatic systems, as well as specific points for degenerative manifestations. Perhaps the most interesting aspect is that many diseases begin to manifest measurable disorders with EAV before exhibiting other clinical manifestations [Leonhardt, 1982].

The EAV measurement system consists essentially (Figure 28) in an instrument which delivers an electrical current of approximately 8 mamps and a potential difference of about 0.5-1 volt to the acupuncture points. The current is conveyed along a circuit consisting of a lead which terminates in a point electrode which is used by the operator to test the various

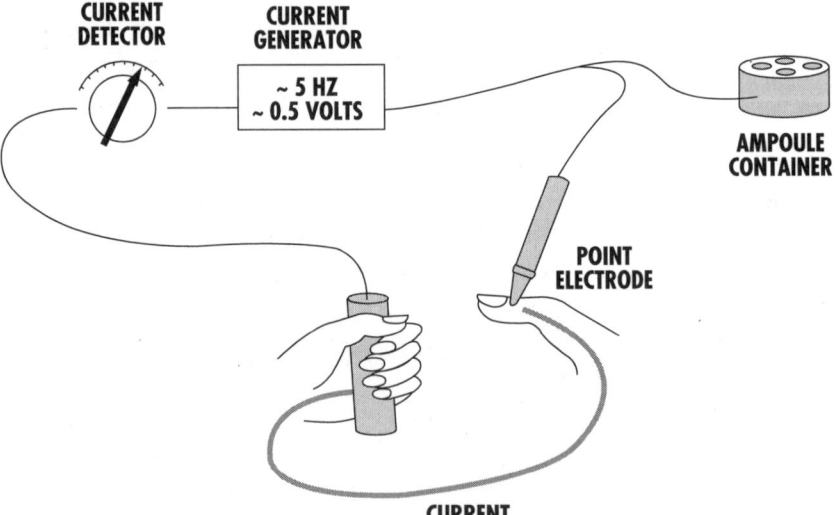

FIGURE 28 Simplified schematic illustration of a circuit for the electronic measurement of the conductivity of acupuncture points [modified from Kroy, 1989].

points, and then by the patient who holds a cylindrical electrode in his or her contralateral hand from which runs a lead returning to an current measurement device and then to a generator. Connected up to the lead that runs to the patient is another lead which runs to a metal ampoule-holder, used for measuring the interference of drugs or other test solutions (see below). On some appliances the ampoule-holder is situated inside the measuring equipment itself.

If the reaction of the body or organ corresponding to the point tested is normal, the electromotive force measured should be approximately 0.8 volts. In practice, the voltage is set in such a way that the ohmmeter registers "50" on an arbitrary scale of 100 units. The current density in these conditions ranges from 5 to 11 µamps.

In the case of diseases affecting the organ corresponding to the point tested, an increase in cutaneous electrical resistance may be measured, and thus a reduction in conductivity. It should be pointed out, however, that a lowering of electrical conductivity is not found in all diseases; in the case of diseases characterized prevalently by inflammatory phenomena there may be an increase in conductivity.

To these characteristic variations in bioelectric indices, which are in themselves of by no means negligible diagnostic interest, another property of the EAV system must be added: in the presence of a lowering of the conductivity index, if an ampoule of a drug with a positive effect on the patient's energetic-informational equilibrium is inserted in the electrical circuit in the ampoule-holder connected up to the electrode via a lead, the point recovers its conductivity and the index returns to the normal level. Conversely, if a healthy subject is being tested and a toxic substance or substance to which the subject reacts pathologically (cf., for instance, allergens) is inserted in the circuit, a previously normal index will drop to pathological levels.

Some type of *interaction* or *interference* would thus be established between the compound inserted in the ampoule-holder and an apparatus (probably consisting in the system of points and meridians envisaged in acupuncture) which controls the cutaneous electrical conductivity in the body. There can be no doubt that, before being accepted within the framework of present-day physiological and pathological knowledge, such a claim requires further testing and considerable substantiatory documentation.

Research in this field today is oriented, on the one hand, towards optimizing the procedures in order to achieve maximum reproducibility of measurements and, on the other, towards establishing the mechanisms whereby changes in conductivity come about as a result of diseases or the effects of drugs and toxic substances.

In view of the importance which EAV may have both for an understanding of the mechanisms of action of homeopathic drugs, and in general in the future of medicine, it is advisable, in this field, too, to refer to a number of the (very few) objective and verifiable experiments conducted. One of the most advanced centers in studies of this type is the Department of

Molecular and Cellular Biology of the University of Utrecht [van Wijk and Wiegant, 1989; van Wijk and van der Molen, 1990; van Wijk, 1991a; van Wijk, 1991b]. These researchers have verified that the parameter which best lends itself to objective measurements of changes in electrical conductivity at acupuncture points is not conductivity in the absolute sense (highly variable from one subject to another and influenced by the state of humidity of the skin or similar factors), but rather the phenomenon of *conductivity loss*: after applying the point electrode to an acupuncture point and maintaining constant pressure, within a few seconds a drop in conductivity is observed, as if a "charging" of the resistance of the point were taking place, or a "blocking" of the flux of electrical charges. This drop can easily be recorded on paper, so as to be able to construct graphs which can be interpreted in both qualitative and quantitative terms.

Loss of conductivity is a phenomenon which always occurs, but is much more rapid in the presence of a pathological perturbation of the system (diseased organ, intoxication). The van Wijk's group has confirmed that, if to an ampoule-holder connected up to the system by means of a lead (see Figure 28) solutions of particular compounds to which the subject reacts are added, the conductivity loss phenomenon is modified, in the sense that it may increase or diminish. To put it in schematically oversimplified terms, the result would be that, if the compound is toxic, it causes a drop in the index on a point which was previously normal as regards conductivity, whereas if the compound is therapeutic it causes a recovery of the index on a point which was previously pathological. In any event, test results of this kind would provide a strong indication that the solution placed in series in the EAV machine-patient-tester-EAV machine circuit *interferes* with the transmission of the electrical current in the circuit itself.

Van Wijk is conducting studies to optimize the EAV system and, above all, in order to distinguish between subjective (e.g. operator biomagnetic ability or sensitivity) and objective factors. In a series of experiments he has carried out the following studies which are briefly summarized here. The tester takes preliminary readings on points of the skin to identify the point or points which show an appropriate electrical response (loss of conductivity) and a good response (recovery of conductivity) to a series of drugs tested by the operator by placing them in the ampoule-holder. Once the optimal point has been identified, the subject swallows 1 ml of liquid containing 0.1 µg of diphenyl. This substance is toxic, but when taken in small quantities, does not cause any particular harm to the body. A few minutes after swallowing the diphenyl, an increased rate of loss of conductivity is registered on the points identified, which is recorded in a tracing with three successive readings. The use of diphenyl in a healthy subject is thus a good method of obtaining repeatable variations which are not subject to the variability encountered in patients suffering from spontaneous diseases, which in a method such as this one prevents statistical assessment of the results achieved.

In these experiments [van Wijk and Wiegant, 1989; van Wijk, 1991a] the authors have demonstrated that this drop in conductivity was made reversible when an ampoule containing a homeopathic dilution of sulphur (*Sulphur* 12x) was inserted in the ampoule-holder. It should be noted that greater or lesser dilutions had no effect and that the effect was registered only if the *Sulphur* 12x was prepared by means of dilution and succussion and not by simple dilution. The authors have explained the phenomenon on the basis of the homeopathic law of similars, in that the symptoms of diphenyl intoxication are similar to those of sulphur intoxication. Clearly, this is an explanation of an analogical and not a scientific type, but the experiment reported nevertheless provides documentary evidence of a specific interaction of *Sulphur* 12x and diphenyl with the electrophysiological system of the human body, as assessed by EAV.

In a subsequent communication, van Wijk reported that the EAV test also works in double-blind conditions, though less efficiently than in an "open" trial (i.e. when the operator or tester knows the type of ampoule inserted) [van Wijk, 1991b]. After recording the conductivity loss due to diphenyl, sealed ampoules of *Sulphur* 12x were inserted in the ampoule-holder and another set of three tracings was recorded. Placebo ampoules (dilutions of alcohol) were then inserted in the ampoule-holder and the conductivity loss rate was re-measured. The operation was repeated many times, first "open" and then "blind," in the sense that an independent observer inserted the ampoules into the ampoule-holder without telling either the tester or the patient. At the end of the experiment the tracings were processed as conductivity loss rate (in μamps/sec) and were compared for the true drug (in this case *Sulphur* 12x) versus placebo.

From these experiments it emerged that *Sulphur* causes recovery of conductivity (i.e. it prevents the loss of conductivity in the first few seconds after application of the point electrode) induced by diphenyl much more than placebo does. In the "open" experiments the difference is striking: with *Sulphur* in the ampoule-holder the loss of conductivity is from 0 to 0.25 μamps/sec, whereas with placebo it is from 1 to 1.75 μamps/sec. In the double-blind experiments, the difference was less marked, in that several false-positive tests were registered (i.e. the placebo had an effect) as well as several false-negatives (i.e. *Sulphur* had no effect), but on the whole the difference was highly significant (see Table 8).

TABLE 8

Effect of Placebo and Sulphur 12x on loss of conductivity induced by diphenyl in a series of double-blind tests

	Placebo	Sulphur 12x
No effect	35 tests	32 tests
Effect (blocking of conductivity loss)	13 tests	39 tests
Statistical difference: $P < 0.005$		

The use of EAV and of similar equipment in the detection of allergies has also been described by others [for a review see Fuller Royal, 1990; Fuller Royal and Fuller Royal, 1991]. The data obtained by means of electrodiagnosis of food allergies have been found to correlate with those obtained using better known methods such as RAST, skin tests, and alimentary provocation tests. Other studies, conducted double-blind [Ali, 1989], have shown that, in subjects suffering from allergies, electro-diagnostic testing shows a 73% correlation with levels of IgE antibodies specific for pollens and house dust.

The EAV test appears to function both with homeopathic and allopathic medicines, being used, for example, to assess the degree of pancreatic damage in diabetic patients and to establish an appropriate insulin dosage [Tsuei et al., 1989; Lam et al., 1990]. One thing is certain: if things were really like this, it would be an important field for development also in the allopathic context, in view of the fact, amongst other things, that the equipment required for such investigations is extremely simple and relatively inexpensive.

The mechanism whereby this interference phenomenon comes about is still obscure, in that very little research has been done to date in this field. In any event, one can hardly fail to appreciate the importance of the phenomenon described, which, once confirmed and accepted, would lead to conclusions such as:

a) The human body presents an increased electrical conductivity of the skin on the acupuncture points.

b) This conductivity is not stable, but is influenced by the state of health or sickness of the subject as a whole and of the organs of the body, which, according to the acupuncture concept, are linked to each of the points.

c) The electrical conductivity can be altered (both positively and negatively) by the introduction of toxic substances or drugs.

d) The alterations of electrical conductivity can be induced not only by the swallowing of the substances themselves, but also by placing ampoules containing solutions of the same substances in an ampoule-holder connected up by a wire to the system.

e) The EAV system makes it possible to demonstrate that the molecules in a solution possess the property of long-range interaction with electromagnetic frequencies.

f) Both homeopathic and allopathic drugs can be tested for their reactivity with the patient, just as allergies to particular substances can be detected by EAV.

Notwithstanding these positive results, many aspects of the EAV methodology are still uncertain, and its reliability as a diagnostic tool should be treated as hypothetical. The most controversial issue has to do with the role of the tester in the overall procedure: it has been shown in "blind" experiments that the tester is somewhat affected by the patient in the fine tuning of his muscular activity and the change in the muscular force applied to the electrode may change the current flux [van Wijk and Wiegant, 1994].

In a different, though related series of experiments, van Wijk's group joined forces with the Endler and Haidvogel group, who had performed the experiments on the effects of high dilutions of thyroxine on frog metamorphosis mentioned in Chapter 4, Section 1. In this latest series of tests, the authors [Endler *et al.*, 1994a] prepared high dilutions of thyroxine (T_4 30x) and, as controls, high dilutions of water (H_2O 30x), according to the rules of homeopathy. The dilutions were sealed in glass ampoules, and codes were applied to the ampoules by independent researchers from the Institute of Zoology of the University of Graz, with the result that the tests were performed blind. The ampoules—obviously sealed—were immersed in different containers in which the animals were being bred at a very precise stage of development (immediately after the complete appearance of the rear limbs and prior to the loss of the tail).

The experiment consisted in counting the number of small frogs that climbed the walls of the breeding containers, and went out of the water. The results (reproduced by five different researchers and making a total of more than 3000 observations) showed that the frogs from the container in which the T_4 30x ampoule was immersed climbed out of the water with a significantly greater frequency than the frogs treated with the H_2O 30x ampoule. Assays of thyroid hormones and iodine on the ampoules and on the ampoule washing fluid ruled out the presence of accidental contamination of the ampoules used in the test. However incredible these results may seem, we mention them here both in order to illustrate the problems with which researchers in the field of homeopathy are coming to grips and on account of their suggestive analogies with the results mentioned above in connection with the EAV tests.

Similar results have been confirmed by the same research team in a more recent communication [Endler *et al.*, 1994c; Endler *et al.*, 1995].

Other clinico-therapeutic experiences deriving from particular applications and variants of EAV have to do with the use of equipment such as MORA (from the initials of its inventors, Dr. Morell and his colleague, the engineer Rasche), for which, however, the reader is referred to other more specific texts [Meletani, 1990].

All these observations, if confirmed and consolidated by further evidence and testing, would indicate that:

a) Information of a nonmolecular nature remains impressed in the water in the process of dilution and dynamization.

b) This information may pass from an ampoule to the body by direct or indirect contact via the water of biological fluids.

c) In suitable experimental conditions, this information may bring about a certain effect which appears to be somehow related (by similarity or antagonism) to the effect of the initial preparation with which the dilution has been prepared.

As regards the diagnostic aspect at least, it is hard to see how electroacupuncture can fail to integrate with conventional diagnostics, being perhaps an extra means of gaining information about the functional disorders of organs or tissues, on previous infections (immunity) or infections in progress, on allergies or forms of food intolerance, on the particular reactivity of a patient to potentially dangerous drugs in cases of idiosyncrasy. Those who use these procedures stress the concept of "functional diagnostics," meaning by this the possibility of detecting homeostatic alterations early compared to anatomico-pathological alterations [Leonhardt, 1982]. If this were true, EAV could be complementary to traditional diagnostics. In the last years some reports confirmed previous positive findings [Krop *et al.*, 1997; Kail, 2001], while others showed that electrodermal devices like vegatest, when utilized under strictly controlled conditions (i.e. double blind), are not reliable as diagnostic tools, at least in allergy testing [Lewith *et al.*, 2001; Semizzi *et al.*, submitted for publication].

7.4 High dilutions, chaos and fractals

After what we have said in connection with complex systems and chaos (Chapter 5, Section 7), and after citing theories and trials in favor of the existence of metamolecular biophysical phenomena, we shall attempt a brief résumé of the situation here in this section.

First of all, we should recall what we have said in connection with the instability of the dynamic systems of the body. The existence of chaos and forms of fractal geometry is also of substantial importance for homeopathy. In fact, the hypothesis currently taking shape in this context claims that the homeopathic remedy, containing a set of specific items of information for a given patient, *may act as an attractor* in a pathophysiological situation with a tendency towards chaos and towards disorganization (disease). When a system is in a state of dys-equilibrium controlled by many factors, i.e. when it presents a behavior pattern characterized by complexity and chaos, a *small amount* of energy should be enough to make it shift one way or the other. The nearer one is to the bifurcation point, and the greater the freedom of choice, the lower will be the energy needed to shift the system in one direction or another.

This concept is well illustrated by going back to the mathematics of dynamic systems and of chaos. Considering the Verhulst algorithm, which has already been presented above (Chapter 5, Section 7.1), it can be demonstrated that the chaotic evolution of the nonlinear "homeostatic" function

$$A_{n+1} = A_n + A_n k (A_{max} - A_n)$$

can be changed to a more orderly evolution by means of very minor changes in the parameters such as changes in the coefficient k or of A_{max}. In fact, Figure 29A shows that a modification of k from 0.56 to 0.57 (i.e. 0.01) induces a dramatic shift from a totally chaotic attractor (where all the values from approximately 1 to 7 are allowed) to a situation where the A values resulting from the iteration are "confined" in three bands of values, arranged in the following sequence: low (A = about 1), medium (A = about 3), and high (A = about 7). The small change in k has forced the function into a new attractor, with characteristics of lower chaoticity, higher predictability, and better harmony. It is worthy of note that in the example given here, this effect is produced only by a small change in k. If the change is too marked, namely 0.02 as in Figure 29B, the function continues to present a chaotic trend.

Figure 29C shows that the modification of k from 0.56 to 0.55 (i.e. a 0.01 decrease in coefficient instead of the 0.01 increase as in Figure 29A) does not affect the chaotic behavior of the attractor. This indicates that the *direction* of the change is not indifferent: in other words, to obtain a specific and "qualitative" change of attractor, we need information that

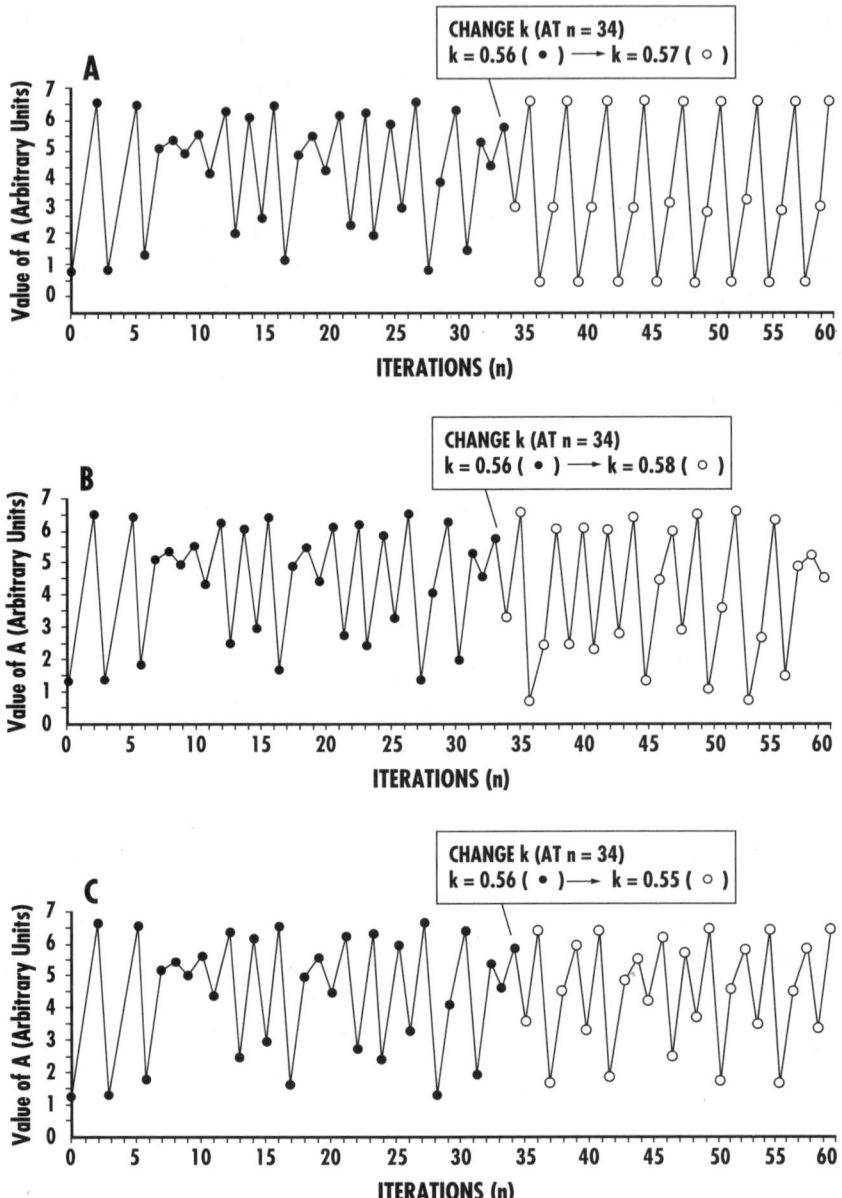

FIGURE 29 Effects of small changes of a constant coefficient in the chaotic behavior of a complex function. The panels show successive changes in the variable "A" in the iterations of the Verhulst algorithm (the formula is in the text). A_{max} and the (initial) A_n in all cases are assumed equal to 5.0 and 1.0, respectively. The changes in the coefficient k introduced at iteration n = 34 are indicated in the panels.

may *direct* the change in the desired way. This information cannot be wholly deduced from the appearance of the chaotic system: for certain values of k, a further increase may cause a return of order, while for other values of k, a further increase may cause an increase in chaos or the onset of chaos starting from an ordered situation (see, for example, Figure 16D - 16E). Owing to the complex behavior of chaotic systems, the outcome of a change in k coefficient cannot be wholly predictable, but has to be tested experimentally. Experience provides information to predict the behavior of complex systems in the proximity of the bifurcation points.

In brief, then, it may be postulated that the homeopathic drug, containing little of the material of the original solute (or none of it, according to the dilution) possesses a high "information content" for the specific case, thanks to the matching of the symptoms ascribed to the drug itself and those of the patient (law of similars). This information content will be capable of forcing the body homeostasis into a different attractor, or a different system of attractors, *in the specific direction dictated by the remedy*. In other words, this information, supplied in critical conditions of sensitivity of the system, will represent an adjustment towards a given type of behaviour, something like a "catalyst of order," or "pacemaker."

The information received, amplified and processed by one or more regulatory systems, might counteract the disorder induced by the pathological factor that has perturbed the normal homeostasis of the body. If we are referring to the field of high dilutions, it is clear that such "attractive" information must be based on the permanence of the image of the original compound, or of an image related to it. What we mean by "image" here is not merely spatial geometry, but potentially a spatio-temporal order as well in the form (form = in*form*ation and memory) of a certain oscillation frequency of the molecular dipoles or proton exchanges at hydrogen bond level.

It has been seen, in earlier sections of this chapter, that this "permanence of information" is now more than a simple hypothesis, even if its physical basis still remains highly uncertain. It has been demonstrated that such a phenomenon is *not absurd* in principle and that various models have also been proposed by competent researchers in the field.

It is worthwhile here re-examining, in particular, the problem of metamolecular information from the point of view of chaos and fractals. The relationship between these new mathematical theories (and experiences) and homeopathy can hardly fail to be extremely close both because the communication of information from the solute to the solvent is nothing other than the transition of water from disorder to a partial order, and because the dilution/dynamization processes may be regarded as resembling fractal dynamics. Other investigators have pointed out how the language of mathematics of nonlinear dynamics contains concepts that describe homeopathic observations [Garner and Hock, 1991; Shepperd, 1994; Teut, 2001]. Another important factor contributing to the effect of ultra-low doses of drugs of ultra-low physical energies on biological systems is stochastic resonance [Torres and Ruiz, 1996], a well known physical phenomenon according to which a signal may be amplified by the noise, instead of being masked by it [Wiesenfeld and Moss, 1995].

7.4.1 Transition from disorder to coherence

On dissolving a given compound in water, the compound "informs" the collectivity of the water molecules near to it, organizing them in such a way that as a whole they take on a configuration that reflects that of the compound itself. This is well known in chemistry, being due essentially to hydrophobic forces and to weak forces of attraction and repulsion of charges. It has also been seen that the nearest water molecules, thus reorganized, communicate in turn, via hydrogen bonds and probably also via electromagnetic vibrations related to the coherent motion of the dipoles, with other nearby molecules and so on up to a certain distance.

These modifications of the water are, however, a measure of "transfer of form," without this necessarily involving any chemical change in the water molecules *per se* (at least as regards the molecules not immediately in contact with the compound in solution), consisting only in a broad-ranging reorganization. According to the conventional view, successive dilutions entail a progressive reduction in the number of molecules of the solute up to its disappearance and up to the simultaneous disappearance of the reorganization form of the water already produced.

In homeopathic theory, by contrast, the solute, thanks to the succussion at the time of dilution, is believed to communicate an "excess" of information to the water compared to that strictly related to the molecular concentration of the solute itself. The reorganization of the molecular relationships is thought to take on a trend similar to that considered apropos of the Bénard cells (Chapter 5, Section 8.1): the water molecules, subjected to a given flow of energy, take on collective behavior patterns; in other words, a *coherence regimen* is set up in large domains of the water molecules. Obviously, these collective behavior patterns do not consist in macroscopic movements of masses of water, but in coherent vibrations of the molecular magnetic dipoles or of the protons involved in the hydrogen bonds between numerous adjacent water or ethanol molecules. Moreover, how this regimen can be maintained over time is somehow bound up with the possibility that the collective movements may in some way be isolated from the surrounding molecular chaos. As illustrated above, there is no univocal theory on this point, but the hypotheses put forward in earlier sections of this chapter (superradiance, NMR) appear suggestive.

7.4.2 Fractal dynamics

Various experiments have suggested that the biological activity of homeo-pathic dilutions does not diminish or increase regularly with increasing dilutions, but follows a "pseudosinusoidal" trend, with peaks of activity and troughs of inactivity. The most evident example is in Figure 1 (page 68), taken from the famous experiment performed by Benveniste's research team [Davenas *et al.*, 1988], but similar trends have also been reported by others [Poitevin *et al.*, 1985; Davenas *et al.*, 1987; Boiron and Belon, 1990; Poitevin, 1990; Sainte-Laudy *et al.*, 1991; Garner and Hock, 1991]. It can be seen that the activity causing basophil degranulation is present at the 9 log dilution (corresponding by and large to the homeopathic 9x dilution), and then drops to a minimum level at the 11 log dilution, only to pick up again and rise to a peak at the 15 log dilution, thereafter descending again, and so on. It will be noted that the recurrence pattern of the peaks is not regular, but chaotic and unpredictable, but at the same time it must be admitted that this recurrence exists, i.e. that the effective information re-presents itself after a number of log dilutions. According to the logic of current chemical reasoning, such a trend appears thoroughly and quite definitely absurd, but in the light of new knowledge of chaotic phenomena and the nonlinearity of many biological mechanisms perhaps some kind of underlying logic can be traced.

If we are prepared to give credence to such paradoxical results, one ques-tion inevitably springs to mind: how can information disappear and then reappear? Where did the information go in the mean time, while the inac-tive dilutions were being done, between one peak and another? To answer this question the fractal "line of reasoning" may come in handy. In fact, if we are to take the results of the experiments seriously, we have to admit that the specific information of the compound dissolved is not completely "dissipated" in the course of the successive dilutions, even when the dilu-tions are inactive. Evidently there exists some mechanism of transmission and storage of the information in the course of the dilutions such that the next dilution following an active dilution may give rise to a form (or vibra-tional frequency) differing from the previous one (and for this reason inac-tive), but capable, after a few steps of further diversification, of causing the original (active) information to "reappear." The dilutions, then, would not produce a loss of information (increased entropy), but only a change and variety of forms, which in turn may regenerate the starting form. Such behavior is reminiscent of what we have seen apropos of the mathematical iterations that generate fractals (see Chapter 5, Section 7, and Figures 16 and 17).

The repetitive waves of appearance and disappearance of activity may therefore represent chaotic oscillations of the result of a process of transfer of information from one dilution to the next. This, then, would be a phenomenon similar to the "recurrent regularity" typical of chaotic systems and fractals (see Chapter 5, Section 7).

If this is how things were, it would be easier to put into perspective the problem of the poor reproducibility of results, often seen in experimental trials in this field. The low reproducibility may depend on many factors related to the materials and methods used, but it is quite clear that if we postulate the existence of intrinsically chaotic mechanisms in the process of information transfer, the nonreproducibility should be viewed in a new light. In fact, wherever chaos and complexity play a significant role it is only to be expected that *minimal variations in the conditions of the experiment will express themselves in the form of substantial variations in the results* (cf., too, the discussion in Chapter 5, Section 8).

For instance, anyone wishing to repeat an experiment such as the one conducted by Benveniste's team (see Figure 1) should absolutely not expect to find the same activity peaks and inactivity troughs for the same dilutions, nor to observe the same phenomenon in all the experiments performed. On the other hand, there has to be a certain type of reproducibility in scientific research (e.g. the appearance of peaks at certain dilutions, at least in a significant number of cases and the nonappearance of peaks in control experiments with untreated water). This has been confirmed by Davenas (personal communication) and by other experiments reported in Chapter 4, as well as by EAV tests.

The hypothesis has been advanced [Gardner and Hock, 1991] that the successive dilutions and dynamizations performed in the preparation of a homeopathic remedy introduce an element of *information gain*, as is observed in the Mandelbrot sets with successive iterations (see Figure 17). It is suggested that low dilutions (few iterations) produce poor definition of details and carry rough and imprecise information, whereas high dilutions (many iterations) are characterized by better definition of details, as can be seen in the profiles of the Mandelbrot sets. If the dilutions/iterations are few, the image is "blurred," whereas, if they are repeated many times, the image is precise and, surprisingly, "reappears," i.e. it is reproduced in detail in subsets and in subsets of subsets. The image of a certain structure (in the case of homeopathy, the mother tincture) reappears in a "similar" form in successive dilutions, practically to infinity.

Such a phenomenon may basically be responsible for the fact that in classic homeopathy the high dilutions are regarded as more specific and profound in their therapeutic effect if there is perfect matching of the symptoms of the patient and the remedy, i.e. if the "*details*" of the analogy have emerged clearly from the homeopathic history-taking. In practice, the fewer the symptoms shared by the patient and the remedy, the lower will be the dilutions used; the more symptoms they have in common, the higher will be the dilutions prescribed.

Our aim in referring to these aspects is also to stress that a scientific approach to homeopathy in future will require the joint contribution of several disciplines, including mathematics, geometry and computer sciences. In general terms, the suggestions we are making here emphasize the fact that those researchers who are prepared to engage in the study of the unsolved, complex problems of biology and physics (including the study of homeopathic high dilutions) must begin to include the dimensions of chaos and the fractals in their conceptual, and possibly also in their experimental armamentarium. Chaos should appear less daunting to scientists today than it did in the past, because, thanks to the discovery of fractal geometry, we are beginning to come to grips with a number of rules of behavior which allow a certain degree of predictability.

We shall attempt here to summarize the main points dealt with in order to construct a number of hypotheses which constitute the frame of reference for putting homeopathy into rational and experimentally viable perspective, particularly that part of homeopathy relating to the use of high (metamolecular) dilutions. Hypotheses are essential to the evolution of knowledge. Only a patient, multidisciplinary effort will contribute towards clarifying, at least in part, the mysteries of the infinitely small. The hypotheses set forth here also refer to theories proposed by other authors [Vithoulkas, 1980; Tetau, 1985; Callinan, 1986; Rubik, 1990; Popp, 1990a; Popp, 1990b; Ullman, 1991a; Schulte and Endler, 1994; Schiff, 1995; Bastide and Lagache, 1997; Bastide, 1998; Vallance, 1998; Taddei Ferretti and Marotta, 1998; Schulte, 1999; Schwartz *et al.*, 2000].

7.5

Discussion on high-dilution homeopathy

The main difficulty of homeopathy using dilutions which enter into the "metamolecular" domain consists in the fact that it apparently contradicts the biomedical model dominant today, namely the biochemical-molecular model. In a highly diluted homeopathic preparation, very few or no molecules at all of the drug are present, and thus it proves impossible to explain, in terms of present-day pharmacological knowledge, how such a preparation can have any effect.

Nevertheless, a new vision of matter and life, more compatible with the possible *modus operandi* of homeopathy, is emerging on the frontiers of science, particularly from the fields of quantum physics and mathematical theories and research which have yet to be systematized. Organisms are seen as highly regulated, complex, dynamic systems which display a characteristic meta-stability around certain homeostatic levels. This meta-stability is the net result of continual oscillations, rhythms, networks, amplifications and feedback cycles. Living systems are "suspended" between order and chaos; they partake of these two fundamental characteristics of matter and exploit them in a manner designed to promote survival. Order and chaos are to be found at all levels of homeostasis, from the molecule to the human mind. We cannot see how these new perspectives can fail to have an impact on the new orientations and trends in medicine. Medical theory, methodology and technology have always proceeded hand in hand with the general scientific theory and socio-economic situations of the times.

Homeopathy is witnessing a revival in the present age, marked, as it is, by a staggering increase in scientific knowledge, accompanied by the awareness of a substantial degree of indeterminacy of reality. This is not tantamount, as many people are inclined to believe, to resorting to para-psychological or esoteric paradigms to escape the anguish of chaos and lack of trust or confidence in the modern health system. It is instead more likely that most of the success of homeopathy depends precisely on its original basic assumptions, which are at one and the same time realistic in theory and empirical in content.

Realism in this case coincides with humility and practicality; this was expressed by Hahnemann himself when he said, not without a sense of the paradoxical (for which he was to pay dearly): "Of such learned reveries (to which the name of *theoretic medicine* is given, and for which special professorships are instituted) we have had quite enough, and it is now high time that all who call themselves physicians should at length cease to deceive suffering mankind with mere talk, and begin now, instead, for once to act, that is, really to help and to cure" (note to paragraph 1 of the *Organon*). Certainly, we cannot fully endorse this statement today (otherwise we should never have set about writing this book). It is also true, however, that the arguments discussed and documented here appear to bear witness to the *substantial soundness* of Hahnemann's position, which methodologically takes into account the complexity of the human being and of human disease.

7.5.1 Oscillations and resonance

We have extensively illustrated the fact that living creatures are open systems far from equilibrium, subject to regulatory apparati which cannot necessarily be represented by linear equations, and thus are capable of perceiving minimal perturbations, particularly when they are predisposed to such sensitivity, possibly by the very pathological process itself. New evidence from electromagnetism studies lends support to the possibility that living systems respond to extremely weak magnetic fields, and particularly to specific frequencies. At the same time, studies regarding the physics of water suggest, or at least do not rule out, the possibility that water itself may act as a store and vehicle for electromagnetic oscillations. The tradition and new experimental evidence stemming from acupuncture and related techniques demonstrate that an individual with a molecular or functional disorder presents an imbalance of electromagnetic homeostasis which appears to be exploitable for diagnostic purposes and reversible if treated by specific stimulation.

Disease may therefore be regarded not only as a functional or molecular-structural abnormality, as in the classic view, but also (and not by way of contrast) as a disturbance of an entire network of electromagnetic communications based on long-range interactions between elements (molecules, nerve centers, organs, to mention but a few) which oscillate at frequencies which are coherent and specific and thus capable of resonance. This would be a *disturbance of internal oscillators and their communications*. Our knowledge is still too scanty to say whether or not these oscillators can be identified with certain nerve centers in particular (the ability to oscillate at characteristic frequencies is typical, though not exclusively so, of nerve centers) or with the collective behavior of nerve centers and/or other tissues or cells.

A disturbance of oscillation and of the communication associated with it may be brought back to a state of equilibrium by means of *syntonization or tuning, i.e. by means of a change in frequency imposed by interaction with another oscillator.* According to this notion, the homeopathic remedy might act in the patient as an external guide frequency.

The phenomenon of resonance is well known in physics, where it occurs in many fields: acoustics, mechanics, and electromagnetism, as well as nuclear physics. By virtue of this phenomenon, a system which is characterized by its own oscillation frequency can enter into vibration if stimulated (subjected to sound waves, electromagnetic waves, or mechanical vibrations according to the nature of the system) by frequencies close to those peculiar to the system itself. If the system is already oscillating, the resonance may greatly increase the amplitude of the oscillation, whenever the waves overlap, while the opposite may also occur, namely an arrest of oscillation, if the interaction is between two waves of the same frequency but opposite in phase. Of course, biological systems are characterized by very complex oscillatory frequencies, in keeping with the complexity of their components. For resonance phenomena to occur, the frequencies do not need to overlap exactly; it is enough for there to be matching of one or more harmonics (harmonics are the simplest components into which periodic functions produced by their overlap can be broken down); the harmonics of a given periodic system all have frequencies which are multiples of the fundamental frequency, called the first harmonic.

Resonance, then, is a way whereby information is transmitted between two *similar* systems (as regards vibrational or harmonic frequencies) without structural modifications and without the passage of matter. These linkage phenomena between oscillators, which generate synchronism and cooperativity, are of paramount importance in many physiological functions, particularly in the nervous system, but also in the cells regulating cardiac rhythm, in the cells secreting insulin in the pancreas, in the ciliated epithelia, and in the involuntary contractions of smooth muscle [Breithaupt, 1988; Engel *et al.*, 1992; Strogatz and Stewart, 1993].

Therefore, a dynamized and potentized homeopathic drug might be regarded as a small amount of matter containing elements oscillating in phase (coherently), capable of transmitting these oscillatory frequencies, via a process of resonance, to biological fluids (in turn mostly made up of water), but also to complex "metastable" structures, subject to nonlinear behavior patterns and capable in turn of oscillating (macromolecules, α-helixes, membranes, filamentous structures, receptors). There would thus be the possibility of a link between drug frequencies and oscillators present in the living organism perturbed by the disease.

Even signals which are extremely small, but which are endowed with highly specific information and are capable of resounding in unison with the recipient system, could act as regulators, if it is admitted that the dysregulated system or systems are in a state of precarious equilibrium, near to the "*bifurcation*" point, where the choice whether to move in one direction or the other is related to minimal fluctuations on the border between order and chaos. The new concepts emerging from chaos studies tell us that at this "border" minimal variations in the conditions of the system (such as those induced even by a very small oscillatory resonance) may play a decisive role in the subsequent evolution of the system itself. In a variety of systems, the "butterfly effect" may be used to control chaos, on condition that the parameters to be controlled and changed are well known [see also Shinbrot *et al.*, 1993; Schiff *et al.*, 1994; Moss, 1994].

7.5.2 Bifurcations

Where are these "bifurcations" sensitive to minimal doses and, presumably, to metamolecular information? They may be found in the behavior of any complex system, from single molecules to cells and to the whole body. Here we consider specifically the bifurcations occurring in the dynamic progression of diseases.

As illustrated previously (Chapter 5, Section 1 and Chapter 6, Section 2.4), the story and intimate nature of a pathological process present various phases or aspects which integrate one another in sequences in time and space. If we are referring to the majority of diseases, which are not exclusively of genetic origin, what usually appears as the "disease" according to the traditional diagnostic criterion is the last phase, consisting in precise biochemical and anatomical abnormalities. Before this, however, there are at least three other phases:

a) *From health to the initial disorder*

Starting from an ideal state of health, we have the very first stage in which an initial disorder, mostly nonapparent apart from a number of very indistinct symptoms or variations in very subtle parameters, makes the body susceptible to perturbations induced by external agents. The subject cannot be defined as a sick person, but is more predisposed to falling sick than normal and has a tendency to fall sick. In this stage we could, for instance, include those who are subject to overwork (stress) or to an unbalanced diet, those who smoke, who are exposed to low doses of ionizing radiation, or who present particular genetic characteristics making them statistically "at risk" (heterozygous carriers of autosomal recessive diseases, a number of HLA groups, race, etc.).

To what extent this disorder is "normal," in the sense that it is a simple reversible oscillation of a state of equilibrium, and to what extent it is "pathological," in the sense that it generates disease in the presence of other perturbing factors, is an extremely subtle and hazy issue, so much so indeed that the same situations, which may even be quite severe, are supported as a normal burden of life by some people, whereas they are regarded as serious diseases by others (often defined as imaginary or psychosomatic illnesses). Clearly, at this level the balance between normal and pathological is extremely precarious, and the subsequent course of the disease can come down on side or the other according to shifts in minor factors.

It has been said (Chapter 5, Section 8) that the body may be seen as a system of flux and that, in the domain of complexity, variations in the flow of energy can induce turbulence:

$$\text{Complexity} + \text{energy flow} \longrightarrow \text{turbulence}$$

Diseases, in the initial stages, can be regarded as turbulence phenomena in the metastable equilibrium that we call health. The order of the system changes, but the parameters, matter and energy making up the system do not necessarily change with it. We have seen and understood that disease presents a component related to imbalances in the electromagnetic homeostasis of the body, based on forms of communication or regulation mediated by frequency and vibrational signals. View from this angle, the homeopathic drug, which is rich in information though lacking in material substance, might positively act as an order-carrying factor and guide the body towards a new or pre-existing pattern of behavior.

b) *The reactive phase*
A second bifurcation is to be found in the reactive phase of homeostatic biological systems. As extensively documented above, these systems - particularly the inflammatory and immune systems, but also the liver detoxification systems, the hemostatic system, and others - are "two-faced," i.e. they bring about healing, but they also cause damage.

To what extent, in each individual case, the damage prevails over the restoration of the state of health or vice versa, depends on subtle variations in the behavior of the homeostatic system itself. In particular, the fate of the reaction depends on the "choice" that the system has to make between the price to pay, in terms of toxicity and suffering, and the guarantee of success of the operation in terms of survival of the body. For instance, in the presence of a lesion of the surface of a blood vessel, the hemostatic system comes into action to block the risk of hemorrhage and to initiate repair (clotting, platelet aggregation, increase in connective tissue and vascular musculature). Yet, through the same effector mechanisms a pathological event can occur: the hemostatic system entirely blocks the circulation of the blood in the vessel (thrombosis, atherosclerosis).

What is it that "tips the scale" in favor of the positively-directed action rather than the unnecessary and frankly pathological one? It is the complexity of the multiplicity of mechanisms involved. A "choice" of this type depends, in fact, both on the individual elements involved (receptors, concentration of mediators, presence of exogenous chemical substances) and on the type of coordination available, on a "centralized" control system that assesses the information coming in from the various regions and elements involved and regulates accordingly the various responses.

Thus, at the level of such a bifurcation, the outcome of the reaction may depend on an item of information that is *significant in terms of the coordination* of the reaction system or systems. Since such coordination is guaranteed by cybernetic networks such as the nervous and hemato-hormonal systems, but also by the acupuncture regulation system and perhaps by other information networks as yet to be identified (exchanges of frequencies by means of water or biopolymers, cf. Bistolfi, 1989), the result is that an item of metamolecular information that reaches these systems and is decoded by them may be useful in the optimal "choice" of reaction to the damage.

c) *Adaptation?*

A third phase of the disease process, in which another very critical moment of decision presents itself, is when the reactive systems fail to cope with the situation and rapidly restore the original state. At this point adaptation may set in, which is a semipermanent modification which, on the one hand, reduces the symptoms, but, on the other, may lead to various consequences, including deposition of toxins, hyperplasia, shifting of the receptor sensitivity threshold and biochemical and anatomical changes that "defer the problem" for lengthy periods or shift the pathological consequences from one organ to another. This has already been mentioned in the chapter on the complexity of diseases (Chapter 5, Section 5.1). Adaptation makes it possible to *live with* the disease, but also constitutes, in a certain sense, a renunciation of complete healing. At this point, too, homeopathy and homotoxicology, as therapies aimed at "re-arousing" the reactive capacity, may be of decisive importance.

Homeopathy should therefore act on the initial "decision-taking" levels of the body's repair and defense systems. When a disease reaches the stage where gross biochemical and anatomical consequences of the disease process are present, we are entering a field in which there would appear to be a much greater indication for the use of strong therapies such as surgery, replacement therapy, or the use of drugs at high doses, though even here a possible contribution of homeopathy should not be ruled out (provided at least some of the homeostatic control systems can intervene).

Even as referring to the diagnostic sphere, it is clear that the more a disease claims attention in terms of biochemical and anatomical abnormalities, logically the greater will be the tendency to resort to laboratory investigations and diagnostic imaging techniques, whereas a homeopathic "diagnostic work-up" aimed at capturing the subtle differences in personality and symptoms between one patient and another would make very little sense. Conversely, however, conventional diagnostic means can achieve very little within the framework of the initial subtle changes in complex homeostatic equilibria, or, even if they manage to pinpoint individual variations in biochemical or functional parameters, yield no criteria for "reconstructing" the picture as a whole and thus for implementing a complete therapy.

In conclusion, then, homeopathy is not opposed to the conventional approach even in the context of these considerations: homeopathy is concerned with the very early, subtle, global, and individual stages of the disease process, whereas conventional medicine tends to intervene at more anatomical and biochemical levels. Depending upon the level at which they operate, different methodologies of both diagnostic and therapeutic type are adopted, which should be fully integrated in the patient's best interests.

7.5.3 Integrated approach and specificity

Nobody today, even on the conventional medicine front, would deny the fact that when treating a disease we have to aim at putting the real situation of the patient as a whole into proper perspective. This precept is undoubtedly accepted theoretically by the advocates of any type of therapeutic approach, whether homeopathic, allopathic, or otherwise, but in practice it is hard to apply to actual cases. Despite the good intentions, the doctor is obliged, in his diagnostic and therapeutic efforts, to split off the disease process from the host body and to concentrate all his or her attention and therapy on the organ, cell or molecule. Though in many cases this will prove immediately effective, in others it fails to resolve the situation and above all to allow implementation of a complete therapy, because it is unable to influence all the levels of imbalance that have led to the disease and modulate its course. To achieve this ideal, almost utopian goal we currently lack both the "diagnostic" and therapeutic means.

In this connection, the route traced by the homeopathic method is suggestive in view of its tendency to consider not only the details, but also the "central core" of the patient's abnormal condition, as it may be perceived by the physician on the basis of the detailed study of the patient's "history," analysis of his or her type of constitution, attention to neurological and also psychological symptoms, and consideration of physiological peculiarities (tastes and aversions for certain foods, neurovegetative functions, etc.) and of the patient's reactivity to environmental stimuli (heat, cold, meteorological and seasonal changes, and so on).

Homeopathy is a *"probe"* into complex systems. Despite all the limitations related to difficulties in rendering the homeopathic approach objective, it is clear that it entails an attempt to "explore" the patient's medical history at the level of the neuroendocrine system and thus to calibrate some form of therapeutic intervention at this level, too. Homeopathy and homotoxicology regard inflammation as a "symptom" (i.e. as a signal or message) and not as a "disease," and they regard this symptom as the expression of an alteration of the relationship between subject and environment and/or between systems in the same subject. In the light of what we have said about the complexity of living systems, these concepts appear to be of great topical interest, quite apart from the difficulties encountered in rationalizing and perhaps even in demonstrating everything that homeopathy claims.

Homeopathy used with ultra-diluted drugs is thus a tentative approach to the bioenergetic regulation of the human body, utilizing a physical-biochemical interface due to the extreme sensitivity of biological systems to this type of regulation. The strength of the method consists in the fact that it attempts to achieve the maximum possible degree of *specificity* of the exogenous regulatory intervention. As stated earlier, the effective doses will be lower, the more specific the stimulus and the more sensitive the target system. If we admit that information is contained in metamolecular form in the homeopathic remedy, this information may also act in a metamolecular manner in the bioenergetic target system.

How can the maximum specificity of information be achieved, if we know so little about such bioenergetic systems? The answer is implicit in what was outlined in Chapter 6 of this book: *through the application of the law of similars*. This fundamental principle, based, as it is, essentially on the observation of *effects* (i.e. on comparison of the effects of the drug with those of the disease), is in a certain sense independent of any knowledge of the mechanism which causes the effects and thus also applies to the metamolecular level, once we have admitted the existence of the latter.

Homeopathic reasoning is based more on analogy than on inductive thinking. The use of analogy (identification of similarity) is justified on theoretical grounds on the basis of the fact that the various elements of reality are interlinked, because they all derive from the same evolutionary process; in nature, we find the result of a growth of items of information which are always kept "in contact" with one another (cf. fractals). Animals have always lived in contact with vegetable substances and minerals, and it is for this reason that a molecule contained in a flower may be "similar" to molecules contained in the animal, and there may therefore be a transfer of information.

Information is transferred only between similars, or between opposites, or in any event between elements that are capable of interacting as a result of affinity of structure or of vibrational frequencies (harmony, resonance, coherence). Analogical reasoning consists in grasping this basic principle. Reality has grown like a fractal and resembles a hologram: the complex contains the simple form, and the simple form contains the program of the complex.

The "secret" of homeopathy lies in the meticulous gathering of information both in the proving phase and in the homeopathic history-taking phase. This information can come from the hidden depths of the homeostatic regulatory system under investigation, but is still information. In the homeopathic method it is used directly in the therapeutic intervention, trusting in the fact that the body will know how to receive, decode and utilize this informational input for the purposes of restoring the lost equilibrium.

Going over from collecting data to implementing therapy, regardless of the diagnosis in the classic sense, might seem to be a leap in the dark, in which one gives up any attempt to rationalize the pathophysiological picture. In actual fact, this leap in the dark applies only to those who use homeopathy as an alternative to rigorous, scientific clinical reasoning; this alternative was comprehensible once when such reasoning was practically impossible. Today, this is no longer the case: homeopathic thinking can and must integrate with scientific reasoning regarding the known mechanisms of disease, because, as we have seen, the similarity can be rationalized and understood also at more precise and profounder levels than those relating merely to the symptoms.

There is no valid reason for excluding from the gathering of symptoms the execution of laboratory tests and diagnostic imaging; indeed, there are excellent reasons for using them, in view of the fact that any increase in knowledge does nothing but enhance the "image" of the disease and thus facilitates therapeutic decisions. The problem rather is of a practical nature: we should review the classic pathogenetic pictures of the various homeopathic remedies, integrating them with the most up-to-date knowledge. This will involve repeating large-scale provings in healthy subjects and clinical trials in groups of patients, or the design and conduct of new trials with newly identified compounds.

Another "secret" of homeopathy is that it deals with the human being as a whole, devoting the maximum attention to symptoms of a psychological type and those peculiar to each individual subject (individualization). In this way, it achieves a very substantial measure of specificity, inasmuch as it is now well known that the response to drugs can vary on the basis of the characteristics of the individual user.

If to these considerations we add the fact that we are witnessing a convergence of the homeopathic and the acupuncture approaches (particularly as regards EAV, but also over other by no means marginal aspects, such as biorhythms, the analysis of symptoms, disease etiology, and diet), it will be appreciated that the ability to gather information is gaining in strength also in technological terms. If it were true, as the studies presented above appear to suggest, that the sensitivity of a given patient to a given compound can be detected by measuring the currents travelling along the meridians, we would thus have another key to penetrating the "sanctuary" of biological and pathological information. Gathering information, such as knowing, for instance, whether a certain patient is allergic to or intolerant of a certain compound, or knowing whether a certain drug restores the balance or produces electrical dysequilibrium would be an undeniable step forward from the point of view of diagnosis and therapy.

An interpretation of homeopathy such as that presented here reconciles the "integrated" view, which considers the complexity of the human being in all his or her components, with the "reductionist" view, which considers the single organ, cell, or molecule. In fact, there cannot be a contrast between the whole and the fragment which this whole contains. On this basis, the controversy between homeopathy and allopathy, as if only the latter were "scientific," actually appears quite anachronistic. As we have seen in other sections of this book (Chapter 6, Sections 2.6 and 2.7), homeopathy and allopathy have different and specific indications, though in many cases they can usefully be combined.

The biophysical paradigm has been developed in recent years by several authors [see for a review Schulte, 1999], but there is still not consensus on the so-called memory of water, nor is there a consistent theory explaining the mechanism of action of high-potency homeopathic medicines. Based on the lack of agreement on the physical bases [Walach *et al.*, 1999] and on the negative results of some clinical trials and provings carried on under strictly blind conditions, a non-local interpretation of the high-potency homeopathy has also been suggested [Walach, 2000].

Further insights and discussions on the implications of dynamic systems theory for the understanding of homeopathic effects are reported in the second appendix of this book and in other recent reviews [Elia, 1999; Ruiz *et al.*, 1999; Schwartz *et al.*, 2000; Widakowich, 2000].

8 Prospects

The experiments, results, theories and speculation reported in this book do not lend themselves to easy conclusions. On the other hand, all due caution is warranted in science when it comes to drawing conclusions. The aim of the authors may be regarded as achieved if what they have written has shed light on a series of new insights and aroused interest in the subject.

The practice of homeopathy is spreading and, slowly but surely, the theoretical and experimental basis on which this practice must necessarily rest is gaining ground. Given the present state of our knowledge, it is no longer possible to dismiss the issue of homeopathy as if were some kind of awkward fossil of medical science. A vast body of experimental evidence, as problematical and controversial as that of any other new field of research, bears witness with increasing consistency to the substantial convergence emerging between the traditional principles of homeopathy and new insights in the fields of immunology, biology and physics.

Modern science is becoming increasingly oriented towards tackling various aspects of the complexity of nature, and medicine cannot escape this tendency. Molecular analysis and systems integration must go hand in hand if we are to avoid the risk of slipping into reductionism as an end in itself. Homeopathy, on the strength of a centuries-old empirical tradition while, at the same time, representing a frontier field of research, will certainly have a future in this context. This therapeutic method, in fact, *appears made to measure for tackling the complexity of disease*, in that it originated and has subsequently developed for the precise purpose of achieving a reasoned selection of remedies in the virtual absence of any kind of certainty as to the "intimate nature" of diseases.

As we have extensively explained, despite its "holistic" vocation, homeopathy cannot be indicated for all diseases, because in those cases where the cause and mechanism of the disease itself are well known and clear, "exact" science can demonstrate which are, or may be, the appropriate remedies (in many cases the theoretically effective remedies are known but are not applicable). In many other pathophysiological situations, however, in those cases where the cause and mechanism lie in the complex dynamic interplay of many factors, which in themselves are not pathological, but are a source of disease on account of their harmful interactions, homeopathy may prove a highly effective instrument. In point of fact, its few theoretical principles, its strong measure of realism, and its very substantial body of experience (albeit with all the methodological shortcomings outlined above) have enabled homeopathy to survive on the borders of scientific medicine and to present itself anew today as a valid counterpart.

From what has been said, however, there emerges a need for the utmost caution. Classic homeopathy is simple in its traditional principles, but difficult in its applications, particularly owing to the great variety of diseases and human beings. To claim that all the issues raised by homeopathy have been clarified would be an unobjective and, above all, a hazardous conclusion if applied indiscriminately in the practical clinical sphere. It is one thing to talk about theories, hypotheses and the results of experimental models, and quite another to transfer these to human subjects.

The practical application of homeopathy, as it is often practiced at the level of medicine of the masses, has little to do with what we have been talking about in this treatise. There is a tendency to transform homeopathy into a kind of *universal remedy* for all cases in which conventional medicine fails, or to consider homeopathy as a *useful placebo*, because it helps to restore the doctor-patient relationship. The former tendency is misleading and wrong-headed, while the latter is limiting, but there are sound reasons, both of a commercial and socio-cultural nature, for fostering and pursuing both. If homeopathy were to remain confined to these two positions, it would betray its origins and its basic aims.

The so-called "alternative" forms of medicine contain an appreciable dose of methodological uncertainty and for this reason can easily be used beyond the bounds of any kind of scientific logic. In the ocean of present-day ignorance as to the causes and therapies of many diseases, it is all too easy to find any number of empirical and intuitive approaches which no-one can readily demonstrate as being either beneficial or harmful. What emerges from the present study suggests that homeopathy can be addressed on a rational, objective and experimental basis and that it is now possible - much more so today than it once was - to use the knowledge and methodologies of conventional medicine and modern biomedical research also to investigate this controversial discipline.

In this field, scientific research may have a basic role to play in distinguishing between certainties and hypotheses, between what is plausible and what has been demonstrated, in objectivating and measuring as much as possible, in rationalizing concepts, in establishing limits of applicability, in refining materials and methodologies, and in controlling the quality of experimental trials and products.

The main lines of research from which we can expect future development of the scientific theories outlined herein are the following:

a) *Research into the physicochemical properties of water* and of water-alcohol solutions. In particular, it would be important to consolidate the NMR evidence (and that provided by other physical spectroscopic methods such as ultraviolet, infra-red and Raman-laser spectroscopy) so as to be able to have methods capable of detecting any possible changes produced in the solvent by dilution and dynamization. In the first place, this would provide methods for the objective "analysis" of information transfer and for studying its stability, mechanisms and variations in a scientific manner.

b) *Design and development of experimental models* of cells, isolated organs and animals for studying the possible biological effects of homeopathic remedies (at the various dilutions) in a rigorous, reproducible and standardizable manner. The standardization of the reagent preparation procedures and the repetition of the results obtained to date in different laboratories should be one of the primary objectives to be achieved in the near future.

c) *Pharmacological and biochemical studies of the active ingredients* used in homeopathy, for the purposes of identifying the possible targets in the patient's body at molecular, cellular, or some other level. Quite apart from the issue of high dilutions, it would be important in itself to work right through from the empirical identification of the remedies (as per the homeopathic tradition) to a definition of the mechanism of action on a pathophysiological and pharmacological basis.

d) *Controlled clinical trials*, which constitute a decisive aspect also of homeopathic research. Gearing methodologies to the particular demands of the homeopathic method makes it possible to draw reliable conclusions as to the efficacy of a remedy or series of remedies in the treatment of a disease or series of diseases. Needless to say, from controlled clinical trials we should not expect a definitive "confirmation" or "condemnation" of homeopathy as such, but only an extensive series of results of varying degrees of reliability and positive or negative outcomes, as in all fields of modern medicine. From these results, obtained patiently and methodically by various research teams, we can expect a better definition of the field of applicability of homeopathy, a more rational choice of remedies and dosages, and a clearer knowledge of any interference or synergisms between the homeopathic method and conventional medicine.

e) *Classic homeopathic experimentation*. The edifice of homeopathy, according to its classic tenets, can never be regarded as complete. New substances, both natural and synthetic, can be continually introduced into the homeopathic pharmacopoeia, after being tested in healthy subjects (proving) and in patients (clinical confirmation). The materia medicas and repertories can and must be updated, amended with the removal of any errors, and made easier to consult and use. In view of the vast amount of material accumulated over the years by the homeopathic tradition, there can be no doubt that in this process of implementation and revision a fundamental contribution will be made by the increasingly widespread use of internationally linked and coordinated computer systems.

As can be seen, many different disciplines can contribute to the study of the principles of homeopathy and to the definition of the experiments to be conducted to test their validity. In this book we have reviewed many of the lines of research already embarked upon or so far only sketchily developed. Of course, we have not been able to clarify various issues in detail, particularly in the field of biophysics, which is beyond the sphere of competence of the authors. This book, then, should be viewed mainly as a contribution made to these issues by General Pathology, a discipline by its very nature oriented towards forms of synthesis and integration rather than towards the analysis of individual details. The existence, in this field, of some form of overall, synthetic thinking, which at the same time is critical and rigorous, may help to direct the efforts of investigators in a coherent and productive manner for medicine in the future, which will be neither official nor alternative, but only medicine, if possible increasingly geared to meeting the challenges of new diseases.

The fields of research open to investigators are therefore multiple and extremely broad-ranging. The various health authorities should realize this and promote suitable research projects on these topics, with greater conviction and commitment than has been the case to date. If research in this field is worthwhile, it necessarily follows that adequate resources must urgently be devoted to it.

It would also be desirable if, without forgoing a proper measure of caution and graduality in their interventions, academic circles would abandon the scepticism which has so far characterized their attitude towards homeopathy and which sometimes expresses itself as out and out hostility. If this subject were in some way included in the university syllabus, two important objectives would be achieved: first and foremost, newly graduated doctors would be better informed as to the possible indications or contraindications of homeopathic remedies, which the patients often take as self-medication. It is undeniable that a knowledge of homeopathy would also be useful for doctors who do not intend to use it in their specific sector. Moreover, young researchers would have an incentive to undertake studies in this field, which, as things stand in the universities today, may seem useless or even counterproductive for the purposes of a university career. One of the mechanisms which favor research, in fact, is the evaluation of scientific qualifications and curricula in applications for university posts or promotion. If homeopathy "does not exist" in the university, research will hardly be developed in this setting, or at least not to a degree comparable with that of other disciplines.

The implications of research in homeopathy are very far-reaching. From a general point of view, our very understanding of biological and physiological reality could be greatly extended by it. The phenomenon of the effects of microdoses prepared according to homeopathic procedures may also have spin-off applications in botany, veterinary science and in the study of ecosystems. In medicine, the specific, rationalized use of small doses (or high dilutions) of specific substances for stimulating or restoring the balance of endogenous defense and repair systems of the human body may complement, increase and even in some cases replace the present technological approach. It would appear increasingly necessary for the problems posed by modern diseases to receive high level technological and scientific responses, but also responses based on a new awareness of the complex relationship between the human being and the environment and on a rational use of resources.

A homeopathic theory which also aims to become a scientific theory in the modern sense of the term, without relinquishing its basic principles, should incorporate in the body of its teaching the issues pertaining to the new frontiers which we have attempted to present and discuss in this review. In view of the multiplicity of factors involved in such an updating process—conduct of research studies and their results, forms of socio-economic conditioning, evolution of scientific paradigms—it is by no means easy to foresee at what a rate and to what extent this may come about. It seems clear, however, that a more fruitful dialogue between homeopathy and modern biomedical science will be to the advantage not of one side or the other, but of medicine itself, whose only true mission is and always has been *"to restore the sick to health, to cure, as it is termed"* (*Organon*, paragraph 1).

References

Aabel S. (2000) No beneficial effect of isopathic prophylactic treatment for birch pollen allergy during a low-pollen season: A double-blind, placebo-controlled clinical trial of homeopathic Betula 30c. *Br. Hom. J.* 89: 169.

Aabel, S., Fossheim, S., Rise, F. (2001) Nuclear magnetic resonance (NMR) studies of homeopathic solutions. *Br. Hom. J.* 90: 14.

Adey, W.R. (1988) Physiological signalling across cell membranes and cooperative influences of extremely low frequency electromagnetic fields. In: *Biological Coherence and Response to External Stimuli* (H. Frohlich, ed.) Springer-Verlag, Berlin, p. 148.

Adler, M. (1999) Efficacy and safety of a fixed-combination homeopathic therapy for sinusitis. *Adv. Ther.* 16: 103.

Aissa, J., Litime, M.H., Attias, E., Allal, A., Benveniste, J. (1993) Transfer of molecular signals via electronic circuitry. *FASEB J.* 7: A602 (3489).

Albertini, H., Goldberg, W. (1986) Evaluation d'un traitement homéopathique de le névralgie dentaire. Bilan de 60 observations dentaires in recherches en homéopathie. *Fondat. Franc. Rech. Homéopath.* Lyon, p 75.

Alberts, B., Bray, D., Lewis, J., Raff, M., Roberts, K., Watson, J.D. (1989) *Molecular Biology of the Cell. 2nd edition.* Garland Publ., New York.

Albrecht-Buehler, G. (1990) In defense of "nonmolecular" cell biology. *Int. Rev. Cytol.* 120: 191.

Albrecht-Buehler, G. (1991) Surface extension of 3T3 cells towards distant infrared light sources. *J. Cell. Biol.* 114: 493.

Aldrich, T.E., Easterly, C.E. (1987) Electromagnetic fields and public health. *Environ. Health Perspect.* 75: 159.

Algrain, M., Arpin, M., Louvard, D. (1993) Wizardry at the cell cortex. *Curr. Biol.* 3: 451.

Ali, M. (1989) Correlation of IgE antibodies with specificity for pollen and mold allergy with changes in electrodermal skin responses following exposure to allergens. *Am. J. Clin. Pathol.* 91: 357.

Allen, H.C. (1910) *The Materia Medica of the Nosodes.* Boericke & Tafel, Philadelphia.

Amodeo, C., Dorfman, P., Ricciotti, F., Tetau, M., Veroux, P.F. (1988) Evaluation de l'activité d'Arnica 5CH sur les troubles veineux après perfusion prolongée. *Cah. Biother.* 98: 77.

Anagnostatos, G.S., Vithoulkas, G., Garzonis, P., Tavouxoglou, C. (1991) A working hypothesis for homeopathic microdiluted remedies. *Berlin J. Res. Homoeopathy* 1 (3): 141.

Anagnostatos, G.S. (1994) Small water clusters (chlatrates) in the preparation process of homoeopathy. In: *Ultra High Dilution* (P.C. Endler and J. Schulte, eds.). Kluwer Acad. Publ., Dordrecht, p. 121.

Anderson, L.A., Phillipson, J.D. (1982) Mistletoe—the magic herb. *Pharmaceut. J.* 229: 437.

Andreoli, V. (1991) Follia e biologia. *Le Scienze (Italian edition of Sci. Am.)* 275: 44.

Arcieri, G. (1988) *Introduzione alla Medicina Cibernetica e Quantistica.* Nuova Ipsa Editore, Palermo.

Arecchi, F.T., Arecchi, I. (1990) *I Simboli e la Realtà.* Jaca Book, Milano.

Arend, W.P., Dayer, J.M. (1990) Cytokines and cytokine inhibitors or antagonists in rheumatoid arthritis. *Arthr. Rheum.* 33: 305.

Attena, F. (1991) Omeopatia e memoria dell'acqua. Fondamenti scientifici e considerazioni sociologiche. *Feder. Medica* 44: 36.

Attena, F., Del Giudice, N., Verrengia, G., and Granito, C. (2000) Homoeopathy in primary care: Self-reported change in health status. *Complement Ther. Med.* 8: 21.

Aubin, M. (1984) Elements de pharmacologie homéopathique. *Homéopathie Francaise* 72: 231.

Aulagnier, G. (1985) Action d'un traitement homéopathique sur la reprise du transit post opératoire. *Homéopathie* 6: 42.

Aulas, J.J., Chefdeville, F. (1984) Etude historique et critique des sources de la Matière Médicale homéopathique. Origines et développements de la Matière Médicale hahnemannienne. *Encycl. Med. Chir. (Paris), Homéopathie* 38080 (A10).

Bach, J.F. (1988) Immunotherapy of autoimmune diseases. *Rec. Prog. Med.* 79: 343.

Balsano, F., Bonomo, L., Di Perri, T., Grassi, C., Guidi, G., Muiesan, G., Zanussi, C. (1988) Effetto di un composto glicoproteico estratto da Klebsiella pneumoniae sul decorso clinico di infezioni acute delle vie aeree in pazienti affetti da bronchite cronica. *Rec. Prog. Med.* 79: 73.

Balzarini, A., Felisi, E., Martini, A., and De Conno, F. (2000) Efficacy of homeopathic treatment of skin reactions during radiotherapy for breast cancer: A randomised, double-blind clinical trial. *Br. Hom. J.* 89: 8.

Bannister, W.H., Federici, G., Heath, J.H., Bannister, J.V. (1986) Antioxidant systems in tumor cells: the levels of antioxidant enzymes, ferritin, and total iron in a human epatoma cell line. *Free Rad. Res. Comms.* 1: 361.

Barros, J., Pasteur, St. (1984) *Omeopatia, Medicina del Terreno.* F. Palombi Editori (original edition: *Homeopatia, Medicina del Terreno.* E. Bibl. Universitad Central de Venezuela, Caracas 1977).

Bascands, J.L., Cabos-Boutot, C., Manuel, Y., Girolami, J.P. (1990) Pretreatment with low doses of cadmium (Cd) protects rat mesangial cells agaist the direct toxic effect of cadmium. *J. O.M.H.I.* 3: 9.

Bass, D.A., Olbrantz, P., Szejda, P., Seeds, M.C., McCall, C.E. (1986) Subpopulations of neutrophils with increased oxidative product formation in blood of patients with infection. *J. Immunol.* 136: 860.

Bassett, C.A.L., Pawluk, R.J., Pilla, A.A. (1974) Augmentation of bone repair by inductively coupled electromagnetic fields. *Science* 184: 575.

Bastide, P., Aubin, B., Baronnet, S. (1975) Etude pharmacologique d'une preparation d'Apis mel. (7CH) vis-à-vis de l'erytheme aux rayons U.V. chez le cobayes albinos. *Ann. Hom. Fr.* 17 (3): 289.

Bastide, M., Doucet-Jaboeuf, M., Daurat, V. (1985) Activity and chronopharmacology of very low doses of physiological immune inducers. *Immunol. Today* 6: 234.

Bastide, M., Daurat, V., Doucet-Jaboeuf, M., Pelegrin, A., Dorfman, P. (1987) Immunomodulatory activity of very low doses of thymulin in mice. *Int. J. Immunotherapy* 3: 191.

Bastide, M. (1989) Report on research on very low dose effects. In: *Signals and Images.* Proceedings of 3rd Symposium of International Group on Very Low Dose Effects. Atelier Alpha Bleue, Paris, p 7.

Bastide, M. (1994) Immunological examples on ultra high dilution research. In: *Ultra High Dilution* (P.C. Endler and J. Schulte, eds.). Kluwer Acad. Publ., Dordrecht, p. 27.

Bastide, M. and Lagache, A. (1997) A communication process: A new paradigm applied to high-dilution effects on the living body. *Altern. Ther. Health Med.* 3: 35.

Bastide, M. (1998) Information and communication in living organisms. In: *Fundamental research in ultra high dilution and homeopathy,* (J. Schulte, et al., ed.). Dordrecht: Kluwer Acad. Publ. pp. 229–39.

Bayr, G. (1986) A model for homeopathic drug tests including statistical analysis. *Brit. Hom. J.* 75: 80.

Beardsley, T. (1991) Ingegneria genetica per i vaccini anti AIDS. *Le Scienze (Italian edition of Sci. Am.)* 278: 8.

Beauvais, F., Bidet, B., Descours, B., Hieblot, C., Burtin, C., Benveniste, J. (1991) Regulation of human basophil activation. I. Dissociation of cationic dye binding from histamine release in activated human basophils. *J. Allergy Clin. Immunol.* 87: 1020.

Bellavite, P. (1988) The superoxide-forming enzymatic system of phagocytes. *Free Rad. Biol. Med.* 4: 225.

Bellavite, P. (1990a) Ricerca in omeopatia: Dati, problemi e prospettive. *Ann. Ist. Sup. Sanità* 26: 179.

Bellavite, P. (1990b) Moderne interpretazioni patogenetiche dell'infiammazione acuta. *Riv. Ital. Omotossicol.* VIII (3): 12.

Bellavite, P., Chirumbolo, S., Signorini, A., Bianchi, I., Dri, P. (1991a) Simultaneous measurement of oxidative metabolism and adhesion of human neutrophils and evaluation of multiple doses of agonists and inhibitors. In: *Ultra Low Doses* (C. Doutremepuich, ed.). Taylor and Francis Ltd., London, p. 93.

Bellavite, P., Chirumbolo, S., Signorini, A., Bianchi, I. (1991b) Effects of various homeopathic drugs on superoxide production and adhesion of human neutrophils. *5th GIRI Meeting*, Paris, Abs. 1.

Bellavite, P., Chirumbolo, S., Guzzo, P. and Lechi, C. (1991c) Homologous priming and adaptation of neutrophils treated with chemotactic peptides. *5th GIRI Meeting*, Paris, Abs. 2.

Bellavite, P., Chirumbolo, S., Lippi, G., Guzzo, P., Santonastaso, C. (1993a) Homologous priming in chemotactic peptide stimulated neutrophils. *Cell Biochem. Funct.* 11: 93.

Bellavite, P., Chirumbolo, S., Lippi, G., Andrioli, G., Bonazzi, L., Ferro, I. (1993b) Dual effects of formylpeptides on the adhesion of endotoxin-primed human neutrophils. *Cell. Biochem. Funct.* 11: 231.

Bellavite, P., Lippi, G., Signorini, A., Andrioli, G., Chirumbolo, S. (1993c) Nonlinear dose-dependent metabolic and adhesive responses of human neutrophils to chemotactic agents. In: *Omeomed92* (C. Bornoroni, ed.). Editrice Compositori, Bologna, p. 135.

Bellavite, P., Carletto, A., Biasi, D., Caramaschi, P., Poli, F., Suttora, F., Bambara, L.M. (1994) Studies of skin-window exudate human neutrophils. Complex patterns of adherence to serum-coated surfaces in dependence on FMLP doses. *Inflammation* 18: 575.

Belon, P., Cumps, J., Ennis, M., Mannaioni, P. F., Sainte-Laudy, J., Roberfroid, M., and Wiegant, F. A. C. (1999) Inhibition of human basophil degranulation by successive histamine dilutions: Results of a European multi-centre trial. *Inflamm. Res.* 48: S17.

Bentwich, Z., Weisman, Z., Topper, R., Oberbaum, M. (1993) Specific immune response to high dilutions of KLH; transfer of immunological information. In: *Omeomed92* (C. Bornoroni, ed.). Editrice Compositori, Bologna, p. 9.

Benveniste, J. (1981) The human basophil degranulation test as an in vitro method for the diagnosis of allergies. *Clin. Allergy* 11: 1.

Benveniste, J. (1988) Letter. *Nature* 334: 291.

Benveniste, J. (1991a) Defence of diluted water (letter). *Nature* 353: 787.

Benveniste, J. (1991b) Commentary. *Homint R. & D. Newsletter* 2: 3.

Benveniste, J., Davenas, E., Ducot, B., Cornillet, B., Poitevin, B., Spira, A. (1991a) L'agitation de solutions hautement diluées n'induit pas d'activité biologique spécifique. *C.R. Acad. Sci. Paris* 312: 461.

Benveniste, J., Davenas, E., Ducot, B., Spira, A. (1991b) Basophil achromasia by dilute ligand: a reappraisal. *FASEB J.* 5: A3706.

Benveniste, J., Arnoux, B., Hadji, L. (1992) Highly dilute antigen increases coronary flow of isolated heart from immunized guinea pigs. *FASEB J.* 6: A1610.

Benveniste, J., Ducot, B., Spira, A. (1994a) Memory of water revisited (letter). *Nature* 370: 322.

Benveniste, J., Aissa, J., Litime, M.H., Tsangaris, G.Th., Thomas, Y. (1994b) Transfer of the molecular signal by electronic amplification. *FASEB J.* 8 (4): Abs. 2304.

Benveniste, J. (1994) Further biological effects induced by ultra high dilutions. Inhibition by a magnetic field. In: *Ultra High Dilution* (P. C. Endler and J. Schulte, eds.). Kluwer Acad. Publ., Dordrecht, p. 35.

Berezin, A.A. (1990) Isotopical positional correlations as a possible model for Benveniste experiments. *Medical Hypotheses* 31: 43.

Berezin, A.A. (1991) Diversity of stable isotopes and physical foundations of homeopathic effect. *Berlin J. Res. Homeopathy* 1: 85.

Berezin, A.A. (1994) Ultra high dilution effect and isotopic self-organisation. In: *Ultra High Dilution* (P.C. Endler and J. Schulte, eds.). Kluwer Acad. Publ., Dordrecht, p. 137.

Berkowitz, C.D. (1994) Homoeopathy: keeping an open mind. *Lancet* 344: 701.

Bernard, C. (1973) *Introduzione allo Studio della Medicina Sperimentale.* Feltrinelli Editore, Milano.

Berridge, M., Galione, A. (1988) Cytosolic calcium oscillators. *FASEB J.* 2: 3074.

Berry, R. S. (1990) When the melting and freezing points are not the same. *Sci. Am.* 263 (2): 50.

Bertani, S., Lussignoli, S., Andrioli, G., Bellavite, P., and Conforti, A. (1999) Dual effects of a homeopathic mineral complex on carrageenan-induced oedema in rats. *Br. Hom. J.* 88: 101.

Betti, L., Brizzi, M., Nani, D., and Peruzzi, M. (1997) Effect of high dilutions of Arsenicum album on wheat seedlings from seed poisoned with the same substance. *Br. Hom. J.* 86: 86.

Bianchi, I. (1987) *Argomenti di Omotossicologia. Vol. I.* Guna Editore, Milano.

Bianchi, I. (1990) *Argomenti di Omotossicologia, Vol. II.* Guna Editore, Milano.

Biasi, D., Bambara, L.M., Carletto, A., Caraffi, M., Serra, M.C., Chirumbolo, S. (1993) Factor-specific changes of the oxidative metabolism of exudate human neutrophils. *Inflammation* 17: 13.

Bildet, J., Guere, J.M., Saurel, J., Aubin, M., Demerque, D., Quilichini, R. (1975) Etude de l'action de differentes diluitions de Phosphorus sur l'hepatite toxique du rat. *Ann. Hom. Fr.* 17 (4): 425.

Bildet, J., Dupont, H., Aubin, M., Baronnet, S., Berjon, J.J., Gomez, H., Manlhiot, J.L. (1981) Action in vitro de dilutions infinitésimales de Phytolacca Americana sur la transformation lymphoblastique à la phytohemagglutinine. *Ann. Hom. Fr.* 23 (3): 102.

Bildet, J., Bonini, F., Gendre, P., Aubin, M., Demarque, D., Quilichini, R. (1984a) Etude au microscope électronique de l'action de diluitions de phosporus 15 CH sur l'hepatite toxique du rat. *Homéopathie Francaise* 72: 211.

Bildet, J., Aubin, M., Baronnet, S., Berjon, J.J., Gomez, H., Manlhiot, J.L. (1984b) Resistance de la cellule hepatique du rat aprés une intoxication infinitésimale au tetrachlorure de carbone. *Homéopathie Francaise* 72: 175.

Bildet, J., Guyot, M., Bonini, F., Grignon, M.C., Poitevin, B., Quilichini, R. (1990) Demonstrating the effects of Apis mellifica and Apium virus dilutions on erythema induced by U.V. radiation on guinea pigs. *Berlin J. Res. Homeopathy* 1: 28.

Birnboim, H.C. (1986) DNA strand breaks in human leukocytes induced by superoxide anion, hydrogen peroxide and tumor promoters are repaired slowly compared to breaks induced by ionizing radiation. *Carcinogenesis* 7: 1511.

Bistolfi, F., Olzi, E., Asdente, M. (1985) *Campi Magnetici e Cancro.* Edizioni Minerva Medica, Torino.

Bistolfi, F. (1989) *Radiazioni Non Ionizzanti, Ordine, Disordine e Biostrutture.* Edizioni Minerva Medica, Torino.

Blandina, P., Brunelleschi, S., Fantozzi, R., Giannella, E., Mannaioni, P.F., Masini, E. (1987) The antianaphylactic action of histamine H_2-receptor agonists in the guinea-pig isolated heart. *Br. J. Pharmac.* 90:459.

Blaser, K., de Weck, A.L. (1982) Regulation of the IgE antibody response by idiotype-anti-idiotype network. *Prog. Allergy* 32: 203.

Boiron, J., Abecassis, J., Cotte, J., Bernard, A.M. (1981) L'étude de l'action de diluitions hannémanniennes de chlorure mercurique sur l'index mitotique de cultures de cellules animales. *Ann. Hom. Fr.* 23 (3): 43.

Boiron, J., Belon, P. (1990) Contributions of fundamental research in homoeopathy. *Berlin J. Res. Homoeopathy* 1: 34.

Bonavida, B., Safrit, J., Tsuchitani, T., Zighelboim, J. (1991) Overcoming tumor cell resistance by low doses of recombinant tumor necrosis factor and drug. In: *Ultra Low Doses* (C. Doutremepuich, Ed.). Taylor and Francis, London, p. 27.

Boon, T. (1993) Teaching the immune system to fight cancer. *Sci. Am.* 268 (3): 32.

Bordes, L.R., Dorfman, P. (1986) Evaluation de l'activité antitussive du sirop Drosetux: Etude en double aveugle versus placebo. *Cahiers d'Otorhinolaryngologie* 21: 731.

Bornoroni, C. (1991) Synergism of action between indoleacetic acid (IAA) and highly diluted solution s of $CaCO_3$ on the growth of oat coleoptiles. *Berlin J. Res. Homeopathy* 1 (4/5): 275.

Both, G. (1987) Zur prophylaxe und therapie des metritis-mastitis-agalactie (MMA)—komplexes des schweines mit biologischen arzneimitteln. *Biologische Tiermedizin* 4: 39.

Bouchaier, F. (1990) Alternative medicines: A general approach to the french situation. *Complem. Med. Res.* 4: 4.

Bourne, H.R., Melmon, K.L., Lichtenstein, M. (1971) Histamine augments leukocyte adenosine 3'-5'-monophosphate and blocks antigenic histamine release. *Science* 173: 743.

Bradley, G.W., Clover, A. (1989) Apparent response of small cell lung cancer to an extract of mistletoe and homoeopathic treatment. *Thorax* 44: 1047.

Braunwald, E. (1991) Cellular and molecular biology of cardiovascular disease. In: *Harrison's Principles of Internal Medicine* (Wilson et al., eds.). McGraw-Hill, Inc, N.York, p. 835.

Breithaupt, H. (1988) Biological rhytms and communication. In: *Electromagnetic bio-information* (Popp, F.A. *et al.*, eds.). Urban & Schwarzenberg, Munchen, p. 18.

Brigo, B. (1987) Le traitment homéopatique de la migraine: une étude de 60 cas, controlée en double aveugle. *Journal of Liga Med. Hom. Int.* 1: 18.

Brigo, B., Masciello, E. (1988) *Omeopatia, Medicina Non Violenta*. Ed. Boiron, Milano.

Brigo, B., Serpelloni, G. (1991) Homeopathic treatment of migraines: A randomized doubleblind controlled study of sixty cases. *Berlin J. Res. Homeopathy* 1 (2): 98.

Brigo, B. (1990) *Fitoterapia e Gemmoterapia nella Pratica Clinica. III.* Edizioni La Grafica Briantea, Como.

Briheim, G., Stendahl, O., Coble, B.I., Dahlgren, C. (1988) Exudate polymorphonuclear leukocytes isolated from skin chambers are primed for enhanced response to subsequent stimulation with the chemoattractant fMet-Leu-Phe and C3 opsonized yeast particles. *Inflammation* 12: 141.

Brizzi, M., Nani, D., Peruzzi, M., Betti L. (2000) Statistical analysis of the effect of high dilutions of arsenic in a large dataset from a wheat germination model. *Br. Hom. J.* 89: 63.

Brodde, O.E., Michel, M.C. (1989) Disease states can modify both receptor number and signal transduction pathways. *Trends Pharmacol. Sci.* 10: 383.

Bryant, P. (1993) Towards the cellular functions of tumour suppressors. *Trends Cell Biol.* 3: 31.

Bullock, T.H. (1977) Electromagnetic sensing in fish. *Neurosci. Res. Program. Bull.* 15: 17.

Byrn, C., Olsson, I., Falkheden, L., Lindh, M., Hösterey, U., Fogelberg, M., Linder, L.E., Bunketorp, O. (1993) Subcutaneous sterile water injections for chronic neck and shoulder pain following whiplash injuries. *Lancet* 341: 449–452.

Byus, C.V., Lundak, R.L., Fletcher, R.M., Sadey, W.R. (1984) Alterations in protein kinase activity following exposure of cultured lymphocytes to modulated microwave fields. *Bioelectromagnetics* 5: 34.

Cadossi, R., Bersani, F., Cossarizza, A., Zucchini, P., Emilia, G., Torelli, G., Franceschi, C. (1992) Lymphocytes and low-frequency electromagnetic fields. *FASEB J.* 6: 2667.

Cadwgan, T.M., Benjamin, N. (1993) Evidence for altered platelet nitric oxide synthesis in essential hypertension. *J. Hypertension* 11:417.

Calabrese, E.J., McCarthy, M.E., Kenyon, E. (1987) The occurrence of chemically induced hormesis. *Health Phys.* 52: 531.

Calabrese, E. J. and Baldwin, L. A. (2000) The marginalization of hormesis. *Hum. Exp. Toxicol.* 19: 32.

Callens, E., Debiane, H., Santais, M.C., Ruff, F. (1993) Effects of highly diluted beta2-adrenergic agonists on isolated guinea pig trachea. *Brit. Hom. J.* 82: 123.

Callinan, P. (1986) L'énergie vibratoire et l'homme. Un modèle pour le mode d'action de l'homéopathie. *Homéopathie francaise* 74: 355.

Cambar, J., Cal, J.C. (1982) Etude des variations circadiennes de la dose léthale 50 du chlorure mercurique chez la souris. *C.R. Acad. Sci. (Paris)* 294: 149.

Cambar, J., Desmouliere, A., Cal, J.C., Guillemain, J. (1983) Mise en évidence de l'effet protecteur de dilutions homéopathiques de Mercurius corrosivus vis-à-vis de la mortalité au chlorure mercurique chez la souris. *Ann. Hom. Fr.* 25 (5): 160.

Cambar, J., Guillemain, J. (1985) La chronobiologie: ses applications thérapeutiques et son intérèt dans le cadre de l'homéopathie. *Cah. Biothér.* 88: 53.

Campbell, A.C.H. (1980) Thuja—a drug picture based on provings. *Brit. Hom. J.* 69: 182.

Campbell, J.H., Taylor, M.A., Beattie, N., McSharry, C., Aitchison, T., Carter, R., Stevenson, R.D., Reilly, D.T. (1990) Is homoeopathy a placebo response? A controlled trial of homoeopathic immunotherapy in atopic asthma. *Am. Rev. Resp. Dis.* 141: A24.

Candegabe, M. E. and Carrara, H. C. (1997) *Approssimazione al Metodo Pratico e Preciso della Omeopatia Pura.* Venezia: Centro Internaz. della Grafica.

Capsoni, F., Minonzio, F., Venegoni, E., Ongari, A.M., Meroni, P.L., Guidi, G., Zanussi, C. (1988) In vitro and ex vivo effect of RU 41740 on human polymorphonuclear leukocyte function. *Int. J. Immunopharmac.* 10: 121.

Carrel, A. (1950) Il ruolo futuro della medicina. In: *Medicina Ufficiale e Medicine Eretiche.* Bompiani. Original edition (1945): Le ròle futur del la médecine. In: *Médecine officielle et médecines hérétiques.* Plon, Paris, vol.1, p. 345.

Casaril, M., Gabrielli, G.B., Dusi, S., Nicoli, N., Bellisola, G., Corrocher, R. (1985) Decreased activity of liver glutathione peroxidase in human epatocellular carcinoma. *Eur. J. Cancer Clin. Oncol.* 21: 941.

Catt, K.J., Balla, T. (1989) Phosphoinositide metabolism and hormone action. *Annu. Rev. Med.* 40: 487.

Cazin, J.C., Cazin, M., Gaborit, J.L., Chaoui, A., Boiron, J., Belon, P., Cherruault, Y., Papapanayotou, C. (1987) A study of the effect of decimal and centesimal dilutions of Arsenic on the retention and mobilisation of Arsenic in the rat. *Human Toxicology* 6: 315.

Cazin, J.C., Cazin, M., Chaoui, A., Belon, P. (1991) Influence of several physical factors on the activity of ultra low doses. In: *Ultra Low Doses* (C. Doutremepuich, ed.). Taylor and Francis, London, p. 69.

Cerutti, P.A. (1991) Oxidant stress and carcinogenesis. *Eur. J. Clin. Invest.* 21: 1.

Chapman, E.H., Weintraub, R.J., Milburn, M.A., Pirozzi, T.O., Woo, E. (1999) Homeopathic treatment of mild traumatic brain injury: A randomized, double-blind, placebo-controlled clinical trial. *J. Head Trauma Rehabil.* 14: 521.

Charette, G. (1982) *La Materia Medica Omeopatica Spiegata*. IPSA Editore, Palermo.

Cheek, T.R. (1991) Calcium regulation and homeostasis. *Curr. Opin. Cell Biol.* 3: 199.

Chen, L., Ashe, S., Brady, W.A., Hellstrom, I., Hellstrom, K.E., McGowan, P., Ledbetter, J.A., Linsley, P.S. (1992) Costimulation of antitumor immunity by the B7 counterreceptor for the T lymphocyte molecules CD28 and CTLA-4. *Cell* 71: 1093.

Cherruault, Y., Guillez, A., Sainte-Laudy, J., Belon, Ph. (1989) Etude mathematique et statistique des effets de dilutions successives de chlorhydrate d'histamine sur la réactivité des basophiles humains. *Bio-Sciences* 7: 63.

Chevrel, J.P., Saglier, J., Destable, M.D. (1984) Reprise du transit intestinal en chirurgie digestive. *Presse Med.* 13: 833.

Chiabrera, A., Grattarola, M., Parodi, G., Marcer, M. (1984) Interazione tra campo elettromagnetico e cellule. *Le Scienze (Italian edition of Sci. Am.)* 192: 78.

Chibeni, S.S. (2001) On the scientific status of homeopathy. *Br. Hom. J.* 90: 92.

Chirila, M., Hristescu, S., Manda, G., Neagu, M., Olinescu, A. (1990a) The action of succussed substances on the human lymphocytes and PMN granulocytes in vitro stimulated with phytohaemagglutinin (PHA) and zymosan opsonized. In: *Proc. 4th GIRI Meeting*, Paris, Abs. 11.

Chirila, M., Hristescu, S., Manda, G., Neagu, M., Olinescu, A. (1990b) The action of succussed substance on the proliferative response of human lymphocytes in vitro stimulated with phytohaemaglutinin. In: *Proc. II Congr. Int. O.M.H.I.*, Ediciones Tecnico Cientificas, Mexico, p. 23.

Chirumbolo, S., Signorini, A., Bianchi, I., Lippi, G., Bellavite, P. (1993) Effects of homeopathic preparations of organic acids and of minerals on the oxidative metabolism of human neutrophils. *Brit. Hom. J.* 82: 237.

Chou, Y., Tao, M., Qiou, M. (1991) Influence of acupuncture on the induction of interferon by peripheral leukocytes of asymptomatic hepatitis B virus carriers (ASC). *Int. J. Acupunct.* 2: 255.

Cristea, A., Nicula, S., and Dare, V. (1997) Pharmacodynamic effects of very high dilutions of Belladonna on the isolated rat duodenum. In: *Signals Images*, (M. Bastide, ed.) pp. 161. Dordrecht: Kluwer. pp. 161.

Cier, A., Boiron, J., Vingert, C., Braise, J. (1966) Sur le traitement du diabéte expérimental par des dilutions infinitésimales d'alloxane. *Ann. Hom. Fr.* 8: 137.

Citro, M. (1992) TFF: Un'alchimia elettronica. Basi teoriche e dati preliminari. *Empedocle* (IPSA ed., Palermo) 10 (2-3): 39.

Citro, M., Pongratz, W., Endler, P.C. (1993) Transmission of hormone signals by electronic circuitry. In: *Science Innovation 93, Meeting of the American Association for the Advancement of Science*, Boston.

Citro, M., Smith, C.W., Scott-Morley, A., Pongratz, W., Endler, P.C. (1994) Transfer of information from molecules by means of electronic amplification. Preliminary studies. In: *Ultra High Dilution* (P.C. Endler and J. Schulte, eds.). Kluwer Acad. Publ., Dordrecht, p. 209.

Clegg, J.S. (1982) Alternative views on the role of water in cell function. In: *Biophysic of Water* (F. Franks and S. Mathias, eds.). Wiley & Sons Ltd., New York, p. 365.

Cohen, S., Tyrrel, D.A.J., Smith, A.P. (1991) Psychological stress and the susceptibility to the common cold. *N. Engl. J. Med.* 325: 606.

Cohen, I.R. (1991) Autoimmunity to chaperonins in the pathogenesis of arthritis and diabetes. *Annu. Rev. Immunol.* 9: 567.

Colas, H., Aubin, M., Picard, Ph., Lebecq, J.C. (1975) Inhibition du test de transformation lymphoblastique (TTL) à la phytohemagglutinine (PHA) par phytolacca americana en diluition homéopathiques. *Ann. Hom. Fr.* 17 (6): 629.

Colin, P. (2000) An epidemiological study of a homeopathic practice. *Br. Hom. J.* 89: 116.

Collier, J., Vallance, P. (1991) Importanza fisiologica dell'ossido d'azoto. *Brit. Med. J. (Italian edition)* 15: 285.

314   The Emerging Science of Homeopathy

Conforti, A., Signorini, A., Bellavite, P. (1993) Effects of high dilutions of histamin and other natural compounds on acute inflammation in rats. In: *Omeomed92* (C. Bornoroni, ed.). Editrice Compositori, Bologna, p. 163.

Conti, P., Gigante, G., Cifone, M.G., Alesse, E., Ianni, G.F., Reale M., Angeletti, P.U. (1983) Reduced mitogenic stimulation of human lymphocytes by extremely low frequency electromagnetic fields. *FEBS Lett.* 162: 156.

Cossarizza, A., Monti, D., Bersani, F., Cantini, M., Cadossi, R., Sacchi, A., Franceschi, C. (1989) Extremely low frequency pulsed electromagnetic fields increase cell proliferation in lymphocytes from young and aged subjects. *Biochem. Biophys. Res. Commun.* 160: 692.

Coulter, H.L. (1976) *Guida alla Medicina Omeopatica.* EDIUM Editrice, Milano.

Cramer, F. (1993) *Chaos and Order. The Complex Structure of Living Systems.* VCH Verlagsgesellschaft, Weinheim (Ger.)

Crapanne, J.B. (1985) Conduite des essais cliniques multicentriques in homéopathie. *Homéopathie* 1: 19.

Cristea, A., Nicula, S., ad Dare, V. (1997) Pharmacodynamic effects of very high dilutions of Belladonna on the isolated rat duodenum. In: *Signals and Images*, edited by M. Bastide, pp 161. Kluwer, Dordricht.

Croquette, V. (1991) Determinismo e caos. In: *Il Caos. Le Leggi del Disordine* (G. Casati, ed.). Le Scienze S.p.A., Milano, p. 34.

Crutchfield, J.P., Farmer, J.D., Packard, N.H., Shaw, R.S. (1986) Chaos. *Sci. Am.* 255: 38.

Cucherat, M., Haugh, M. C., Gooch, M., and Boissel, J. P. (HMRAG: Homeopathic Medicines Research Advisory Group) (2000) Evidence of clinical efficacy of homeopathy: A meta-analysis of clinical trials. *Eur. J Clin. Pharmacol.* 56: 27.

Dalgleish, A.G. (1994) Cancer vaccines. *Eur. J. Cancer* 30A: 1029.

Dantas, F. and Rampes, H. (2000) Do homeopathic medicines provoke adverse effects? A systematic review. *Br. Hom. J.* 89, Suppl 1: S35.

Datta, S., Mallick, P., Bukhsh AR. (1999) Efficacy of a potentized homoeopathic drug (Arsenicum Album.) in reducing genotoxic effects produced by arsenic trioxide in mice: Comparative studies of pre-, post- and combined pre- and post-oral administration and comparative efficacy of two microdoses. *Complement. Ther. Med.* 7: 62.

Datta, S., Mallick, P., Bukhsh, A.R. (1999) Efficacy of a potentized homoeopathic drug (Arsenicum Album.) in reducing genotoxic effects produced by arsenic trioxide in mice: II. Comparative efficacy of an antibiotic., actinomycin D alone and in combination with either of two microdoses. *Complement. Ther. Med.* 7: 156.

Daurat, V., Dorfman, P., Bastide, M. (1988) Immunomodulatory activity of low doses of interferon a,b in mice. *Biomed & Pharmacother.* 42: 197.

Davenas, E., Poitevin, B., Benveniste, J. (1987) Effect on mouse peritoneal macrophages of orally administered very high dilutions of silica. *Eur. J. Pharmacol.* 135: 313.

Davenas, E., Beauvais, F., Amara, J., Robinson, M., Miadonna, A., Tedeschi, A., Pomeranz, B., Fortner, P., Belon, P., Sainte-Laudy, J., Poitevin, B., Benveniste, J. (1988) Human basophil degranulation triggered by very dilute antiserum against IgE. *Nature* 333: 816.

Dawey, R.W. (1988) Homoeopathy and the contemporary complementary medical scene. *Homoeopathy* 38: 115.

de Caro, G., Gentili, L., Lucentini, P. (1990) Isoproterenol induced salivary gland enlargement is influenced in the rat by ultradiluted solutions of eldoisin. In: *Proc. 4th GIRI Meeting*, Paris, Abs. 23.

De Gerlache, J., Lans, M. (1991) Modulation of experimental rat liver carcinogenesis by ultra low doses of the carcinogens. In: *Ultra Low Doses* (C. Doutremepuich, ed.) Taylor and Francis, London, p. 17.

Delbancut, A., Dorfman, P., Cambar, J. (1993) Protective effect of very low concentrations of heavy metals (cadmium and cisplatin) against cytotoxic doses of these metals on renal tubular cell cultures. *Brit. Hom. J.* 82: 123.

Del Giudice, N., Del Giudice, E. (1984) *Omeopatia e Bioenergetica*. Cortina International, Verona.

Del Giudice, E., Preparata, G., Vitiello, G. (1988a) Water as a free electric dipole laser. *Phys. Rev. Lett.* 61: 1085.

Del Giudice, E., Doglia, S., Milani, M., Vitiello, G. (1988b) Structures, correlations and electromagnetic interactions in living matter: Theory and applications. In: *Biological Coherence and Response to External Stimuli* (H. Frohlich, ed.). Springer-Verlag, Berlin, p. 49.

Del Giudice, E. (1990) Collective processes in living matter: A key for homeopathy. In: *Homeopathy in Focus*. VGM (Verlag fur Ganzheitsmedizin) Essen, p. 14.

Demangeat, J.L., Demangeat, C., Gries, P., Poitevin, B., Constantinesco, A. (1992) Modifications des temps de relaxation RMN a 4 MHz des protons du solvant dans les très hautes dilutions salines de Silice/Lactose. *J. Med. Nucl. Biopy.* 16 (2): 135.

De Togni, P., Bellavite, P., Della Bianca, V., Grzeskowiak, M., Rossi, F. (1985) Intensity and kinetics of the respiratory burst of human neutrophils in relation to receptor occupancy and rate of occupation by formyl-methionyl-leucyl-phenylalanine. *Biochim. Biophys. Acta* 838: 12.

Dewdney, A.K. (1991) Bellezza e profondità degli insiemi di Mandelbrot e di Julia. *In Il Caos. Le Leggi del Disordine.* (G. Casati, ed.). Le Scienze S.p.a., Milano, p. 122.

Diaz, M.O., Rubin, C.M., Harden, A., Ziemin, S., Larson, R.A., Le Beau, M.M., Rowley, J.D. (1990) Deletions of interferon genes in acute lymphoblastic leukemia. *N. Engl. J. Med.* 322: 77.

Di Concetto, G. (1989) Medicina cinese e medicina occidentale: possibilità di una sintesi. *Dimensioni dello Sviluppo* 4: 159.

Dinarello, C.A. (1991) Inflammatory cytokines: interleukin-1 and tumor necrosis factor as effector molecules in autoimmune diseases. *Curr. Opin. Immunol.* 3: 941.

Dinarello, C.A. (1994) Blocking interleukin-1 receptors. *Int. J. Clin. Lab. Res.* 24: 61.

Dittmann, J., Harisch G. (1996)Characterization of differing effects caused by homeopathically prepared and conventional dilutions using cytochrome P450 2E1 and other enzymes as detection systems. *J. Altern. Complement. Med.* 2: 279.

Dittmann, J., Kanapin, H., Harisch, G. (1999) Biochemical efficacy of homeopathic and electronic preparations of D8 potassium cyanate. *Forsch. Komplementarmed.* 6: 15.

Dorfman, P., Lasserre, M.N., Tétau, M. (1987) Préparation à l'accouchement par homéopathie. Expérimentation en double insu versus placebo. *Cah. Biother.* 94: 77.

Dormandy, T.L. (1983) An approach to free radicals. *Lancet* 2: 1010.

Doucet-Jaboeuf, M., Guillemain, G., Piechaczyk, M., Karouby, Y., Bastide, M. (1982) Evaluation de la dose limite d'activité du facteur thymique serique. *C.R. Acad. Sc. Paris* 295: 283.

Doucet-Jaboeuf, M., Pelegrin, A., Cot, M.C., Guillemain, J., Bastide, M. (1984) Seasonal variations in the humoral immune response in mice following administration of thymic hormones. In: *Ann. Rev. Chronopharmacology. Vol. 1.* (A. Reinberg et al., eds.). Pergamon Press, Oxford, p. 231.

Doucet-Jaboeuf, M., Pelegrin, A., Sizes, M., Guillemain, J., Bastide, M. (1985) Action of very low doses of biological immunomodulators on the humoral immune response in mice. *Int. J. Immunoparmacol.* 7: 312.

Doutremepuich, C., Pailley, D., Anne, M.C., Hariveau, E., Quilichini, R. (1987a) Platelet aggregation on whole blood after administration of ultra low dosage acetylsalicylic acid in healthy volunteers. *Thrombosis Res.* 47: 373.

Doutremepuich, C., Pailley, D., Anne, M.C., De Seze, O., Paccalin, J., Quilichini, R. (1987b) Template bleeding time after ingestion of ultra low dosages of acetylsalicylic acid in healthy subjects. Preliminary study. *Thrombosis Res.* 48: 501.

Doutremepuich, C., Peillet, D., de Seze, O., Anne, M.C., Paccalin, J., Quilichini, R. (1988) Variation du temps de saignement aprés administration à différentes posologies d'acide acétyl salicylique chez le volontaire sain. *Ann. Pharm. Fr.* 46: 35.

Doutremepuich, C., de Séze, O., Le Roy, D., Lalanne, M.C., Anne, M.C. (1990) Aspirin at very ultra low dosage in healthy volunteers; effects on bleeding time, platelet aggregation and coagulation. *Haemostasis* 20: 99.

Doutremepuich, C., Lalanne, M.C., Ramboer, I., Sertillanges, M.N., De Seze, O. (1993) Platelets/endothelial cells interactions in presence of acetylsalicylic acid at ultra low dose. In: *Omeomed92* (C. Bornoroni, ed.). Editrice Compositori, Bologna, p. 109.

Downer, S.M., Cody, M.M., McCluskey, P., Wilson, P.D., Arnott, S.J., Lister, T.A., Slevin, M.L. (1994) Pursuit and practice of complementary therapies by cancer patients receiving conventional treatment. *Brit. Med. J.* 309: 86.

Dranoff, G., Jaffeee, E., Lazenby, A., Golumbek, P., Levitsky, H., Brose, K., Jackson, V., Hamada, H., Pardoll, D., Mulligan, R.C. (1993) Vaccination with irradiated tumor cells engineered to secrete murine GM-CSF stimulates potent, specific and long lasting antitumor immunity. *Proc. Natl. Acad. Sci. USA* 90: 3539.

Drossou, P., Haralambidou, N., Diamantidis, S. (1990) Homoeopathic treatment of leukaemias. *Homeopathy International* May: 12.

Drost-Hansen, W. (1982) The occurrence and extent of vicinal water. In: *Biophysics of Water* (F. Franks and S. Mathias, eds.). Wiley & Sons Ltd., New York, p. 163.

Dujany, R. (1978) *Omeopatia*. Edizioni Red, Como.

Dwyer, J.M. (1992) Manipulating the immune system with immune globulins. *N. Engl. J. Med.* 326: 107.

Egan, S.E., Weinberg, R.A. (1993) The pathway to signal achievement. *Nature* 365: 781.

Eid, P., Felisi, E., Sideri, M. (1993) Applicability of homoeopathic Caulophyllum thalictroides during labour. *Brit. Hom. J.* 82:245.

Eid, P., Felisi, E., Sideri, M. (1994) Super-placebo ou action pharmacologique? Une etude en double aveugle, randomisée avec un remède homéopathique (Caulophyllum Thalictroides) dans le travail de l'accouchement. *Proc. V Congr. O.M.H.I., Paris*, 20-23 oct. 1994.

Elia, V. and Niccoli, M. (1999) Thermodynamics of extremely diluted aqueous solutions. *Ann. N. Y. Acad. Sci.* 879: 241.

Endler, P.C., Pongratz, W., Van Wijk, R., Kastberger, G., Haidvogl, M. (1991a) Effects of highly diluted succussed thyroxine on metamorphosis of highland frogs. *Berlin J. Res. Homoeopathy* 1 (3): 151.

Endler, P.C., Pongratz, W., Kastberger, G., Wiegant, F.A.C., Haidvogel, M. (1991b) Climbing activity in frogs and the effect of highly diluted succussed thyroxine. *Brit. Hom. J.* 80: 194.

Endler, P.C., Pongratz, W., van Wijk, R., Wiegant, F.A.C., Waltl, K., Gehrer, M., Hilgers, H. (1994a) A zoological example on ultra high dilution research. Energetic coupling between the dilution and the organism in a model of amphibia. In: *Ultra High Dilution* (P.C. Endler and J. Schulte, eds.). Kluwer Acad. Publ., Dordrecht, p. 39.

Endler, P.C., Pongratz, W., Kastberger, G., Wiegant, F.A.C., Schulte, J. (1994b) The effect of highly diluted agitated thyroxine on the climbing activity of frogs. *Vet. Hum. Toxicol.* 36: 56.

Endler, P.C., Pongratz, W., van Wijk, R., Waltl, K., Hilgers, H., Brandmaier, R. (1994c) Transmission of hormone information by non-molecular means. *FASEB J.* 8: Abs.2313.

Endler, P. C., Pongratz, W., Smith, C. W., and Schulte, J. (1995) Non-molecular information transfer from thyroxine to frogs with regard to homeopathic toxicology. *Vet. Hum. Toxicol.* 37: 259.

Engel, A.K., Konig, P., Schillen, T.B. (1992) Why does the cortex oscillate? *Curr. Biol.* 2: 332.

Engel, W.K. (1992) Oral immunosuppression for multiple sclerosis. *Lancet* 339: 64.

Ernst, E. and Pittler, M. H. (1998) Efficacy of homeopathic arnica: A systematic review of placebo- controlled clinical trials. *Arch. Surg.* 133: 1187.

Ernst, E., Rand, J. I., and Stevinson, C. (1998) Complementary therapies for depression: An overview. *Arch. Gen. Psychiatry* 55: 1026.

Eskinazi, D. (1999) Homeopathy re-revisited: is homeopathy compatible with biomedical observations? *Arch. Intern. Med.* 159: 1981.

Evans, W.Ch. (1989) *Trease and Evan's Pharmacognosy*. Thirteen edition. Ballière Tindall, London.

Farné, M. (1990) Lo stress, aspetti positivi e negativi. *Le Scienze (Italian edition of Sci. Am.)* 263: 40.

Fathman, G.G. (1993) Stimulating the lymphocytes. *Curr. Biol.* 3: 558.

Fay, S.P., Domalewski, M.D., Sklar, L.A. (1993) Evidence for protonation in the human neutrophil peptide receptor binding pocket. *Biochemistry* 32: 1627.

Ferley, J.P., Putignat, N., Azzopardi, Y., Charrel, M., Zmirou, D. (1987) Evaluation en médicine ambulatoire de l'activité d'un complexe homéopatique dans la prévention de la grippe et des syndromes grippaux. *Immunologie Médicale* 20: 22.

Ferley, J.P., Zmirou, D., D'Adhemar, D., Balducci, F. (1989) A controlled evaluation of a homoeopathic preparation in influenza-like syndromes. *Brit. J. Clin. Pharmac.* 27: 329.

Fesenko, E. E. and Gluvstein, A.Y. (1995) Changes in the state of water, induced by radiofrequency electromagnetic fields. *FEBS Lett.* 367: 53.

Fesenko, E. E., Geletyuk, V. I., Kazachenko, V. N. and Chemeris, N. K. (1995) Preliminary microwave irradiation of water solutions changes their channel-modifying activity. *FEBS Lett.* 366: 49.

Fields, B.N., Knipe, D.H. (1990) *Virology, Vol. 1, 2nd Ed.* Raven Press, New York.

Fimiani, V., Cavallaro, A., Ainis, O., Bottari C. (2000) Immunomodulatory effect of the homoeopathic drug Engystol-N on some activities of isolated human leukocytes and in whole blood. *Immunopharmacol. Immunotoxicol.* 22: 103.

Finney, J.L. (1982) Towards a molecular picture of liquid water. In: *Biophysics of Water* (F. Franks and S. Mathias, eds.) Wiley & Sons Ltd, N.York, p. 73.

Fisher, P. (1986) An experimental double-blind clinical trial method in homeopathy. *Brit. Hom. J.* 75: 142.

Fisher, P., House, I., Belon, P., Turner, P. (1987) The influence of the homeopathic remedy Plumbum metallicum on the excretion kinetics of lead in rats. *Human Toxicol.* 6: 321.

Fisher, P. (1989) *Research in Homoeopathy*. Edited by Faculty of Homoeopathy, London.

Fisher, P., Greenwood, A., Huskisson, E.C., Turner, P., Belon, P. (1989) Effect of homoeopathic treatment on fibrositis (primary fibromyalgia). *Brit. Med. J.* 299: 365.

Fisher, P. (1990) Negative results. *Brit. Hom. J.* 79: 230.

Fisher, P., Ward, A. (1994) Complementary medicine in Europe. *Brit. Med. J.* 309: 107.

Fletcher, M.P., Halpern, G.M. (1988) Effects of dilutions of bryonia (4-9CH) and lung-histamine (4-9CH) on human neutrophil (PMN) activation responses as assessed by flow cytometry. In: *2nd GIRI Meeting*. Monte Carlo, A20.

Fougeray, S., Moubry, K., Vallot, N., Bastide, M. (1993) Effect of high dilutions of epidermal growth factor (EGF) on in vitro proliferation of keratinocyte and fibroblast cell lines. *Brit. Hom. J.* 82: 124.

Franks, F. (1982) *Water. A Comprehensive Treatise*. Plenum, New York.

Franks, F., Mathias, S.F., (editors) (1982) *Biophysics of Water*. Wiley Intersci. Publ., Chichester.

Frati, L. (1989) Oncogeni e fattori di crescita. In: *Progressi nella Ricerca sul Cancro*. Le Scienze S.p.A., Milano, p. 34.

Freeman, W.J. (1991) The physiology of perception. *Sci. Am.* 264:34.

Friend, S.H., Dryia, T.P., Weinberg, R.A. (1988) Oncogenes and tumour-suppressing genes. *N. Engl. J. Med.* 318: 618.

Friedman, A., Weiner, H.L. (1994) Induction of anergy or active suppression following oral tolerance is determined by antigen dosage. *Proc. Natl. Acad. Sci. USA* 91: 6688.

Frohlich, H. (ed.) (1988) *Biological Coherence and Response to External Stimuli*. Springer-Verlag, Berlin.

Fuller Royal, F. (1990) Understanding homeopathy, acupuncture and electrodiagnosis: Clinical applications of quantum mechanics. *Am. J. Acupuncture* 18: 37.

Fuller Royal, F., Fuller Royal, D. (1991) Scientific support for electrodiagnosis. Relationship to homoeopathy and acupuncture. *Brit. Hom. J.* 80: 166.

Fuller Royal, F. (1991) Proving homoeopathic medicines. *Brit. Hom. J.* 80: 122.

Furst, A. (1987) Hormetic effects in pharmacology: pharmacological inversions as prototypes for hormesis. *Health Phys.* 52: 527.

Fye, W.B. (1986) Nitroglycerin: a homeopathic remedy. *Circulation* 73: 21.

Gabius, S., Beuth, J., Joshi, S.S., Kayser, K., Koch, B., Kratzin, H., Pulverer, G., Vidal, F., Walzel, H., Westernhausen, M., Gabius, H.J. (1992) Galactoside-binding lectin from mistletoe: on the way to clinical trial. In: *Proc. VI GIRI Meeting*, Munchen. Abs. 2.

Gabius, S., Joshi, S.S., Kayser, K., Gabius, H.J. (1992) The galactoside-specific lectin from mistletoe as biological response modifier. *Int. J. Oncol.* 1 (6): 705.

Galva, D. (1991) I campi magnetici domestici contribuiscono al rischio di leucemie. *Medico e Paziente* 2: 14.

Garber, G.E., Cameron, D.W., Hawley-Foss, N., Greenway, D., Shannon, M.E. (1991) The use of ozone-treated blood in the therapy of HIV infection and immune disease: A pilot study of safety and efficacy. *AIDS* 5: 981.

Garner, C., Hock, N. (1991) Chaos theory and homoeopathy. *Berlin J. Res. Homeopathy* 1: 236.

Gassinger, C.A., Wunstel, G., Netter, P. (1981) Klinische Prufung zum Nachweis der terapeutischen Wirksamkeit des homöopatisch en Arzneimittels Eupatorium perfoliatum D2 (Wasserhanf composite) bei der Diagnose "Grippaler infection". *Arzneimittelforschung Drug Res.* 31: 732.

Gaus, W., Walach, H., Haag, G. (1992) The efficacy of classic homeopathic therapy in chronic headache. Study protocol. *Der Schmerz* (Springer-Verlag) 6: 134.

Ghosh, A. (1983) Homoeopathic treatment of osteoarthritis (Letter). *Lancet* I: 304.

Gibson, R.G, Gibson, S.L.M., Mac Neil, A.D., Buchanan, W. Watson (1980) Homeopathic therapy in rheumatoid arthritis: evaluation by double-blind clinical therapeutic trial. *Brit. J. Clin. Pharmac.* 9: 453.

Gibson, S., Gibson, R. (1987) *Homoeopathy for everyone*. Penguin Books Ltd, Harmonsworth (England).

Goetzl, E.J., Sreedharan, S.P. (1992) Mediators of communication and adaptation in the neuroendocrine and immune system. *FASEB J.* 6: 2646.

Goldberger, A.L., Rigney, D.R., West, B.J. (1990) Chaos and fractals in human physiology. *Sci. Am.* 262 (2): 34.

Golde, D.W. (1991) The stem cell. *Sci. Am.* 265 (1): 36.

Golub, E.S. (1984) *Le Basi Cellulari della Risposta Immunitaria*. Zanichelli, Bologna.

Gong, J., Chen, D., Kashiwaba, M., and Kufe, D. (1997) Induction of antitumor activity by immunization with fusions of dendritic and carcinoma cells. *Nature Medicine* 3: 558.

Goodman, R., Shirley-Henderson, A. (1990) Exposure of cells to extremely low-frequency electromagnetic fields: relationship to malignancy? *Cancer Cells* 2: 355.

Goodman Gilman, A., Goodman, L.S., Gilman, A. (1980) *The Pharmacological Basis of Therapeutics*. Macmillan publ. Co., New York.

Goodman Gilman, A., Goodman, L.S., Gilman, A. (1992) *Le Basi Farmacologiche della Terapia*. Zanichelli, Bologna.

Goodyear, K., Lewith, G., and Low, J. L. (1998) Randomized double-blind placebo-controlled trial of homoeopathic 'proving' for Belladonna C30. *J. R. Soc. Med.* 91: 579.

Granata, G. (1990) *Compendio di Omeopatia*. Hoepli Editore, Milano.

Grange, J.M., Denman, A.M. (1993) Microdose-mediated immune modulation. A possible key to a scientific re-evaluation of homoeopathy. *Brit. Hom. J.* 82: 113.

GRECHO (Groupe des Recherches et d'Essais Cliniques en Homéopathie) (1989) Evaluation de deux produits homéopathiques sur la reprise du transit aprés chirurgie digestive. *Presse Med.* 18: 59.

Gregory, J.K., Clary, D.C., Liu, K., Brown, M.G. and Saykally, R.J. (1997) The water dipole moment in water clusters. *Science* 275: 814.

Guajardo, G., Bellavite, P., Wynn, S., Searcy, R., Fernandez, R., and Kayne, S. (1999) Homeopathic terminology: a consensus quest. *Br. Hom. J.* 88: 135.

Guermonprez, M., Pinkas, M., Torck, M. (1985) *Matiére Médicale Homéopathique*. Doin Editeur, Paris.

Guerritore, A. (1987) La natura vivente. *Studium* 4-5: 597.

Guidotti, G.G. (1990) *Patologia Generale*. Casa Editrice Ambrosiana, Milano.

Guillemain, J., Cal, J.C., Desmoulieres, A., Tetau, M., Cambar, J. (1984) Effet protecteur de dilutions homéopathiques de metaux néphrotoxiques vis-à-vis d'une intoxication mercurielle. *Cah. Biothérapie* 81 (suppl.): 27.

Guillemain, J., Douylliez, C., Bastide, M., Cambar, J., Narcisse, G. (1987) Pharmacologie de l'infinitésimal. Application aux dilutions homéopathiques. *Homéopathie* 4: 35.

Gutterman, J.U. (1994) Cytokine therapeutics: Lessons from interferon-alpha. *Proc. Natl. Acad. Sci. USA* 91: 1198.

Gutzwiller, M.C. (1992) Quantum chaos. *Sci Am.* 266: 26.

Hadji, L., Arnoux, B., Benveniste, J. (1991) Effect of dilute histamine on coronary flow of isolated guinea-pig heart. *FASEB J.* 5: A1583.

Haehl, R. (1989) *Samuel Hahnemann. His Life and Work* (reprint edition). B. Jain Publ. Ltd., New Delhi.

Hagglof, B., Blom, L., Dahlquist, G., Lonnberg, G., Sahlin, B. (1991) The Swedish childhood diabetes study: indications of severe psychological stress as a risk factor for type 1 (insulin-dependent) diabetes mellitus in childhood. *Diabetologica* 34: 579.

Hahnemann, C.F.S. (1796) Essay on a new principle for ascertaining the curative powers of drugs, and some examinations of the previous principles. *Hufeland's Journal* 2: 391.

Hahnemann, C.F.S. (1994) *Organon of Medicine*. With explanations by Joseph Reves, edited from the 5th and 6th edition. Homeopress Ltd, Haifa.

Haidvogl, M. (1994) Clinical studies on homoeopathy. The problem of a useful design. In: *Ultra High Dilution* (P.C. Endler and J. Schulte, eds.). Kluwer Acad. Publ., Dordrecht, p. 233.

Halliwell, B. (1987) Oxidants and human disease: some new concepts. *FASEB J.* 1: 358.

Halliwell, B., Gutteridge, J.M.C., Cross, C.E. (1992) Free radicals, antioxidants, and human disease: Where are we now? *J. Lab. Clin. Med.* 119: 598.

Hameroff, S.R. (1988) Coherence in the cytoskeleton: Implications for biological information processing. In: *Biological Coherence and Response to External Stimuli* (H. Frohlich, ed.). Springer-Verlag, Berlin, p. 242.

Harish, G., Kretschmer, M. (1988) Smallest zinc quantities affect the histamine release from peritoneal mast cells of the rat. *Experientia* 44: 761.

Harold, F.M. (1986) *The Vital Force: A Study of Bioenergetics*. W.H. Freeman and Company, New York.

Harrison, H., Fixsen, A., Vickers, A. (1999) A randomized comparison of homoeopathic and standard care for the treatment of glue ear in children. *Complement. Ther. Med.* 7: 132.

Hart, O., Mullee, M.A., Lewith, G. and Miller, J. (1997) Double-blind, placebo-controlled, randomized clinical trial of homeopathic arnica C30 for pain and infection after total abdominal hysterectomy. *J. R. Soc. Med.* 90: 73.

Hashizume, K., Ichikawa, K., Sakurai, A., Suzuki, S., Takeda, T., Kobayashi, M., Miyamoto, T., Arai, M., Nagasawa, T. (1991) Administration of thyroxine in treated Graves' disease. Effects on the level of antibodies to TSH receptors and on the risk of recurrence of hyperthyroidism. *N. Engl. J. Med.* 324: 947.

Hasted, J.B. (1988) Metastable states of biopolymers. In: *Biological Coherence and Response to External Stimuli* (H. Frohlich, ed.). Springer-Verlag, Berlin, p. 102.

Heger, M., Riley, D. S., and Haidvogl, M. (2000) International integrative primary care outcomes study (IIPCOS-2): An international research project of homeopathy in primary care. *Br. Hom. J.* 89 Suppl 1: S10.

Heine, H. and Schmolz, M. (2000) Immunoregulation via 'bystander suppression' needs minute amounts of substances—a basis for homeopathic therapy? *Med. Hypotheses* 54: 392.

Hering, C. (1849) Glonoine, a new medicine for headache. *Am. J. Homoeopathy* 4: 3.

Hill, N., Stam, C., Tuinder, S., and van Haselen, R. A. (1995) A placebo controlled clinical trial investigating the efficacy of a homeopathic after-bite gel in reducing mosquito bite induced erythema. *Eur. J. Clin. Pharmacol.* 49: 103.

Hirst, S.J., Hayes, N.A., Burridge, J., Pearce, F.L., Foreman, J.C. (1993) Human basophil degranulation is not triggered by very dilute antiserum against human IgE. *Nature* 366: 525.

Hochstrasser, B. (1999) Quality of life of pregnant women in homeopathic or mainstream medical type of care and the course of the pregnancy. *Forsch. Komplementarmed.* 6 Suppl 1: 23.

Hofstadter, D.R. (1991) Attrattori strani: enti fra ordine e caos. In: *Il Caos. Le Leggi del Disordine* (G. Casati, ed.) Le Scienze S.p.A., Milano, p. 71.

Holffenbuttel, B.H.R., Van Haeften, T.W. (1993) Non-insulin dependent diabetes mellitus: defects in insulin secretion. *Eur. J. Clin. Invest.* 23: 69.

Hollstein, M., Sidransky, D., Vogelstein, B., Harris, C.C. (1991) p53 mutations in human cancers. *Science* 253: 49.

Hornung, J., Vogler, S. (1990) A documentation project. Clinical studies on unconventional treatment of cancer. *Berlin J. Res. Homoeopathy* 1: 22.

Hornung, J., Griebel, S. (1991) Strutturazione e finalità del progetto: Studi clinici su terapie tumorali non convenzionali. *Riv. Ital. Omotossicol.* IX (3): 37.

Hornung, J. (1991) An overview of formal methodology requirements for controlled clinical trials. *Berlin J. Res. Homeopaty* 1 (4/5): 288.

Hunter, T. (1984) The proteins of oncogenes. *Sci Am.* 251: 60.

Hyltander, A., Korner, U., Lundholm, K.G. (1993) Evaluation of mechanisms behind elevated energy expenditure in cancer patients with solid tumors. *Eur. J. Clin. Invest.* 23: 46.

Ibarra, R. (1991) Chronobiology, a possible explanation for homeopathic aggravation. *Berlin J. Res. Homeopathy* 1 (4/5): 281.

Ingber, D. (1991) Integrins as mechanochemical transducers. *Curr. Opin. Cell. Biol.* 3: 841.

Invernizzi, G., Gala, C. (1989) Aspetti psicologici del problema cancro. In: *Progressi nella Ricerca sul Cancro*. Le Scienze S.p.A., Milano, p. 163.

Jacob, F. (1973) *The Logic of Life: A History of Eredity*. Pantheon, New York.

Jacobs, J., Jimenez, L.M., Gloyd, S.S., Gale, J.L., Crothers, D. (1994) Treatment of acute childhood diarrhea with homeopathic medicine: a randomized clinical trial in Nicaragua. *Pediatrics* 93: 719.

Jacobs, J., Jimenez, L. M., Malthouse, S., Chapman, E., Crothers, D., Masuk, M., and Jonas, W. B. (2000) Homeopathic treatment of acute childhood diarrhea: results from a clinical trial in Nepal. *J Alt. Compl. Med.* 6: 131.

Jacobs, J., Springer, D.A., Crothers, D. (2001) Homeopathic treatment of acute otitis media in children: a preliminary randomized placebo-controlled trial. *Pediatr. Infect. Dis. J.* 20: 177.

Jensen, P. (1990) Use of alternative medicine by patients with atopic dermatitis and psoriasis. *Acta Derm. Venereol. (Stockholm)* 70: 421.

Jerne, N.K. (1974) Towards a network theory of the immune system. *Ann. Immunol.* 125C: 373.

Jonas, W.B., Fortier, A.F., Heckendorn, D.K., Nacy, C.A. (1991) Prophylaxis of tularemia infection in mice using agitated ultra-high dilutions of tularemia-infected tissue. In: *Proc. 5th GIRI Meeting*, Paris, Abs. 21.

Jonas, W. B. and Jacobs, J. (1996) *Healing With Homeopathy: The Complete Guide*. New York: Warner Books.

Jonas W.B. (1999) Do homeopathic nosodes protect against infection? An experimental test. *Altern. Ther. Health Med.* 5: 36.

Jonas, W. B., Linde, K., and Ramirez, G. (2000) Homeopathy and rheumatic disease. *Rheum. Dis. Clin. North Am.* 26: 117.

Jonas, W., Lin, Y. and Tortella, F. (2001) Neuroprotection from glutamate toxicity with ultra-low dose glutamate. *Neuroreport* 12(2):335.

Jones, R.J., Sharkis, S.J., Miller, C.B., Rowinsky, E.K., Burke, P.J., Stratford May W. (1990) Bryostatin 1, a unique biologic response modifier: anti-leukemic activity in vitro. *Blood* 75: 1319.

Julian, O.A. (1979) *Materia Medica of New Homoeopathic Remedies*. Beaconsfield Publ, Beaconsfield.

Julian, O.A., Haffen, M. (1982) *Omeopatia*. Masson Italia Editore, Milano.

Julian, O.A. (1983) *La Materia Medica dei Nosodi*. Nuova Ipsa Editore, Palermo.

Jurgens, H., Peitgen, H.O., Saupe, D. (1990) The language of fractals. *Sci. Am.* 263 (2): 40.

Kail, K. (2001) Clinical outcomes of a diagnostic and treatment protocol in allergy/sensitivity patients. *Altern. Med. Rev.* 6:188.

Kainz, J. T.; Kozel, G.; Haidvogl, M.; Smolle, J. (1996) Homeopathic versus placebo therapy of children with warts on the hands: a randomized, double-blind clinical trial. *Dermatology* 4: 318.

Katz, D.H., Bargatze, R.F., Bogowitz, C.A., Katz, L.R. (1979) Regulation of IgE antibody production by serum molecules. V. Evidence that coincidental sensitization and imbalance in the normal damping mechanism results in "allergic breakthrough". *J. Immunol.* 122: 2191.

Kauffman, S.A. (1991) Antichaos and adaptation. *Sci. Am.* 265 (2): 64.

Kauffman, S.A. (1993) *Origins of Order: Self-Organization and Selection in Evolution*. Oxford University Press, Oxford.

Kaveri, S.V., Dietrich, G., Hurez, V., Kazatchkine, M.D. (1991) Intravenous immunoglobulins (IVIg) in the treatment of autoimmune diseases. *Clin. Exp. Immunol.* 86: 192.

Kell, D.B. (1988) Coherent properties of energy-coupling membrane systems. In: *Biological Coherence and Response to External Stimuli* (E. Frohlich, ed.). Springer Verlag, Berlin, p. 233.

Kelsoe, G., Reth, M., Rajewsky, K. (1981) Control of idiotope expression by monoclonal anti-idiotope expression by monoclonal anti-idiotope and idiotope-bearing antibody. *Eur. J. Immunol.* 11: 418.

Kent, J.T. (1990) *Lectures of Homoeopathic Materia Medica* (Reprint edition). B. Jain Publishers. Pahargani, New Delhi, India.

Kenyon, J.N. (1983) *Modern Techniques of Acupuncture. 3 Vols.* Thorson Publ. Ltd., Wellinborough (U.K.).

Khansari, D.N., Murgo, A.J., Faith, R.E. (1990) Effects of stress on the immune system. *Immunol. Today* 11: 170.

Khorana, H.G. (1993) Two light-transducing membrane proteins: Bacteriorodopsin and the mammalian rhodopsin. *Proc. Natl. Acad. Sci. USA* 90: 1166.

Khuda-Bukhsh, A.R., Banik, S. (1991) Assessment of cytogenetic damage in X-irradiated mice and its alteration by oral administration of potentized homeopathic drug, Ginseng D200. *Berlin J. Res. Homeopathy* 1 (4/5): 254.

Khuda-Bukhsh, A.R., Maity, S. (1991) Alterations of cytogenetic effects by oral administration of a homeopathic drug, Ruta graveolens, in mice exposed to sub-lethal X-irradiation. *Berlin J. Res. Homeopathy* 1 (4/5): 264.

Kief, H. (1988) Die biologische Grundlagen der autohomologen Immunotherapie. *Erfachrungsheilkunde* (Verlag, Heidelberg) 37: 175.

Kief, H. (1991) Die Behandlung der Neurodermitis bei Kleinkindern mit autohomologer Immunotherapie (AHIT). *Natur Heilpraxis* 3: 240.

Kirsch, M. (1989) Rafforzamento immunitario e immunostimolazione attraverso la disintossicazione del mesenchima. *Riv. Ital. Omotossicol.* VII: 5.

Kleijnen, J., Knipschild, P., ter Riet, G. (1991) Clinical trials of homoeopathy. *Brit. Med. J.* 302: 316.

Koenig, P., Swoboda, F. (1987) Acidum succinicum 30x—a drug proving. *Brit. Hom. J.* 76: 19.

Koh, Y.Y., Lim, H.S., Min, K.U., Min, Y.G. (1994) Airways of allergic rhinitics are "primed" to repeated allergen inhalation challenge. *Clin. Exp. Allergy* 24:347.

Kollerstrom, J. (1982) Basic scientific research into the "low dose effect". *Brit. Hom. J.* 71: 41.

Konig, H.L. (1989) Bioinformation. Electrophysical aspects. In: *Electromagnetic Bio-Information* (Popp, F.A. *et al.*, eds.) Urban & Schwarzenberg, Munchen, p. 42.

Koopman G., Arwert, F., Eriksson, A.W., Bart, J., Kipp, A., Van Kruining, H. (1990) In vitro effects of Viscum album preparations on human fibroblasts and tumor cell lines. *Brit. Hom. J.* 79: 12.

Kremer, F., Santo, L., Poglitsch, A., Koschnitzke, C., Behrens, H., Genzel, L. (1988) The influence of low-intensity millimeter waves on biological systems. In: *Biological Coherence and Response to External Stimuli* (H. Frohlich, ed.). Springer-Verlag, Berlin, p. 86.

Krop, J., Lewith, G. T., Gziut, W., and Radulescu, C. (1997) A double-blind, randomized, controlled investigation of electrodermal testing in the diagnosis of allergies. *J. Alt. Compl. Med.* 3: 241.

Kroy, W. (1989). The use of optical radiation for stimulation therapy. In: *Electromagnetic Bio-Information* (Popp, F.A. *et al.*, eds.). Urban & Schwarzenberg, Munchen, p. 200.

Ku, G., Kronenberg, M., Peacock, D.J., Tempst, P., Banquerigo, M.L., Brahn, E., Braun, B.S., Reeve, J.R.Jnr (1993) Prevention of experimental autoimmune arthritis with a peptide fragment of type II collagen. *Eur. J. Immunol.* 23: 591.

Kugler, A., Stuhler, G., Walden, P., et al. (2000) Regression of human metastatic renal cell carcinoma after vaccination with tumor cell-dendritic cell hybrids. *Nature Medicine* 6: 332.

Kuhn, T. (1962) *The Structure of Scientific Revolutions.* University of Chicago Press, Chicago

Kundu, S. N., Mitra, K., and Bukhsh, A. R. (2000) Efficacy of a potentized homoeopathic drug (Arsenicum-album-30) in reducing cytotoxic effects produced by arsenic trioxide in mice: III. Enzymatic changes and recovery of tissue damage in liver. *Complement Ther. Med.* 8: 76.

Kuttan, G., Kuttan, R. (1992) Immunomodulatory activity of a peptide isolated from Viscum Album extract (NSC 635 089). *Immunol. Invest.* 21: 285.

Kumar, V., Sercarz, E.E. (1991) Regulation of autoimmunity. *Curr. Opin. Immunol.* 3: 888.

Lalanne, M.Cl., Doutremepuich, C., de Seze, O., Belon, P. (1990) What is the effect of acetylsalicylic acid at ultra low dose on the interaction platelets/vessel wall? *Thromb. Res.* 60: 231.

Lalanne, M.Cl., de Seze, O., Doutremepuich, C., Belon, P. (1991) Could proteolytic enzyme modulate the interaction platelets/vessel wall in presence of ASA at ultra low doses? *Thromb. Res.* 63: 419.

Lalanne, M.C., Ramboer, I., De Seze, O., Doutremepuich, C. (1992) In vitro platelets/endothelial cells interactions in presence of acetylsalicylic acid at various dosages. *Thromb. Res.* 65: 33.

Lam, F.M.K., Tsuei, J.J., Zhao, Z. (1990) Study on the bioenergetic measurement of acupuncture points for determination of correct dosages of allopathic and homeopathic medicines in the treatment of diabetes mellitus. *Amer. J. Acupunct.* 18: 127.

Lancet (Editorial) (1991) Welcome to ouabain—a new steroid hormone. *Lancet* 338: 543.

Lang, R.A., Burgess, A.W. (1990) Autocrine growth factors and tumorigenic transformation. *Immunol. Today* 11: 244.

Laplantine, F. (1986) *Anthropologie de la maladie.* Payot, Paris.

Lapp, C., Wurmser, L., Ney, J. (1955) Mobilization de l'arsenic fixé chez le cobaye sous l'influence des doses infinitesimales d'arseniate. *Therapie* 10: 625.

Lasne, Y., Duplan, J.C., Fenet, B., Guerin, A. (1989) Contribution à l'approche scientifique de la doctrine homéopathique. *De Natura Rerum* 3: 38.

Lasters, I., Bardiaux, M. (1988) Explanation of Benveniste. *Nature* 334: 385.

Leonhardt, H. (1982) *Fondamenti dell'Elettroagopuntura Secondo Voll.* Piccin Editore, Padova.

Lewith, G. T., Kenyon, J. N., Broomfield, J., and Preston-Hulburt, P. (2001) Is electrodermal testing as effective as skin prick tests for diagnosing allergies? A double blind, randomised block design study. *Br. Med. J.* 322: 131.

Lewith, G., Brown, P.K., Tyrrel, D.A.J. (1989) Controlled study of a homoeopathic dilution of influenza vaccine on antibody titres in man. *Comp. Med. Res.* 3: 22.

Lichtenstein, L.M., Gillespie, E. (1973) Inhibition of histamine release by histamine controlled by H_2 receptor. *Nature* 244: 287.

Lichtenstein, L.M., Gillespie, E. (1975) The effects of the H_1 and H_2 antihistamines on "allergic" histamine release and its inhibition by histamine. *J. Pharmac. Exp. Ther.* 192: 441.

Linde, K., Melchart, D., Eitel, F., Worku, F., Wagner, H. (1991) Critical evaluation of studies on effects of very low doses and high dilutions on experimental intoxications. *Proc. 5th GIRI Meeting*, Paris, Abs. 41.

Linde, K. (1991) *Dosisabhangige Umkehreffekte. Eine Differenzierende Literaturbetrachtung.* Dissertation and der Medizinischen Fakultat der Ludwig-Maximilians-Universitat Munchen. Munchen.

Linde, K., Melchart, D., Jonas, W.B., Worku, F., Wagner, H., Eitel, F. (1993) Criteria-based analyses on experimental and clinical studies on homoeopathy. In: *Omeomed92* (C. Bornoroni, ed.). Editrice Compositori, Bologna, p. 171. Also published in Linde, K. Jonas, W., Melchart, D., et. al., Critical Review and Meta-Analysis of Serial Agitated Dilutions in Experimental Toxicology. *Human & Experimental Toxicology* 13: 481-492.

Linde, K., Clausius, N., Ramirez, G., Melchart, D., Eitel, F., Hedges, L. V., and Jonas, W. B. (1997) Are the clinical effects of homeopathy placebo effects? A meta-analysis of placebo-controlled trials. *Lancet* 350: 834.

Linde, K. and Melchart, D. (1998) Randomized controlled trials of individualized homeopathy: A state-of- the-art review. *J. Alt. Compl. Med.* 4: 371.

Linde, K., Scholz, M., Ramirez, G., Clausius, N., Melchart, D., and Jonas, W. B. (1999) Impact of study quality on outcome in placebo-controlled trials of homeopathy. *J. Clin. Epidemiol.* 52: 631.

Linde, K. and Jobst, K. A. (2000) Homeopathy for chronic asthma. *Cochrane. Database. Syst. Rev.*, CD000353

Linde, K., Jonas W.B., Melchart, D., Willich, S. (2001) The methodological quality of randomized controlled trials of homeopathy., herbal medicines and acupuncture. *Int. J. Epidemiol.* 30: 526.

Ling, G.N., Ochsenfeld, M.M. (1983) Studies on the physical state of water in living cells and model systems. I. The quantitative relationship between the concentration of gelatin and certain oxygen-containing polymers and their influence upon the solubility of water for Na salts. *Physiol. Chem. Phys.* 15: 127.

Ling, G.N., Miller, C., Ochsenfeld, M.M. (1973) The physical state of solutes and water in living cells according to the association-induction hypothesis. *Ann N. Y. Acad. Sci. USA* 204: 6.

Litime, M.H., Aissa, J., Benveniste, J. (1993) Antigen signaling at high dilution. *FASEB J.* 7: A602 (3488).

Liu, D.S., Astumian, R.D., Tsong, T.Y. (1990) Activation of Na$^+$ and K$^+$ pumping modes of (Na,K)-ATPase by an oscillating electric field. *J. Biol. Chem.* 265: 7260.

Lodispoto, A. (1984) *Storia della Omeopatia in Italia: Storia Antica di una Terapia Moderna.* Edizioni Mediterranee, Roma.

Lokken, P.; Straumsheim, P. A.; Tveiten, D.; Skjelbred, P.; Borchgrevink, C. F. (1995) Effect of homeopathy on pain and other events after acute trauma: placebo controlled trial with bilateral oral surgery. *Br. Med. J.* 310: 6992.

Long, L., Ernst, E. (2001) Homeopathic remedies for the treatment of osteoarthritis: A systematic review. *Br. Hom. J.* 90: 37.

Lorenz, E. (1979) Predictability: Does the flap of a butterfly's wings in Brazil set off a tornado in Texas? *Address at the Annual Meeting of the American Association for the Advancement of Science.* Washington (cited in Fuller Royal, 1991).

Luben, R.A., Cain, C.D., Chen, M.Y., Rosen, D.M., Adey, W.R. (1982) Effects of electromagnetic stimuli on bone and bone cells in vitro: inhibition of responses to parathyroid hormone by low-energy, low-frequency fields. *Proc. Nal. Acad. Sci. USA* 79: 4180.

Ludmer, P.L., Selwyn, A.P., Shook, T.L., Wayne, R.R., Mudge, G.H., Wayne Alexander, R., Ganz, P. (1986) Paradoxical vasocostriction induced by acetylcholine in atherosclerotic coronary arteries. *N. Engl. J. Med.* 315: 1046.

Lussignoli, S., Bertani, S., Metelmann, H., Bellavite, P., and Conforti, A. (1999) Effect of Traumeel S, a homeopathic formulation, on blood-induced inflammation in rats. *Compl. Ther. Med.* 7: 225.

Luu, C. (1976) *Etude des Dilutions Homéopathiques par Spectroscopie Raman-Laser. Essai d'Interpretation de Leur Méchanisme d'Action.* Ed. Boiron, Paris.

Lux, W. (1833) *Isopathic der Contagionen.* Ed. Kollmann, Liepzig.

Maddox, J., Randi, J., Stewart, W.W. (1988) "High-dilution" experiments a delusion. *Nature* 334: 287.

Magnavita, N. (1989) Radiazioni elettromagnetiche e rischi per la salute. *The Pratictioner (Italian edition)* 124: 30.

Maiwald, L., Weinfurtner, T., Mau, J., Connert, W.D. (1988) Therapie des grippalen infects mit einem homöopatischen Kombinationspraparat im Vergleich zur Acetylsalicylsaure. *Arzneimittelforschung Drug Res.* 38: 578.

Maiwald, L. (1988) Omotossicologia, una metodica scientificamente comprovata e di sperimentata efficacia. *Riv. Ital. Omotossicol.* VII (1): 2.

Majerus, M. (1991) A critical appraisal of scientific arguments regarding basic research in homeopathy: A comprehensive examination of the francophone literature. *Berlin J. Res. Homeopathy* 1 (4/5): 301.

Male, D., Champion, B., Cooke, A. (1988) *Advanced Immunology.* Gower Med. Publ., London.

Malik, S., Balkwill, F. (1991) Epithelial ovarian cancer: A cytokine propelled disease? *Brit. J. Cancer* 64: 617.

Mandelbrot, B.B. (1982) *The Fractal Geometry of Nature.* W.H. Freeman & Co., New York.

Mansvelt, J.D., Van Amons, E. (1975) Inquiry into the limits of biological effects of chemical compounds in tissue culture. I. Low dose effects of mercure chloride. *Z. Naturtorschung* 30: 643.

Markov, M.S., Todorov, S.I., Ratcheva, M.R. (1975) Biomagnetic effect of the constant magnetic field action on water and physiological activity. In: *Physical and Chemical Bases of Biological Information Transfer* (J. Vassileva-Popova, ed.). Plenum Press, New York, p. 441.

Marx, J. (1991) Testing of autoimmune therapy begins. *Science* 252: 27.

Masini, E., Blandina, P., Brunelleschi, S., Mannaioni, P.F. (1982) Evidence for H_2-receptor-mediated inhibition of histamine release from isolated rat mast cells. *Agents and Actions* 12: 85.

Matthews, D.R. (1991) Physiological implications of pulsatile hormone secretion. *Ann. N. Y. Acad. Sci.* 618: 28.

Mayaux, M.J., Guihard-Moscato, M.L., Schwartz, D., Benveniste, J.,, Coquin, Y., Crapanne, J.B., Poitevin, B., Rodary, M., Chevrel, J.P., Mollet, M. (1988) Controlled clinical trial of homeopathy in postoperative ileus. *Lancet* 1: 528.

Melchart, D., Linde, K., Worku, F., Sarkady, L., Holzmann, M., Jurcic, K., and Wagner, H. (1995) Results of five randomized studies on the immunomodulatory activity of preparations of Echinacea. *J. Alt. Compl. Med.* 1: 145.

Meletani, S. (1990) *Mora Terapia. Teoria e Pratica.* Guna Editore, Milano.

Meletani, S. (1992) Diagnostica e terapia con EAV e Mora nella cardiopatia ischemica e nelle vasculopatie ateromatosiche. *Riv. Ital. Omotossicol.* X (3): 37.

Meyer, T. (1991) Cell signaling by second messenger waves. *Cell* 64: 675.

Meyers, F.H., Jawetz, E., Goldfien, A. (1981) *Farmacologia Medica.* Piccin Editore, Padova.

Meuris, J. (1982) *Omeopatia e Materia Medica. Tipologia Omeopatica e Fondamenti Scientifici.* Edizioni Red, Como.

Milgrom, L.R., King, K.R., Lee, J., Pinkus, A.S. (2001) On the investigation of homeopathic potencies using low resolution NMR T2 relaxation times: An experimental and critical survey of the work of Roland Conte et al. *Br. Hom. J.* 90: 5.

Miller, A., Hafler, D.A., Weiner, H.L. (1991a) Immunotherapy in autoimmune diseases. *Curr. Opin. Immunol.* 3: 936.

Miller, A., Lider, O., Weiner, H.L. (1991b) Antigen driven bystander suppression after oral administration of antigen. *J. Exp. Med.* 174: 791.

Miller, S.D., Tan, L.J., Pope, L., McRae, B.L., Karpus, W.J. (1992) Antigen-specific tolerance as a therapy for experimental autoimmune encephalomyelitis. *Int. Rev. Immunol.* 9: 203.

Minors, D. (1985) Chronobiology. Its importance in Clinical Medicine. *Clin. Sci.* 69: 369.

Mitra, K., Kundu, S. N., and Khuda Bukhsh, A. R. (1999) Efficacy of a potentized homoeopathic drug (Arsenicum Album-30) in reducing toxic effects produced by arsenic trioxide in mice: II. On alterations in body weight, tissue weight and total protein. *Complement Ther. Med.* 7: 24.

Moncada, S., Rees, D.D., Schulz, R., Palmer, R.M.J. (1991) Development and mechanism of a specific supersensitivity to nitrovasodilators after inhibition of vascular NO synthesis in vivo. *Proc. Natl. Acad. Sci. USA* 88: 2166.

Monro, J. (1987) Electrical sensitivities in allergic patients. *Clin. Ecol.* 4: 93.

Montfort, H. (2000) A new homeopathic approach to neoplastic diseases: from cell destruction to carcinogen-induced apoptosis. *Br. Hom. J.* 89: 78.

Moss, V.A., Roberts, J.A., Simpson, H.K.L. (1982) The action of "low potency" homeopathic remedies on the movement of guinea pig macrophages and human leukocytes. *Brit. Hom. J.* 71: 48.

Moss, F. (1994) Chaos under control. *Nature* 370: 596

Mossinger, P. (1973) Die behandlung der Pharingitis mit Phytolacca. *Allgemeine Homopatische Zeitung* 218: 111.

Mossinger, P. (1992) *Omeopatia e Medicina Scientifica.* Nuova Ipsa Editore, Palermo.

Mowat, A.Mcl. (1987) The regulation of immune responses to dietary protein antigens. *Immunol. Today* 8: 93.

Muller, E. (1992) Cresce l'insoddisfazione per la medicina ufficiale? *Il Medico d'Italia* 26: 6.

Murray, A.W., Kirschner, M.W. (1991) What controls the cell cycle. *Sci. Am.* 264 (3): 34.

Muscari-Tomaioli, G., Allegri, F., Miali, E., Pomposelli, R., Tubia, P., Targhetta, A., Castellini, M. and Bellavite, P. (2001) Observational study of life quality in cephalalgic patients under homeopathic treatment. *Br. Hom. J.* 90:189.

Nagpaul, V.M. (1987) Provings—Planning and protocol. *Brit. Hom. J.* 76: 76.

Naum, C.C., Kaplan, S.S., Basford, R.E. (1991) Platelets and ATP prime neutrophils for enhanced O_2^- generation at low concentrations but inhibit O_2^- generation at high concentrations. *J. Leukoc. Biol.* 49: 83.

Nespoli, L., De Amici, M., Rondena, D., Collotti, F., Lanfranchi, A., Maccario, R., Ascione, A., Burgio, G.R. (1987) Valutazione degli effetti di un vaccino polibatterico sul sistema immune. Studio in vitro e in vivo. *Riv. Inf. Ped.* 3: 181.

Nicolis, G., Prigogine, Y. (1991) *La Complessità. Esplorazioni nei Nuovi Campi della Scienza.* Einaudi, Torino (Original edition: *Exploring Complexity. An Introduction.* Piper, Munchen, 1987).

Nishimura S., Sekiya T. (1987) Human cancer and cellular oncogenes. *Biochem. J.* 243: 313.

Nugent, A.M., Onuoha, G.N., McEneaney, D.J., Steele, I.C., Hunter, S.J., Prasanna, K., Campbell, N.P.S., Shaw, C., Buchanan, K.D., Nicholls, D.P. (1994) Variable patterns of atrial natriuretic peptide secretion in man. *Eur. J. Clin. Invest.* 24: 267.

Oberbaum, M., Weisman, Z., Markovich, R., Kalinkovich, A., Bentwich, Z. (1991) Wound healing by homeopathic dilutions of silica in experimental animals. In: *Proc. 5th GIRI Meeting,* Paris, Abs. 23.

Oberbaum, M., Markovits, R., Weisman, Z., Kalinkevits, A., Bentwich, Z. (1992) Wound healing by homoeopathic Silicea dilutions in mice. *Harefuah (J. Israel Med. Ass.)* 123: 78.

Oberbaum, M., Cambar, J. (1994) Hormesis: dose-dependent reverse effects of low and very low doses. In: *Ultra High Dilution* (P.C. Endler and J. Schulte, eds.). Kluwer Acad. Publ., Dordrecht, p. 5.

Oberbaum, M., Yaniv, I., Ben-Gal, Y., Stein, J., Ben-Zvi, N., Freedman, L.S., Branski, D. (2001) A randomized., controlled clinical trial of the homeopathic medication Traumeel/s in the treatment of chemotherapy-induced stomatitis in children undergoing stem cell transplantation. *Cancer* 92: 684.

Ovelgonne, J.H., Bol, A.W.J.M., Hop, W.C.J., van Wijk, R. (1991) Mechanical agitation of very diluted antiserum against IgE has no effect on basophil staining properties. In: *Proc. 5th GIRI Meeting,* Paris, Abs. 17.

Ovelgonne, J.H., Bol, A.W.J.M., Hop, W.C.J., van Wijk, R. (1992) Mechanical agitation of very dilute antiserum against IgE has no effect on basophil staining properties. *Experientia* 48: 504.

Palermo, C., Filanti, C., Poggi, S., and Manduca, P. (2000) Osteogenesis in vitro in rat tibia-derived osteoblasts is promoted by the homeopathic preparation, FMS*Calciumfluor. *Cell Biol. Int.* 23: 31.

Palmerini, C.A., Codini, M., Floridi, A., Mattoli, P., Buffetti, S., Di Leginio, E. (1993) The use of Phosphorus 30 CH in the experimental treatment of hepatic fibrosis in rats. In: *Omeomed92* (C. Bornoroni, ed.). Editrice Compositori, Bologna, p. 219.

Pandiella, A., Beguinot, L., Vicentini, L.M., Meldolesi, J. (1989) Transmembrane signalling at the epidermal growth factor receptor. *Trends Pharmacol. Sci.* 10: 411.

Paterson, J. (1944) Report on Mustard Gas Experiment. *J. Am. Inst. Homeopathy* 37: 47 (cited in Ullman, 1991a).

Pennec, J.P., Aubin, M. (1984) Effect of aconitum and veratrum on the isolated perfused heart of the common heel (Anguilla-anguilla). *Comp. Biochem. Physiol.* 776: 367.

Pennec, J.P., Aubin, M., Manlhiot, J.L., Payreu, B., Scaliger, D. (1984a) Action de differentes diluitions de veratrine sur le coeur isolé et perfusé d'anguille. *Homéopathie Francaise* 72: 245.

Pennec, J.P., Aubin, M., Manlhiot, J.L., Payrau, B., Scaliger, D. (1984b) Action de differentes diluitions de veratrine sur le coeur isolé perfusé de rat. *Homéopathie Francaise* 72: 251.

Perelson, A.S. (1989) Immune Network Theory. *Imunol. Rev.* 110: 5.

Petit, C., Belon, P., Got, R. (1989) Effect of homoeopathic dilutions on subcellular enzymatic activity. *Human Toxicol.* 8: 125.

Piccardi, G., Corsi, M.L. (1938) Sulla precipitazione del carbonato di calcio da acqua dura attivata ("T" od "R") e normale. *Gazz. Chim. Ital.* 68: 287.

Piccardi, G. (1938) Sopra un nuovo fenomeno di natura elettrica e sopra un nuovo effetto presentato dai metalli. *Gazz. Chim. Ital.* 68: 246.

Piccardi, G., Botti, E. (1939) Influenza dell'attivazione "T" ed "R" sui colloidi d'oro. *Gazz. Chim. Ital.* 69: 609.

Pittler, M. H., Abbot, N. C., Harkness, E. F., and Ernst, E. (2000) Location bias in controlled clinical trials of complementary/alternative therapies. *J Clin. Epidemiol.* 53: 485.

Poitevin, B., Aubin, M., Royer, J.F. (1983) Effet de belladonna et ferrum phosphoricum sur la chemiluminescence des polynucleaires neutrophiles humains. *Ann. Hom. Fr.* 25 (3): 5.

Poitevin, B., Aubin, M., Benveniste, J. (1985) Effect d'Apis Mellifica sur la degranulation des basophiles humains in vitro. *Homéopathie Francaise* 73: 193.

Poitevin, B., Aubin, M., Benveniste, J. (1986) Approche d'une analyse quantitative de l'effet d'apis mellifica sur la degranulation des basophiles humains in vitro. *Innov. Tech. Biol. Med.* 7: 64.

Poitevin, B., Davenas, E., Benveniste, J. (1988) In vitro immunological degranulation of human basophils is modulated by Lung histamine and Apis mellifica. *Brit. J. Clin. Pharmacol.* 25: 439.

Poitevin, B. (1988a) Scientific bases of homeopathy. *Conference at the Societé Francaise des Sciences et Techniques Farmaceutiques.* Bordeaux, France.

Poitevin, B. (1988b) Relation generale entre homéopathie et immunoallergologie. *Encycl. Med. Chir. (Paris, France) Homéopathie*: 38255, A 10.

Poitevin, B. (1988c) Recherche experimentale. *Encyclopedie Medico-Chirurgicale (Paris, France). Homéopathie*: 38060 A 30.

Poitevin, B. (1990) Scientific bases of homeopathy. In: *Homeopathy in Focus.* VGM Verlag fur Ganzheitmedizin, Essen, p. 42.

Pollard, T.D., Goldman, R.D. (1992) Cytoplasm and cell motility. Editorial Overview. *Curr. Biol.* 4: 1.

Pollock, J.K., Pohl, D.G. (1988) Emission of radiation by active cells. In: *Biological Coherence and Response to External Stimuli* (H. Frohlich, ed.). Springer-Verlag, Berlin, p. 139.

Polonsky, K.S., Given, B.D., Hirsch, L.J., Tillil, H., Shapiro, E.T., Beebe, C., Frank, B.H., Galloway, J.A., Cauter, E.V. (1988) Abnormal patterns of insulin secretion in non-insulin-dependent diabetes mellitus. *N. Engl. J. Med.* 318: 1231.

Pontieri, G.M., Bernelli-Zazzera, A., Bianchi-Santamaria, A., Gazzaniga, P.P., Russo, M.A., Salerno, A., Santamaria, L., Tolone, G. (1987) *Patologia Generale.* Piccin Ed., Padova.

Pool, R. (1988) Unbelievable results spark a controversy. *Science* 241: 407.

Pool, R. (1990) Is there an EMF-cancer connection? *Science* 249: 1096.

Popova, T. (1991) Homoeopathic aggravation. *Brit. Hom. J.* 80: 228.

Popp, F.A. (1985) *Nuovi Orizzonti in Medicina. La teoria dei Biofotoni.* IPSA Editore, Palermo.

Popp, F.A., Warnke, U., Konig, H.L., Peschla, W. (1989) (editors) *Electromagnetic Bio-information.* Urban and Schwarzenberg, Munchen.

Popp, F.A. (1990a) Some elements of homoeopathy. *Brit. Hom. J.* 79: 161.

Popp, F.A. (1990b) Elements of homeopathy. In: *Homeopathy in Focus.* VGM (Verlag fur Ganzheitsmedizin), Essen, p. 70.

Popper, K. (1969) *Scienza e Filosofia.* Einaudi, Torino.

Pound, A.W., Horn, L., Lawson, T.A. (1973) Decreased toxicity of DMN in rats after treatment with carbon tetrachloride. *Pathology* 5: 233.

Ramelet, A.A., Buchheim, G., Lorenz, P., Imfeld, M. (2000) Homeopathic Arnica in post-operative haematomas: a double-blind study. *Dermatology* 201: 347.

Rastogi, D. P., Singh, V. P., Singh, V., Dey, S. K., and Rao, K. (1999) Homeopathy in HIV infection: A trial report of double-blind placebo controlled study. *Br. Hom. J.* 88: 49.

Reckeweg, H.H. (1981) *Homotoxikologie. Ganzheitsschau einer Synthese der Medizin.* Aurelia Verlag, Baden-Baden.

Reilly, D., Taylor, M.A., Beattie, N.G.M., Campbell, J.H., McSharry, C., Aitchison, T.C., Carter, R., Stevenson, R.D. (1994) Is evidence for homeopathy reproducible? *Lancet* 344 (December 10): 1601.

Richardson-Boedler, C. (1994) Patient-made blood isodes (Nosodes). *Homeopath. Int.* 8: 21.

Righetti, M. (1994) Characteristics and selected results of research on homoeopathy. In: *Ultra High Dilution* (P.C. Endler and J. Schulte, eds.) Kluwer Acad. Publ., Dordrecht, p. 223.

Riley, D. (1994) Contemporary drug provings. *Journal of the American Institute of Homeopathy*, 87, 3: 161.

Riley, D., Fischer, M., Singh, B., Haidvogl, M., Heger, M. (2001) Homeopathy and conventional medicine: An outcomes study comparing effectiveness in a primary care setting. *J. Altern. Complement. Med.* 7: 149.

Rossi, F. (1986) The O_2^- forming NADPH oxidase of the phagocytes: nature, mechanisms of activation and function. *Biochim. Biophys. Acta* 853: 65.

Rowlands, S. (1988) The interaction of living red blood cells. In: *Biological Coherence and Response to External Stimuli* (H. Frolich, ed.) Springer-Verlag, Berlin, p. 171.

Rozengurt, E. (1991) Neuropeptides as cellular growth factors: role of multiple signalling pathways. *Eur. J. Clin. Invest.* 21: 123.

Rubik, B. (1989) Report on the status of research on homoeopathy with recommendations for future research. *Brit. Hom. J.* 78: 86.

Rubik, B. (1990) Homeopathy and coherent excitation in living systems. *Berlin J. Res. Homeopathy* 1: 24.

Rubik, B. (1994) The perennial challenge of anomalies at the frontiers of science. *Brit. Hom. J.* 83:155.

Ruelle, D. (1992) *Caso e Caos.* Bollati Boringhieri, Torino (Original edition: *Hasard et Chaos.* Editions Odile Jacob, Paris, 1991)

Ruiz, G., Torres, J. L., Michel, O., and Navarro, R. (1999) Homeopathic effect on heart rate variability. *Br. Hom. J.* 88: 106.

Ruiz-Vega, G., Perez-Ordaz, L., Proa-Flores, P., Aguilar-Diaz, Y. (2000) An evaluation of Coffea cruda effect on rats. *Br. Hom. J.* 89: 122.

Sachs, A.D. (1983) Nuclear magnetic resonance spectroscopy of homoeopathic remedies. *J. Holistic Med.* 5: 172.

Sachs, L. (1986) Growth, differentiation and the reversal of malignancy. *Sci. Am.* 254 (1): 30.

Sachs, L. (1989) Cell differentiation and tumour suppression. In: *Genetic analysis of Tumour Suppression.* Wiley, Chichester. Ciba Found. Symposium 142: 217.

Sagan, L.A. (1989) On radiation, paradigms and hormesis. *Science* 245: 574.

Sainte Laudy, J., Haynes, D., Gerswin, G. (1986) Inhibition of whole blood dilutions on basophil degranulation. *Int. J. Immunother.* 2: 247.

Sainte-Laudy, J. (1987) Standardisation of basophil degranulation for pharmacological studies. *J. Immunol. Methods* 98: 279.

Sainte-Laudy, J., Sambucy, J.L., Belon, P. (1991) Biological activity of ultra low doses: I/ Effect of Ultra low doses of histamine on human basophil degranulation triggered by D. Pteronyssinus extract. In: *Ultra Low Doses* (C. Doutremepuich, ed.). Taylor & Francis, London, p. 127.

Sainte Laudy, J., Belon, P. (1993) Inhibition of human basophil activation by high dilutions of histamine. *Agents and Actions* 38: C245.

Sander, L.M. (1986) Fractal growth processes. *Nature* 322: 789.

Sander, L.M. (1987) Fractal growth. *Sci. Am.* 256 (1): 82.

Santini, R., Tessier, M., Belon, P., Pacheco, H. (1990) Incidence d'un traitement homéopathique par cuprum 4 CH sur le transit intestinal de la souris: etude preliminaire. *C.R. Soc. Biol.* 184: 55.

Savage, R.H., Roe, P.F. (1977) A double blind trial to assess the benefit of Arnica montana in acute stroke illness. *Brit. Hom. J.* 66: 207.

Savage, R.H., Roe, P.F. (1978) A further double blind trial to assess the benefit of Arnica montana in acute stroke illness. *Brit. Hom. J.* 67: 210.

Schiff, S.J., Jerger, K., Duong, D.H., Chang, T., Spano, M.L., Ditto, W.L. (1994) Controlling chaos in the brain. *Nature* 370: 615.

Schiff, M. (1995) *The Memory of Water. Homeopathy and the Battle of Ideas in the New Science.* Thorsons, London..

Schirmer, K.P., Fritz, M., Jackel, W.H. (2000) Effectiveness of Formica ufa and autologous blood injection in patients with ankylosing spondylitis: A double-blind randomized study. Z. Rheumatol. 59: 321.

Schraub, S. (2000) Unproven methods in cancer: a worldwide problem. *Support. Care Cancer* 8: 10.

Schulte, J., Endler, P.C. (1994) Preliminary elements of a theory on ultra high dilutions. In: *Ultra High Dilution* (P.C. Endler and J. Schulte, eds.). Kluwer Acad. Publ., Dordrecht, p. 245.

Schulte, J. (1999) Effects of potentization in aqueous solutions. *Br. Hom. J.* 88: 155.

Schulz, H. (1888) Uber Hefegifte. *Arch. fuer Physiol.* 42: 517.

Schwartz, G. E., Russek, L. G., Bell, I. R., and Riley, D. (2000) Plausibility of homeopathy and conventional chemical therapy: the systemic memory resonance hypothesis. *Med. Hypotheses* 54: 634.

Scofield, A.M. (1984) Experimental research in homoeopathy. A critical review (two parts). *Brit. Hom. J.* 73: 161.

Sehon, A.H. (1982) Suppression of IgE antibody response with tolerogenic conjugates of allergens and haptens. *Prog. Allergy* 32: 161.

Sekkat, C., Dornand, J., Gerber, M. (1988) Oxidative phenomena are implicated in human T-cell stimulation. *Immunology* 63: 431.

Shaya, S.Y., Smith, C.W. (1977) The effects of magnetic and radiofrequency fields on the activity of lysozyme. *Collective Phenomena* 2: 215.

Shepperd, J. (1994) Chaos theory: implications for homeopathy. *J. Am. Inst. Hom.* 87: 22.

Shinbrot, T., Grebogi, C., Ott, E., Yorke, J.A. (1993) Using small perturbations to control chaos. *Nature* 363: 411.

Shipley, M., Berry, H., Broster, G., Jenkins, M., Clover, A., Williams, J. (1983) Controlled trial of homoeopathic treatment of osteoarthritis. *Lancet* 1: 97.

Shoenfeld, Y., Isenberg, D.A. (1989) The mosaic of autoimmunity. *Immunol. Today.* 10: 123.

Simpson, J. J., Donaldson, I., and Davies, W. E. (1998) Use of homeopathy in the treatment of tinnitus. *Br. J. Audiol.* 32: 227.

Skerret, P.J. (1990) Substance P causes pain, but also heals. *Science* 249: 625.

Smilek, D.E., Wraith, D.C., Hodgkinson, S., Dwivedy, S., Steinman, L., McDevitt, H.O. (1991) A single aminoacid change in a myelin basic protein peptide confers the capacity to prevent rather than induce experimental autoimmune encephalomyelitis. *Proc. Natl. Acad. Sci. U.S.A.* 88: 9633.

Smith, R., Boericke, G.W. (1966) Modern instrumentation for the evaluation of homoeopathic drug structure. *J. Am. Inst. Hom.* 59: 263.

Smith, R.B., Boericke, G.W. (1968) Changes caused by succussion on NMR patterns and bioassay of bradykinin triacetate succussions and dilutions. *J. Am. Inst. Hom.* 61: 197.

Smith, T. (1979) A protocol for provings. *Brit. Hom. J.* 68: 172.

Smith, C.W., Choy, R., Monro, J.A. (1985) Water—friend or foe? *Lab. Pract.* 34: 29.

Smith, C.W. (1988) Electromagnetic effects in humans. In: *Biological Coherence and Response to External Stimuli* (H. Frohlich, ed.). Springer-Verlag, Berlin, p. 205.

Smith, C.W. (1989) Coherent electromagnetic fields and bio-communication. In: *Electro-magnetic Bio-Information* (Popp, F.A. *et al.*, eds.). Urban and Swarzenberg, Munchen, p. 1.

Smith, C.W. (1990) Homeopathy, structure and coherence. In: *Homeopathy in Focus*. VGM Verlag fur Ganzheitsmedizin, Essen, p. 96.

Smith, C.W. (1994) Electromagnetic and magnetic vector potential bio-information and water. In: *Ultra High Dilution* (P.C. Endler and J. Schulte, eds.). Kluwer Acad. Publ., Dordrecht, p. 187.

Smith-Sonneborn, J. (1993) The role of the "Stress Protein Response" in Hormesis. *B.E.L.L.E. Newslett.* 1(3): 4.

Smolle, J., Prause, G., and Kerl, H. (1998) A double-blind, controlled clinical trial of homeopathy and an analysis of lunar phases and postoperative outcome. *Arch. Dermatol.* 134: 1368.

Sommaruga, P. (1992) Modelli frattali di oggetti naturali. *Le Scienze (Italian edition of Sci. Am.)* 282: 36.

Sommerer, J.C., Ott, E. (1993) Particles floating on a moving fluid: a dynamically comprehensible physical fractal. *Science* 259: 335.

Southorn, P.A. (1988) Free radicals in medicine. I. Chemical nature and biologic reactions. *Mayo Clin. Proc.* 63: 381.

Speciani, A. (1991) Tolleranza a basso dosaggio. *NATOM* 6 (1): 56.

Stam, C., Bonnet, M.S., van Haselen, R.A. (2001) The efficacy and safety of a homeopathic gel in the treatment of acute low back pain: A multi-centre, randomised, double-blind comparative clinical trial. *Br. Hom. J.* 90: 21.

Stebbing, A.R.D. (1982) Hormesis: the stimulation of growth by low levels of inhibitors. *The Science of Total Environment* 22: 213.

Stillinger, F.H. (1980) Water revisited. *Science* 209: 451.

Straumsheim, P., Borchgrevink, C., Mowinckel, P., Kierulf, H., and Hafslund, O. (2000) Homeopathic treatment of migraine: A double blind, placebo controlled trial of 68 patients. *Br. Hom. J.* 89: 4.

Strogatz, S.H., Stewart, I. (1993) Coupled oscillators and biological synchronization. *Sci. Am.* 269 (3):1993

Sukul, N.C., Bala, S.K., Bhattacharyya, B. (1986) Prolonged cataleptogenic effects of potentized homoeopathic drugs. *Psychopharmacology* 89: 338.

Sukul, N.C. (1990) Increase in serotonin and dopamine metabilites in mouse hypothalamus following oral administration of Agaricus muscarius 12, a homoeopathic drug. *Science and Culture* 56: 134.

Sukul, N.C., Batuev, A.S., Sabanov, V., Kourzina, N.P. (1991) Neuronal activity in the lateral hypothalamus of the cat and the medial frontal cortex of the rat in response to homoeopathic drugs. *Indian Biologist* 23 (2): 17.

Sukul, N.C., Paul, A., Sinhababu, S.P. (1993) Hypothalamic neuronal responses of rats to homoeopathic drugs. In: *Omeomed92* (C. Bornoroni, ed.). Editrice Compositori, Bologna, p. 1.

Sukul, A., Sinhabau, S. P., and Sukul, N. C. (1999) Reduction of alcohol induced sleep time in albino mice by potentized Nux vomica prepared with 90% ethanol. *Br. Hom. J.* 88: 58.

Sukul, A., Sarkar, P., Sinhababu, S.P., Sukul, N.C. (2000) Altered solution structure of alcoholic medium of potentized Nux vomica underlies its antialcoholic effect. *Br. Hom. J.* 89: 73.

Sukul, N.C., Ghosh, S., Sinhababu, S.P., Sukul, A.J. (2001) Strychnos nux-vomica extract and its ultra-high dilution reduce voluntary ethanol intake in rats. *J. Altern. Complement. Med.* 7: 187.

Swayne, J. (1998) *Homeopathic method.* New York: Churchill Livingstone.

Taddei-Ferretti, C., Marotta, M. (editors) (1998) *High Dilution Effects on Cells and Integrated Systems.* Singapore: World Scientific.

Taylor Reilly, D. (1983) Young doctor's views on alternative medicine. *Brit. Med. J.* 287: 337.

Taylor Reilly, D., Taylor Reilly, M. (1990) Homeopathy and Placebo—A redundant hypothesis? Results from the homeopathic immunotherapy trials—the HIT project. In: *Homeopathy in Focus.* VGM (Verlag fur Ganzheitsmedizin), Essen, p. 83.

Taylor Reilly, D., Taylor Reilly, M., McSharry, C., Aitchinson, T. (1986) Is homoeopathy a placebo response? Controlled trial of homoeopathic potency, with pollen in hayfever as model. *Lancet* 2: 881.

Taylor, M. A., Reilly, D., Llewellyn-Jones, R. H., McSharry, C., and Aitchison, T. C. (2000) Randomised controlled trial of homoeopathy versus placebo in perennial allergic rhinitis with overview of four trial series. *Br. Med. J.* 321: 471.

Taylor Safrit, J., Belldegrun, A., Bonavida, B. (1993) Sensitivity of human renal cell carcinoma lines to TNF, adriamycin, and combination: Role of TNF mRNA induction in overcoming resistance. J. Urol. (Balt.) 149: 1202.

Teixeira, M. Z. (1999) Similitude in modern pharmacology. *Br. Hom. J.* 88: 112.

Teodonio M., Negro, F. (1988) *Colera, Omeopatia e Altre Storie.* Fratelli Palombi Editori, Roma.

Tetau, M. (1985) Recepteurs et homéopathie. *Cah. Biother.* 88: 29.

Tetau, M. (1989) *La Materia Medica Omeopatica Clinica e Associazioni Bioterapiche.* IPSA Editore, Palermo.

Teixeira, M. Z. (1999) Similitude in modern pharmacology. *Br. Hom. J.* 88: 112.

Teut, M. (2001) Homeopathy between vital force and self-organization. *Forsch. Komplementarmed. Klass. Naturheilkd* 8: 162.

Thiel, W., Borho, B. (1991) Die therapie von frischen, traumatischen Blutergussen der Kniegelenke (Hamartros) mit Traumeel N Injectionslosung. *Biol. Medizin* 20: 506.

Thomas, Y., Schiff, M., Belkadi, L., Jurgens, P., Kahhak, L., Benveniste, J. (2000) Activation of human neutrophils by electronically transmitted phorbol-myristate acetate. *Med. Hypotheses* 54: 33.

Thompson, E., Hicks, F. (1998) Intrathecal baclofen and homeopathy for the treatment of painful muscle spasms associated with malignant spinal cord compression. *Palliat. Med.* 12: 119.

Toper, R., Weissman, Z., Oberbaum, M., Bentwich, Z. (1990) Effects of high dilutions of antigens on the generation of specific antibodies In: *Proc. 4th GIRI Meeting*, Paris, Abs. 15.

Torres, J. L. and Ruiz, G. (1996) Stochastic resonance and the homoeopathic effect. *Br. Hom. J.* 85: 134.

Towsend, J.F., Luckey, T.D. (1960) Hormoligosis in pharmacology. *J.A.M.A.* 173: 44.

Trabucchi, M. (1992) La vecchiaia della persona. *Feder. Medica* 4: 137.

Trush, M.A., Seed, J.L., Kensler, T.W. (1985) Oxidant-dependent metabolic activation of polycyclic aromatic hydrocarbons by phorbol ester-stimulated human polymorphonuclear leukocytes: possible link between inflammation and cancer. *Proc. Natl. Acad. Sci. USA* 82: 5194.

Tsong, T.Y. (1989) Deciphering the language of cells. *Trends Biochem. Sci.* 14: 89.

Tsuei, J.J., Lam, F.M.K., Mi, Ming-Pi, Zhao, Z. (1989) Study on bioenergy in diabetes mellitus patients. *Amer. J. Acupunct.* 17: 31.

Turner, P. (1987) Homeopathic medicines and antidotes: Some controlled investigations. *Human Toxicol.* 6: 267.

Uchida, A. (1993) Biological significance of autologous tumor-killing activity and its induction therapy. *Cancer Immunol. Immunother.* 37: 75.

Ugazio, G., Koch, R.R., Rechnagel, R.O. (1972) Mechanism of protection against carbon tetrachloride by prior carbon tetrachloride administration. *Exp. Mol. Path.* 16: 281.

Ullman, D. (1991a) *Discovering Homeopathy: Medicine for the 21th Century*. North Atlantic Books, Berkeley.

Ullman, D. (1991b) The international homeopathic renaissance. *Berlin J. Res. Homeopathy* 1 (2): 118.

Ullman, D. (1996) *The Consumer's Guide to Homeopathy*. New York: Putnam.

Vakil, A.E., Vakil, V.E., Nanabhai, A.S. (1988) A study of serum electrolyte and thyroid hormone changes in iodum provers. *Brit. Hom. J.* 77: 152.

Vallance, A. K. (1998) Can biological activity be maintained at ultra-high dilution? An overview of homeopathy, evidence, and Bayesian philosophy. *J. Alt. Compl. Med.* 4: 49.

Vandvik, I.H., Hoyeraal, H.M., Fagertun, H. (1989) Chronic family difficulties and stressful life events in recent onset of juvenile arthritis. *J. Rheumatol.* 16: 1088.

van Haselen, R. A. and Fisher, P. A. (2000) A randomized controlled trial comparing topical piroxicam gel with a homeopathic gel in osteoarthritis of the knee. *Rheumatology* 39: 714-719.

van Haselen, R.A., Fisher, P. (1990) Analysing homoeopathic prescribing using the READ classification and information technology. *Brit. Hom. J.* 79: 74.

van Rossum, J.M., de Bie, J.E.G.M. (1991) Chaos and illusion. *Trends Pharm. Sci.* 12: 379.

van Wassenhoven, M. (2000) Official recognition of homeopathy in Belgium. *Br. Hom. J.* 89: 59

van Wijk, R., Wiegant, F.A.C. (1989) *Homeopathic Remedies and Pressure-induced Changes in the Galvanic Resistance of the Skin*. VSM Geneesmiddlen bv, Alkmaar (The Netherlands).

van Wijk, R., van der Molen, C. (1990) Biological effects and physical characteristics of potentiated high dilutions of sulphur. In: *Homeopathy In Focus*. VGM (Verlag fur Ganzheitsmedizin), Essen.

van Wijk, R. (1991a) Fundamental research on the effect of agitated extreme dilutions on human physiological response. *Homint Res. and Dev. Newsletters* 2 (2): 3.

van Wijk, R. (1991b) Double-blind testing of homeopathic remedies using Electro-Acupuncture (EAV) and diphenyl induced conductivity loss. *Homint Res. and Dev. Newsletters* 2 (3): 1.

van Wijk, R., Wiegant, F.A.C. (1994) Physiological effects of homoeopathic medicines in closed phials; a critical evaluation. In: *Ultra High Dilution* (P.C. Endler and J. Schulte, eds.). Kluwer Acad. Publ., Dordrecht, p. 81.

Varela, F.J., Coutinho, A. (1991) Second generation immune networks. *Immunol. Today* 12: 159.

Varmus, H. (1989) An historical overview of oncogenes. In: *Oncogenes and the molecular origins of cancer* (R.A. Weinberg, ed.). Cold Spring Harbor Lab. Press, p. 3.

Verschuuren, J.J.G.M., Graus, Y.M.F., Van Breda Vriesman,P.J.C., Tzartos, S., de Baets, M.H. (1991) In vivo effects of neonatal administration of antiidiotype antibodies on experimental autoimmune myastenia gravis. *Autoimmunity* 10: 173.

Vickers, A.J., Fisher, P., Smith, C., Wyllie, S. E., and Rees, R. (1998) Homeopathic Arnica 30x is ineffective for muscle soreness after long-distance running: A randomized, double-blind, placebo-controlled trial. *Clin. J. Pain* 14: 227.

Vickers, A. J. (1999) ABC of complementary medicine: Homoeopathy. *Br. Med. J.* 319: 1115.

Vickers, A. J. (1999) Independent replication of pre-clinical research in homeopathy: a systematic review. *Forsch. Komplementarmed.* 6: 311.

Vickers, A. J. and Smith, C. (2000) Homoeopathic Oscillococcinum for preventing and treating influenza and influenza-like syndromes. *Cochrane. Database. Syst. Rev.*, CD001957.

Vickers, A.J., van Haselen, R.A., Heger, M. (2001) Can homeopathically prepared mercury cause symptoms in healthy volunteers? A randomized., double-blind placebo-controlled trial. *J. Altern. Complement. Med.* 7: 141.

Vile, R. (1990) Tumour suppressor genes. *Brit. Med. J. (Italian edition)* 12: 25.

Vithoulkas, G. (1980) *The Science of Homeopathy.* Grove Press Inc., N. York.

Vo, T.K., Druez, C., Delzenne, N., Taper, H.S., Roberfroid, M. (1988) Analysis of antioxidant defense systems during rat hepatocarcinogenesis. *Carcinogenesis* 9: 2009.

Voll, R. (1975) Twenty years of electroacupuncture diagnosis in Germany. A progress report. *Am. J. Acupuncture* 3: 7.

Wagner, H. (1985) Neue Untersuchungen uber die immunostimulierende Wirkung einiger pflanzlicher Homöopathica. *Biologische Medizin* 2: 399.

Wagner, H., Kreher, B., Jurcic, K. (1988) In vitro stimulation of human granulocytes and lymphocytes by pico- and femtogram quantities of cytostatic agents. *Arzneimittelforschung Drug Res.* 38: 273.

Wagner, H. (1988) Studi immunologici in vitro e in vivo con farmaci vegetali a bassi dosaggi. *Riv. Ital. Omotossicol.* VI (3): 13.

Wagner, H., Kreher, B. (1989) Cytotoxic agents as immunomodulators. In: *Proceedings of 3rd Meeting of International Group on Very Low Dose Effects*. Atelier Alpha Bleue, Paris, p. 31.

Walach, H. (1993) Does a highly diluted homoeopathic drug act as a placebo in healthy volunteers? Experimental study of Belladonna 30C in double-blind crossover design—a pilot study. *J. Psychosomatic Res.* 37: 851

Walach, H., Haeusler, W., Lowes, T., Mussbach, D., Schamell, U., Springer, W., Stritzl, G., Gaus, W., and Haag, G. (1997) Classical homeopathic treatment of chronic headaches. *Cephalalgia* 17: 119.

Walach, H., van Asseldonk, T., Bourkas, P., Delinick, A., Ives, G., Karragiannopoulos, C., Van Wassenhoven, M., and Witt, C. (1999) Electric measurement of ultra-high dilutions: A blinded controlled experiment. *Brit. Hom. J.*, 87: 3.

Walach, H. (2000) Magic of signs: A non-local interpretation of homeopathy. *Br. Hom. J.* 89: 127.

Walach, H. and Guthlin, C. (2000) Effects of acupuncture and homeopathy: Prospective documentation. Interim results. *Br. Hom. J.* 89 Suppl 1: S31.

Walach, H., Koster, H., Hennig, T., Haag, G. (2001) The effects of homeopathic bella-donna 30CH in healthy volunteer: A randomized, double-blind experiment. *J. Psychosom. Res.* 50: 155.

Walach, H., Lowes, T., Mussbach, D., Schamell, U., Springer, W., Stritzl, G., Haag, G. (2001) The long-term effects of homeopathic treatment of chronic headaches: One year follow-up and single case time series analysis. *Br. Hom. J.* 90: 63.

Walleczek, J., Liburdy, R.P. (1990) Nonthermal 60-Hz sinusoidal magnetic-field exposure enhances $45Ca^{2+}$ uptake in rat thymocytes: dependence on mitogen activation. *FEBS Lett.* 271: 157.

Walleczek, J. (1992) Electromagnetic effects on cells of the immune system: the role of calcium signaling. *FASEB J.* 6: 3177.

Ware, J.A., Heistad, D.D. (1993) Platelet-endothelium interactions. *N. Engl. J. Med.* 328: 628.

Watanabe, T., Kondo, K., Oishi, M. (1991) Induction of in vitro differentiation of mouse erytroleukemia cells by genistein, an inhibitor of tyrosine protein kinases. *Cancer Res.* 51: 764.

Weaver, J.C., Astumian, R.D. (1990) The response of living cells to very weak electric fields: the thermal noise limit. *Science* 247: 459.

Weiner, H.L., Friedman, A., Miller, A., Khoury, S.J., Al-Sabbagh, A., Santos, L., Sayegh, M., Nussenblatt, R.B., Trentham, D.E., hafler, D.A. (1994) Oral tolerance: Immuno-logic mechanisms and treatment of animal and human organ-specific autoimmune dis-eases by oral administration of autoantigens. *Annu. Rev. Immunol.* 12: 809.

Weingartner, O. (1990) NMR-Features that relate to homoeopathic sulphur-potencies. *Berlin J. Res. Homeopathy* 1: 61.

Weingartner, O. (1992) *Homoopatische Potenzen.* Springer-Verlag, Berlin.

Weiser, M., Strosser, W., Klein, P. (1998) Homeopathic vs conventional treatment of ver-tigo: A randomized double-blind controlled clinical study. *Arch. Otolaryngol. Head Neck Surg.* 124: 879.

Weiser, M., Gegenheimer, L.H., Klein, P. (1999) A randomized equivalence trial compar-ing the efficacy and safety of Luffa comp.-Heel nasal spray with cromolyn sodium spray in the treatment of seasonal allergic rhinitis. *Forsch. Komplementarmed.* 6: 142.

Weisman, Z., Topper, R., Oberbaum, M., Bentwich, Z. (1991) Immunomodulation of spe-cific immune response to KLH by high dilution of antigen In: *Proc. 5th GIRI Meeting,* Paris, Abs. 19.

Weitberg, A.B., Weitzman, S.A., Destrempes, M., Latt, S.A., Stossel, T.P. (1983) Stimu-lated human phagocytes produce cytogenetic changes in cultured mammalian cells. *N. Engl. J. Med.* 308: 26.

Weitzman, S.A., Weitburg, A.B., Clark, E.P., Stossel, T.P. (1985) Phagocytes as carcino-gens: malignant transformation produced by human neutrophils. *Science* 227: 1231.

Wharton, R., Lewith, G. (1986) Complementary medicine and the general pratictioner. *Brit. Med. J.* 292: 1498.

Whitacre, C.C., Gienapp, I.E., Orosz, C.G., Bitar, D.M. (1991) Oral tolerance in experi-mental autoimmune encephalomyelitis. III. Evidence for clonal anergy. *J. Immunol.* 147: 2155.

Whiteford, M. B. (1999) Homeopathic medicine in the city of Oaxaca, Mexico: Patients' perspectives and observations. *Med. Anthropol. Q.* 13: 69.

Whitmarsh, T. E., Coleston-Shields, D. M., and Steiner, T. J. (1997) Double-blind ran-domized placebo-controlled study of homoeopathic prophylaxis of migraine. *Cephalal-gia* 17: 600.

Widakowich, J. (2000) Pharmacodynamic principles of homeopathy. *Med. Hypotheses* 54: 721.

Wiegant, F.A.C. (1994) Memory of water revisited (letter). *Nature* 370: 322.

Wiesenauer, M., Haussler, S., Gaus, W. (1983) Pollinosis-Therapie mit Galphimia glauca. *Fortschr. Med.* 101: 811.

Wiesenauer, M., Gaus, W. (1985) Double-blind trial comparing the effectiveness of the homeopathic preparation Galphimia potentisation D6, Galphimia dilution 10⁻⁶ and placebo on pollinosis. *Arzneimittelforschung Drug Res.* 35: 1745.

Wiesenauer, M., Gaus, W., Bohnacker, U., Haussler, S. (1989) Wirksamkeitsprufung von homöopatische Kombinationspräparaten bei Sinusitis. Ergebnisse einer randomisierten Doppelblindstudie unter Praxisbedingungen. *Arzneimittelforschung Drug Res.* 39: 620.

Wiesenauer, M. and Ludtke, R. (1996) A metaanalysis of the homeopahic treatment of pollinosis with Galphimia glauca. *Forsch. Komplementarmed.* 3: 230.

Wiesenfeld, K. and Moss, F. (1995) Stochastic resonance and the benefits of noise: From ice ages to crayfish and squids. *Nature* 373: 33.

Williams, L.T. (1991) Growth factors. In: *Harrison's Principles of Internal Medicine* (Wilson, J.D. *et al.*, eds.). 12th edition McGraw-Hill, New York, p. 60.

Williamson, A.V., Mackie, W.L., Crawford, W.J., Rennie, B. (1991) A study using Sepia 200c given prophylactically postpartum to prevent anoestrus problems in the dairy cow. *Brit. Hom. J.* 80: 149.

Winsa, B., Adami, H.O., Bergstrom, R., Gamstedt, A., Dahlberg, P.A., Adamson, U., Jansson, R., Karlsson, A. (1991) Stressful life events and Graves' disease. *Lancet* 338: 1475.

Winston, J. (1989) A brief history of potentizing machines. *Brit. Hom. J.* 78: 59.

Wolff, S. (1989) Are radiation-induced effects hormetic? *Science* 245: 575.

Wurmser, L., Ney, J. (1955) Mobilisation de l'arsenic fixé chez le cobaye, sous l'action de doses infinitesimales d'arseniate de sodium. *Therapie* 10: 625.

Wybran, J. (1988) Immunoregulatory agents: synthetic compounds, microbial extracts, Chinese herbs neuropeptides and intravenous immunoglobulins. *Curr. Opinion Immunol.* 1: 275.

Wynn, S.G. (1998) Studies on use of homeopathy in animals. *J. Am. Vet. Med. Assoc.* 212: 719.

Yakir, M., Kreitler, S., Brzezinski, A., Vithoulkas, G., Oberbaum, M., Bentwich, Z. (2001) Effects of homeopathic treatment in women with premenstrual syndrome: A pilot study. *Br. Hom. J.* 90: 148.

Yost, M.G., Liburdy, R.P. (1992) Time-varying and static magnetic fields act in combination to alter calcium signal transduction in the lymphocyte. *FEBS Lett.* 296: 117.

Youbicier-Simo, B.J., Boudard, F., Mekaouche, M., Bastide, M., Bayle, J.D. (1993) Effects of embrionic bursectomy and in ovo administration of highly diluted bursin on adenocorticotropic and immune responses of chickens. *Int. J. Immunother.* 9: 169.

Young, T.M. (1975) NMR studies of succussed solutions: a preliminary report. *J. Am. Inst. Hom.* 68: 8.

Zala, M. (1994) L'homoéopathie n'agit-elle que par un effet placebo? *Cah. Group Hahnemann. Doct. P. Schmidt* 31:121

Zell, J., Connert, W.D., Mau, J., Feuerstake, G. (1988) Behandlung von akuten Sprunggelenksdistorsionen. Doppelblindstudie zum Wirksamkeitsnachweis eines Homöopatischen Salbenpraparats. Fortschr. Med. 106: 96.

Zorian, E.V., Larentsova, L.I., Zorian, A.V. (1998) The use of antihomotoxic therapy in dentistry. *Stomatologiia (Mosk)* 77: 9.

Basic Research and Homeopathy
An Update

Introduction

Research in homeopathy may be divided into two main fields: *clinical* research, which tries to answer the great question: does homeopathy work (the problem of efficacy and effectiveness), and *basic* research, which tries to answer the great question of how it works (the problem of the putative action mechanisms). Existing controversy in the discipline of homeopathy strongly suggests a need to conduct further clinical trials and observational studies to establish whether reproducible therapeutic effects of homeopathic treatments can be unequivocally demonstrated.[1] At the same time, there is need for a theory or, at any rate, for viable hypotheses, to provide reasonable explanations for the effects observed.

The controversy surrounding homeopathic treatments stems in part from the seeming lack of a plausible mechanism that explains purported therapeutic effects of ultra-low-dose or high-dilution remedies. In fact, the scientific validity of a therapeutic method does not depend so much on its success rate as on the fact that the clinical results should be consistent with a pathophysiological, biochemical, and pharmacological theory or rationale. As reported by Kleijnen et al. in their seminal review on clinical trials in homeopathy, "the amount of positive evidence even among the best studies came as a surprise to us. Based on this evidence we would readily accept that homeopathy can be efficacious, if only the mechanism of action were more plausible."[2]

It is only through patient, unrestricted, and methodical research conducted on several planes—clinical, laboratory, epidemiological, and physicochemical—that we shall be able to shed light on the many issues that so far remain unsolved. Homeopathic medicine is now incorporating modern medical methods (clinical trials, statistics, computer programs in repertorization, laboratory studies, animal studies). Now several models explaining some of the claims of homeopathy are available.

There are two main theoretical tenets underlying homeopathy: the principle of *similars* and the use of high dilutions called *potencies*. The principle of similars states that patients with particular signs and symptoms can be cured if given a drug that produces similar symptoms in healthy individuals.[3] As is well known, the homeopathic tradition has developed a method of serial dilution and dynamization (i.e. dilution followed by succussion) that increases the "potency" of the drugs, and this theory has been one of the main obstacles for the acceptance of homeopathy. Moreover, other important tenets of homeopathy are linked to its "holistic" approach to health and disease (Figure 1). These three aspects of homeopathy are strictly related to each other.

Other points upon which traditional homeopathy is based include *Hering's Law* (that during the correct healing process of a given disease, symptoms disappear from the interior to the exterior of the body, from top to bottom, and starting from the last symptoms in the time sequence of appearance), the principle of homeopathic aggravation, the use of single remedies, and the discussed theory of *miasms*.[4]

These great assumptions are being investigated utilizing different experimental systems, making use of human subjects, animals, cells, or chemical solutions. The literature describing such research is rapidly growing.

One could wonder how to choose the experimental system and the level of investigation. In scientific research the level of choice, and as a consequence, the possibility of obtaining relevant results, is dictated by personal interest, technical feasibility, previous experience and, finally, by fortuitous factors.

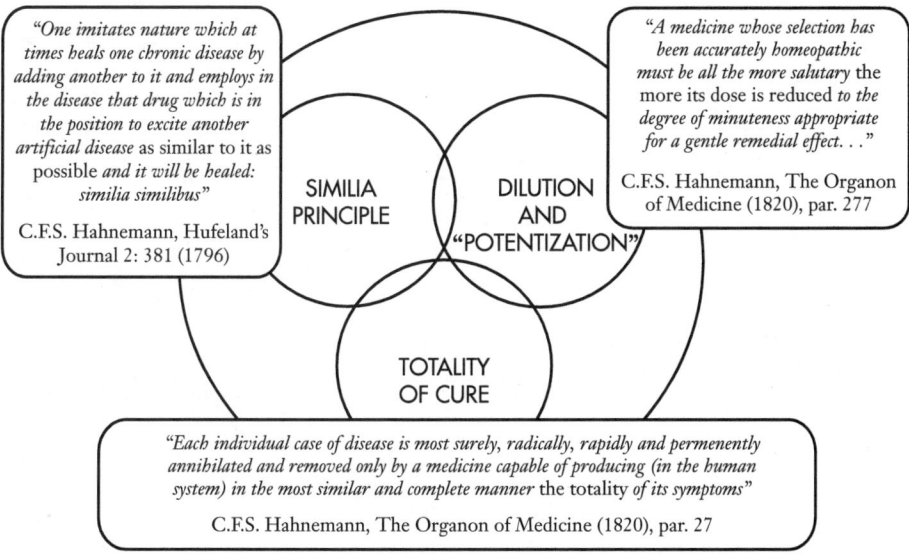

"One imitates nature which at times heals one chronic disease by adding another to it and employs in the disease that drug which is in the position to excite another artificial disease as similar to it as possible *and it will be healed: similia similibus*"

C.F.S. Hahnemann, Hufeland's Journal 2: 381 (1796)

SIMILIA PRINCIPLE

DILUTION AND "POTENTIZATION"

"A medicine whose selection has been accurately homeopathic must be all the more salutary the more its dose is reduced *to the degree of minuteness appropriate for a gentle remedial effect...*"

C.F.S. Hahnemann, The Organon of Medicine (1820), par. 277

TOTALITY OF CURE

"Each individual case of disease is most surely, radically, rapidly and permanently annihilated and removed only by a medicine capable of producing (in the human system) in the most similar and complete manner the totality of its symptoms"

C.F.S. Hahnemann, The Organon of Medicine (1820), par. 27

FIGURE 1 The Major Tenets of Homeopathy

"Conventional" basic research in a number of fields of modern biomedical science may be of interest to homeopathic doctors because studies in those fields may provide important evidence for the clarification of one of more of the above-mentioned tenets of homeopathy. In other words, basic research relevant to homeopathy cannot be defined as "homeopathic research," because scientific research has a wider aim than strict medical definition. Homeopathy is a clinical method, a method of cure and of selection of drugs. The study and understanding of its putative action mechanism(s) is neither homeopathic nor allopathic; it is part of the actual development of biomedical science.

In current scientific literature a substantial body of evidence and examples may be extrapolated to topics such as the principle of similarity or the problem of microdose effects, not because homeopathic issues were formulated as a starting hypothesis or discussed as a possible corollary, but because these studies can document and clarify a number of specific aspects of the biochemical regulatory mechanisms that may underlie the observed paradoxical homeopathic phenomena (Figure 2).

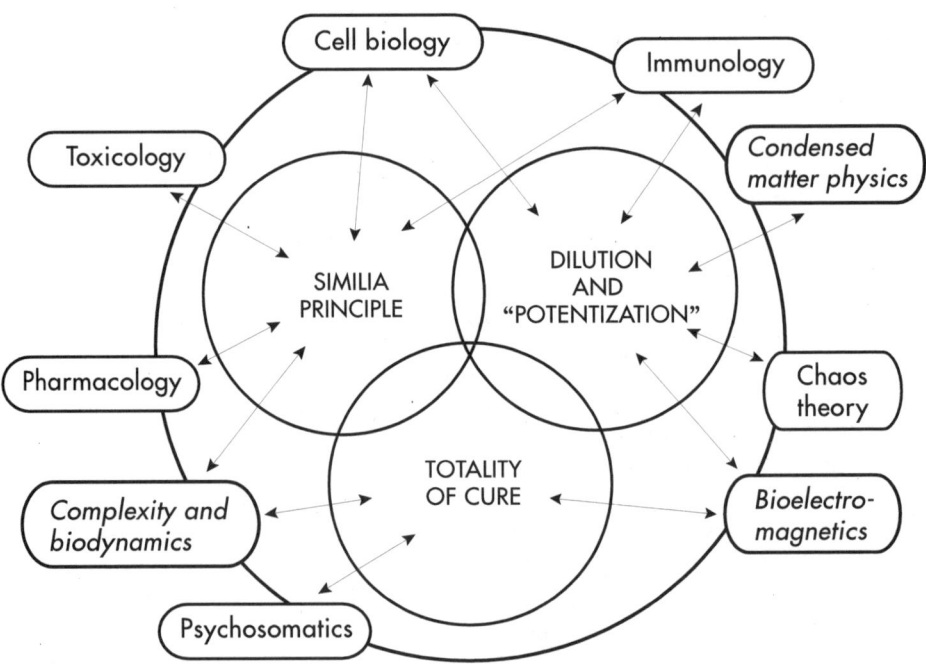

FIGURE 2 Science Fields Involved in Basic Research on Homeopathy

The problems raised by homeopathy are very wide and complex, so no single experiment can clarify everything. We don't have a "theory of everything." Instead, the discipline of homeopathy is being assembled like a puzzle or a mosaic whose pieces are progressively being laid in the right places, and where all the little pieces are important for the realization of the whole image.

It is also important to underline the fact that the scientific puzzle represented by homeopathic claims is now becoming a trigger for the research in these fields. For example, studies sponsored by homeopathic drug companies with the aim of understanding the mechanisms of the *simile* effect, have produced results that have general interest in the fields of immunology, toxicology, and cardiovascular pharmacology.

Before entering into details of some specific experiments, here is a summary of our working hypothesis on the action mechanism of homeopathy. This hypothesis has four main parts:

- Homeopathic medicines may have either chemical (ultra-low-dose) or physical (high-dilution) nature, or both.
- Medicine chosen according to the simile principle may be perceived as harmful by specific biological systems that play a crucial role in the dynamics of the disease.
- Specificity of information may be based on the sensitization of the receiver, on the complexity of the remedy picture, and on the low-dose or high-dilution of the medicine.
- The reaction of the body to the specific "harmful" information may shift the global disequilibrium of the ill person toward a new attractor that is proximal to the health state.

Another important preliminary point is the distinction between very-low dose and high-dilution effects. Both fields fully belong to homeopathy, provided that the medicine is prescribed according to the similia principle and according to a holistic clinical approach. From a scientific standpoint, the mechanism(s) underlying the *similia law* and the effect of microdoses of drugs can be investigated and understood independently of the so-called "high-dilution" or "high-potency" effect.[5] The similia principle is the foundational principle of homeopathy and the *conditio-sine-qua-non* of its definition. Hahnemann originated this system by utilizing low doses of drugs that were available at his time. The principle of *dynamization* or *potentization*, was established in subsequent years, after a number of experimental trials. Moreover, even now the major portion of the market of homeopathic medicines in Europe is represented by medicines containing ponderal doses of active principles.

Here we focus on the similia principle and on the problem of doses, while in Appendix 2 we deal with the problem of the holistic conception of homeopathy.

Similia principle

The similia principle is the basis of homeopathic medicine. It can be formulated as follows:
- Every biologically active substance (drug or remedy) produces characteristic symptoms in healthy bodies which are susceptible to being in some way perturbed by that substance.
- Every sick body expresses a series of characteristic symptoms which are typical of the pathological alteration of that particular subject.
- The healing of a sick body may be obtained by targeted administration of the drug which produces a similar symptom picture in healthy bodies.

The old principle of similarity was formulated as a general "law" on the basis of empirical evidence and analogical reasoning, but this kind of formulation does not allow any progress in the search of the possible mechanism of the alleged therapeutic effects.

Early attempts to empirically investigate the principle of similarity can be traced back to the years around the end of the nineteenth century, when H. Schulz published a series of papers that examined the activity of various kinds of poisons (iodine, bromine, mercuric chloride, arsenious acid, etc.) on yeast, showing that almost all these agents have a slightly stimulatory effect on the yeast metabolism when given in low doses.[6] He then came into contact with the psychiatrist R. Arndt, and together they developed a principle that later became known as the *Arndt-Schulz law*, stating that weak stimuli slightly accelerate vital activity, medium strong stimuli raise it, strong ones suppress it and very strong ones arrest it.[7] Similar observations were reported by several other authors in the 1920s, and from their findings one can conclude that the phenomenon of inverse, or biphasic effects of different doses of the same substance was well known before the era of molecular medicine.[8]

Hormesis

The occurrence of dual effects (both stimulatory and inhibitory) caused by the same agent when used at different doses or for different times has been described in various experimental systems and has been often called *hormoligosis*, or *hormesis*.[9] In 1960 Townsend and Luckey surveyed the field of classic medical pharmacology for examples of hormetic effects and published a wide list of substances known to be capable of causing an inhibition at high concentrations and stimulation at low concentrations.[10] In general, such cases fell into three categories: those involving muscular response, those involving respiration, and those involving transmission of nerve impulses.

Whole-body exposure to low-dose ionizing radiation appears to decrease overall cancer incidence. The data come from at least eight large studies of populations exposed to various forms of radioactive material and from more limited studies of occupational and environmental exposures to plutonium, radium, and radon.[11] Earlier experiments with animals strongly support the protective effect that apparently exists in humans. The combined evidence points to the presence of *no-adverse-effect* thresholds and of hormesis, or beneficial effects, at doses below those thresholds.

In general, these hormetic effects can be documented by a *reverse-u dose-response plot* or even more complex *dose-response curves*. Another possibility is to find a time-course of an intoxication experiment where a high dose causes progressive death of a biological system, a low or intermediate dose causes first a decrease of viability, followed by a recovery and an increase over the basal levels. Rather than being an exception, non-linearity between dose and response are the rule in biological systems. It might even be anticipated that at some doses a response opposite to that seen at high doses could be elicited. Such nonlinearity with dose has multiple implications for numerous aspects of biomedical research on aging and for experimental design.[12]

Despite the substantial development and publication of highly reproducible toxicological data, the concept of hormetic dose-response relationships was never integrated into the mainstream of toxicological thought. Review of the historical foundations of the interpretation of the bioassay and assessment of competitive theories of dose-response relationships lead to the conclusion that multiple factors contributed to the marginalization of hormesis during the middle and subsequent decades of the twentieth century. These factors include the following:

- The close association of hormesis with homeopathy led to the hostility of modern medicine toward homeopathy, thereby creating a guilt-by-association framework and the carryover influence of that hostility in the judgments of medically-based pharmacologists/toxicologists toward hormesis.
- The emphasis of high-dose effects of drugs linked with a lack of appreciation of the significance of the implications of low-dose effects.

- The lack of an evolutionary-based mechanism(s) to account for hormetic effects.[13]

Hormetic effects, which have undoubted importance for the understanding of the similia principle, have been investigated using a number of experimental systems, a few of which are described below.

Laboratory models

The similia principle has been investigated making use of a number of laboratory models. The most important data have been collected using models based on the activation of human basophils, lymphocytes, fibroblasts, renal cells, granulocytes, and vegetable cells.

- The study of basophils has been important mainly for the evidence of high-dilution effects and for the evidence of anti-inflammatory action of histamine.
- Lymphocytes have been used to show the effect of very low doses of interferons and of homeopathic drugs like *Phytolacca*.
- Fibroblasts and renal cells have been used to show the protective effect of very low doses of toxicant on the cellular toxicity exerted by high doses of the same stimulants.
- Granulocytes and platelets have been used for testing homeopathic drugs *in vitro* and for testing the mechanisms of inverse effects from a biological standpoint.

A review of the literature is beyond the scope of this appendix, so we refer here to only a few representative studies and to some of our recent results. More detailed accounts have been reported elsewhere.[14]

In synthesis:

- Dozens of papers report stimulatory or inhibitory effects of homeopathic drugs *in vitro*.
- Most effects on cell systems have been obtained using low doses or very low doses.
- A few groups have reported effects using high dilutions (we mean beyond Avogadro's number), but these effects have not been reproduced by all laboratories.
- The homeopathic similia principle can be found to be operative also at cellular and molecular level.
- Conventional biochemistry, immunology, and cell biology are providing further support for the effect of very low doses.
- Bioelectromagnetics and dynamic systems theory are getting new insights into biological information and communication.

So we are at a good point, but there are also many aspects of the principle that wait for clarification.

An important series of experiments conducted by French groups has shown that very low doses of histamine and of an extract of honeybee (*Apis mellifica*) significantly inhibit basophil degranulation induced by various stimulants.[15] It is worth noting that when delivered to tissue at normal dosages both histamine and honeybee venom have powerful pro-inflammatory irritant properties. Therefore, these experiments clearly illustrate the application of the principle of similarity in an experimental model: a substance that is known to stimulate inflammation at conventional doses is able to inhibit the cell responsible for many phenomena of the acute inflammatory process.

We have developed various models where the functional responses of human blood neutrophils are manipulated *in vitro* in order to express typical inversions of responses on varying the doses of the compounds.

Our first series of experiments in this field was carried out at the beginning of the 1990s. We tested the effects of a large series of compounds at various dilutions on superoxide anion (O_2^-) on blood neutrophils and their adhesion to serum-coated plastic surfaces. This study required a large experimental effort that was sustained in past years by our group and mainly by Dr. Chirumbolo. The data have been published in *The British Homeopathic Journal* in 1993.[16] Superoxide was significantly inhibited by *Manganum phosphoricum* D6 and D8 (33.1 ± 7.35 % and 39.2 ± 5.3 % inhibition of the activity, respectively), and *Magnesium phosphoricum* D6 and D8 (28.3 ± 16.5 % and 30.5 ± 7.4 % inhibition). *Acidum malicum* D4 (53.8 ± 25.8 % stimulation), *Acidum fumaricum* D4 (53.7 ± 33 % stimulation), *Acidum citricum* D3 and D4 (92.0 ± 10.2 % and 9.5 ± 9 % inhibition) stimulated cell metabolism. These effects were highly reproducible in separate experiments. Adhesion function was not modified by any of the tested compounds, suggesting a specificity of the effects on cell metabolism. In the course of the various experiments, *Phosphorus* and *Magnesia phosphorica* often presented inhibitory effects, even at very high dilutions (greater than D15). In five separate experiments done with leukocytes from five different blood donors, we observed the inhibitory effects of certain ultra-high dilution of phosphorus, having done all the right controls to exclude artifacts, but these effects did not always appear at the same dilutions, thus making any statistical assessment of the phenomenon a difficult matter.

In a further series of experiments we found another interesting phenomenon of inversion of effects in the response of human neutrophils to bacterial products. Results showed that pretreatment of neutrophils with low doses of the bacterial peptide fMLP increases their functional responsiveness to high doses (a phenomenon that we called *homologous priming*), while the pretreatment with high doses of fMLP decreases their responsiveness to a second treatment with high doses (a typical example of stress-induced receptor down-regulation or *receptor desensitization*).[17] A second finding regarding the granulocyte behavior under specific conditions of stimulation was that high doses of fMLP induce a marked *increase* of cell adhesion to serum-coated plastic surfaces; on the other hand, after pretreatment of neutrophils with the bacterial endotoxin (LPS), in these conditions a low dose of fMLP *inhibits and reverses* the LPS-induced adhesion.[18]

The phenomenon of inversion of effect, according to the precedent state of the cell, was found not only using LPS-treated cells, but also using inflammatory cells, i.e. cells that were harvested from an experimental inflammatory skin exudate.[19] We harvested human neutrophils from inflammatory exudates of skin. We observed that these cells have a tendency to adhere to serum protein-coated culture tubes. Addition of high doses of the peptide fMLP causes a marked *increase* of cell adhesion to serum-coated plastic surfaces; on the other hand, in these conditions a low dose of fMLP *inhibits and reverses* adhesion.

In brief, the chemotactic agent fMLP, which is considered to be an activator of neutrophil adhesion, paradoxically inhibits the same cell response at low doses when used in preactivated cells. We also investigated the mechanism of this phenomenon and found that low doses of fMLP stimulate an increase in cyclic AMP (cAMP) and that addition of cAMP plus theophylline to the LPS-treated neutrophils inhibits the adhesion.[20] Therefore, it is highly conceivable that the phenomenon of inversion of effect in our model system, that is the inhibition of cell adhesion caused by low doses of fMLP, is due to the increase in cAMP triggered by low doses of the cell agonist.

Low potencies of a homeopathic drug extract (*podophyllum*) have specific stimulating effects on the activation of neutrophil metabolism. We made various dilutions of this compound, and then we tested it on our system. Purified *podophyllotoxin* caused a stimulatory (priming effect) on the oxidative metabolism of human neutrophils, the same effect at doses of 0.1–10 µg/ml, while doses higher than 100 µg/ml of *podophyllotoxin* inhibited the respiratory burst, so that pure toxin showed a typical *biphasic* dose-response curve.[21] Low doses have an effect that is similar to the priming effect of TNF-a. Our findings demonstrate that the same toxin causes enhancement of oxidative metabolism at low doses and inhibition at high doses. The interest of this drug comes also from the fact that it is used also by conventional pharmacology at much higher doses as an inhibitor of cell proliferation and appears to be efficacious against condilomata of the skin.

(Low doses are those that are contained in the homeopathic preparation, high doses—the toxic ones—are the doses that are contained in the allopathic preparation.) Homeopathic doses cause a typical hormesis effect. We obtained similar effects using *colchicine*. Both drugs act at the level of cytoskeleton, by inducing a partial disassembly of microtubule network.

Hormesis is a special application of the similia principle at the biological and physiopathological level, but it is important to say that this kind of inverse effect does not represent the *only* explanation of homeopathic effects, which may have further and more complex implications at the level of whole human organism.

As mentioned above, in the biomedical literature there are many reports about specific compounds that exhibit dual effects (positive and negative), according to different doses employed or to different conditions of testing. For example, these paradoxical effects have been reported using prostaglandins, amyloid b-protein, oxygen free radicals, nitric oxide, neuropeptides, cytokines, insulin, acetylcholine, thrombin and many other compounds.[22] We mention these findings in order to draw attention to the complexity of these forms of regulation and to the existence of a subtle balance of opposite actions in all similar homeostatic systems composed by networks of multiple cell types and signals. This complexity is so great that some investigators have found it useful to apply mathematical models to the description of systems such as the immune network. These models have shown that effective regulation of immune disorders can be accomplished with the same antigen or the same lymphocytes that are responsible for the induction of the disease, providing that the doses or the protocols of administration are changed.

Other evidence of inversion of effects on *in vitro* models comes from testing different doses of anti-inflammatory drugs (diclofenac) on human platelets.[23]

Animal models

Several animal models have revealed nonlinear or even opposite responses to the same drugs or to immunoregulatory agents. By plotting the immune response to antigens in laboratory animals versus the doses of antigen used to pretreat the animals we find that the immune response is depressed (state of tolerance) both in animals receiving very low doses and in animals receiving high doses of antigen. Intermediate doses, however, cause a greater response.[24]

Our group at Verona University explored the applications of the similia principle using two models. The first one showed that high dilutions of histamine are able to modulate the inflammation caused by high doses of histamine in rats.[25] A second rat model was developed by our group, showing that injection of low doses of immune adjuvant (based on killed *Mycobacterium butyricum*) into the peritoneum of rats is capable of preventing and curing the arthritis induced by the injection of high doses of the same adjuvant into the paw.[26] We have also shown that protection by low-dose immune adjuvant is associated with reduction of the pro-inflammatory IL-6 cytokine, with increase of antibodies against Mycobacterium and with increase of circulating nitric oxide derivatives (a possible compensation mechanism).[27]

This is a further example of the induction of tolerance with low doses of antigens, an immunomodulation procedure that has been extensively exploited in recent years for treatment of a number of conditions in humans. We can only mention here a few examples of human therapies, which may be regarded as a special application of the similia principle at the molecular level: the use of bacterial endotoxins as immunostimulants, the treatment of immune disorders with immunoglobulins, of multiple sclerosis with oral myelin, of rheumatoid arthritis with oral collagen, of recurrent bronchitis with bacterial extracts, of allergic diseases with nasal allergens, of cancer with cancer vaccines made with tumor extract or tumor protein components, and of immune disorders with peptides binding to T-cell receptors or to HLA.[28] Most of these therapies are still at the experimental stage, but their existence confirms the increasing acceptance and use of the principle of similarity in modern medicine.

A few years ago researchers at the Harvard Medical School in Boston observed that the autoreactivity of T-cells is managed by the immune system in at least two different ways that are dependent upon the concentration of the antigen they encounter. If they come in contact with high concentrations of a self-antigen, they are deleted (killed), but when given low doses they undergo a special kind of active inhibition (called *bystander suppression*).[29] Other authors have suggested that this type of regulation induced by very low substance concentrations could serve as a model to explain the way in which at least some homeopathic pharmaceuticals mediate their therapeutic effects.[30] The use of sublingual immunotherapy is a typical field where the boundaires of homeopathy (isopathic approach) and of conventional immunology often overlap.[31]

Carrageenan oedema, a classical experimental model commonly used to test activity of anti-inflammatory drugs, was used by our group to evaluate the therapeutic activity of a low-potency mineral complex (MC).[32] The MC was administered in the right plantar surface of albino rats 60 minutes before, simultaneously, and 30 minutes after injection of carrageenan, an irritant that causes a local, transitory increase of fluid volume. The administration of the MC 60 minutes before the injection of carrageenan primed the animal to enhanced inflammatory response to the irritant. The administration of MC contemporarily to carrageenan did not modify the kinetic response and the extent of the oedema, while the administration of the MC 30 min after the induction of the oedema significantly reduced the early phase of the inflammatory reaction. This indicated that the therapeutic action of this MC is not due to conventional anti-inflammatory effect but to activation of endogenous regulatory mechanisms, a phenomenon that may be regarded as a simple application of the similia rule.

Working models of inversion of effects

The investigation of the scientific bases of the principle of similarity, at least as concerns its biological applications, may be facilitated by the formulation of working hypotheses and rational models.

For this purpose we suggest that this principle, in its fundamental meaning, may be traced back to the principle of *inversion of effects*: "biologically active compounds may cause inverse or paradoxical effects on a complex homeostatic system when either the doses of the compound, or the methods of preparation and of administering, or the sensitivity of the target system are changed."

Such an expression of the principle of similarity can be used as an operative definition of an extensive series of biological phenomena ranging from the cellular to the clinical level, the common basis of which may be the versatile adaptability of living systems to external stresses.

This means that a compound (or a treatment) that—according to current knowledge—is considered an inhibitor works as a stimulant, or, the other way around, a stimulant causes inhibitory effects.

Inverse effects that are the biological basis of the homeopathic effect can have various explanations and can be due to various mechanisms, such as the following:

- various receptors (different affinity and different coupling with effectors);
- gating theory (signal transduction);
- heat shock proteins (stress proteins, chaperonins);
- oral tolerance;
- stimulation of counter-regulation at central nervous system level;
- regulation of gene expression;
- regulation of stressed homeostatic networks.

In order to find some explanation of the involved mechanism, we focused on signal transduction and developed a working model that we called *gating theory* , analogous to the role of gating by cyclic AMP in signal transduction pathways.[33] The concept of gating means that in the sequence of signal transmission inside the cell, some signals have a controlling function—gating—that may enhance or block other signals. A gating pathway can positively or negatively regulate information flow through the transmittal pathway and may be activated by intracellular or extracellular signals.

We wanted to find an explanation for inverse effects on adhesion. We tried to find an explanation for how is it possible that a well-known stimulant of adhesion (the bacterial peptide fMLP) becomes an inhibitor of adhesion of LPS-treated cells.

The main assumptions of the model are the following:

- In normal neutrophils, low doses of fMLP induce an increase of cAMP, but not of cell adhesion.
- High doses induce also increase of adhesion.
- The activation mechanism of adhesion by fMLP requires signal transduction pathways different from those necessary for cAMP. In particular, it has been shown that high doses of fMLP induce a rapid and massive activation of phospholipid breakdown, which is a suitable signal for triggering adhesion and oxidative metabolism.
- The increase of cAMP is a signal functionally opposite to that of a high-dose fMLP signal, thus forming a kind of homeostatic balance, a kind of "brake" that prevents a harmful overactivation.

When we use neutrophils that have been previously in contact with LPS, we are in this situation:

- In the absence of fMLP, LPS induces a significant adhesion without increase of cAMP, and low doses of fMLP stimulate cAMP and inhibit adhesion by means of the gating mechanism.
- When high doses of fMLP are used, this inhibition is bypassed and adhesion increases.

Let us draw an analogy using the similia principle. LPS-treated cells represent the "disease" of the leukocyte *in vitro* system, assuming that bacterial LPS mimics the pathological condition. Addition of fMLP represents the therapeutic simile, because this agent causes *similar* pathological effects (adhesion) when tested at high doses in a healthy system (that is on control neutrophils) and therapeutic effects (inhibition of adhesion) when tested in a sick (LPS-treated) system. Clearly this only represents one of a number of possible explanations of apparently paradoxical phenomena that have been described in cell systems.

We were convinced of the general validity of the similia law when we observed some apparently paradoxical phenomena in neutrophils. Our experiments were not designed to investigate homeopathy, but the results drew us to conceive a synthesis between cell biology and homeopathy. Starting from the particular field that we knew so well and directly, we came to consider the general meaning of these phenomena in biological systems.

A different model, based on heat-shock proteins (HSP), has been proposed by the Dutch group of Roeland van Wijk and Fred Wiegant.[34] According to this theory, environmental stress, pathological conditions, and physiological conditions may threaten the organism through different routes (respiration, nutrition, absorption by the skin, etc.). When these toxic compounds or pathological conditions damage cells, one of the most important consequences is damage to cell proteins, which are denatured and may, for example, precipitate in anomalous form inside the cytoplasm. This kind of damage is also called *proteotoxicity*. In response to this damage caused to its proteins, the cells, all the cells, react by utilizing so-called *heat-shock proteins* (HSP). These proteins capture the denatured proteins and neutralize them before they can threaten the functioning of the overall cell metabolism. Therefore, HSP are regarded as the main system protecting the cell from the changes in protein constituents. They are, in other words, a mechanism of self-recovery. Today's knowledge of cell biology gives reasonable insight into the events at cellular level that may be considered analogous to many other processes of self-recovery

In the cytoplasm, HSP exist in a complex relationship with the heat-shock factor (HSF). When protein is utilized for the recovery process, the heat-shock factor is detached and migrates to the nucleus, where it binds to a heat-shock element that in turn activates the transcription of the gene for heat-shock proteins. We have, in a few words, a homeostatic system at the cellular level: the greater the requirement for heat-shock proteins, the greater their production by the cell.

However, a problem arises if this homeostatic system works in a condition of suboptimal response. Several conditions can lead to suboptimal cellular stress response, cell toxicity, and death: excess of toxic load, hormonal and metabolic imbalance that reduces the expression of nuclear HSP or HSF, and damage to cell protein synthetic machinery or energetic supply, with consequent suboptimal HSP synthesis. Such a condition of the cell, in which the reaction to the threat is not optimal, may be considered pathological. The cell could then be considered a "sick system" with the damage insufficiently compensated for.

Here the question is whether compensation can be increased and whether the development of resistance can be stimulated, and if so, how. Van Wijk suggests that self-recovery will be stimulated with a smaller dose of the substance responsible for disturbing the system in the first place. In practice, this author has shown that self-recovery is defined on the cellular level as supplementing the arsenal of protective proteins, stimulating resistance for the disturbing agent and temporarily stimulating proliferation in compensation for cell death.[35]

The model based on the heat-shock proteins is important because it helps us to understand how a toxic compound could become therapeutically useful and protective. In brief, a low dose of a toxic agent would act according to two possible mechanisms:

- increase of available HSP by favouring its detachment from HSF;
- increase of expression of HSP mRNA.

The gating theory proposed by us and the HSP theory proposed by van Wijk are not alternative but complementary. While the model based on gating at the level of signal transduction helps us to understand the experiments showing the inverse effects of biological compounds which are not toxic, but have regulatory properties through the action on receptors and transduction systems, this model based on HSP attempts to account for results in experiments where the investigators have used homeopathic doses of toxic compounds like arsenic, cadmium, mercury, phosphorus to protect cells,[36] plants,[37] and even laboratory animals[38] from intoxication by high doses of the same or similar toxic compounds. (However, it should be mentioned that this protection model did not work using *Plumbum metallicum* as potential protective agent against plumbum intoxication in rats.[39])

It is worth note once again that these results are not *an explanation for homeopathy*, but a demonstration of *how the homeopathic concept of similia principle can be explained in a precise experimental model*. Every model has a value, which necessarily is limited to the phenomena that it tries to explain. Probably in our experimental model of inversion of effects the production of HSP is not involved, because the effect is very rapid and does not require protein synthesis.

The following is a summary of the experimental evidence for the similia principle/inversion of effects:

- Stimulation or protection by low doses of toxic compounds (typical hormesis effect) on cell and animal models.
- Inhibition of specific cellular activities by low doses of stimulating compounds.
- Inhibition or protection of autoimmunity by low doses of antigen;
- paradoxical effects of drugs.
- Therapeutic effects of low doses/high dilutions of toxic compounds in humans (classical homeopathy).

Based on these findings, we can expect *inversion of effects* to be obtained in three fundamental ways:

- By changing the *doses* of the compound or the duration of the application of the treatment: for example, high doses or long lasting application may be inhibitory, low doses and short treatment may be stimulatory (as we will see later, also the opposite may be possible, according to the experimental systems employed).
- By applying the same dose or the same treatment to a system that may present different *states of sensitivity* or of responsiveness, the same compound may cause stimulatory, growth-promoting effects on a healthy/unperturbed, system and inhibitory, suppressing effects of the same variable when applied to a diseased/previously perturbed system.
- By administering the same compound (or two similar compounds) through different means: one way (e.g. parenteral injection) could cause activation or increased response; the other way (e.g., oral administration) could cause suppression or tolerance.

A relevant point of the model concerns the concept of *sensitivity* of the system under treatment. Modern cell biology and immunology have shown that the sensitivity of biological systems (and of individuals) to a given treatment may vary considerably according to a number of factors ranging from genetic predisposition to environmental conditioning, and to previous experience.

The problem of dilution/dynamization

Homeopathic medicines are used in very-low doses, in ultra-low doses, or even in high dilutions-dynamizations. The concept of dose is obviously related to the receiver system, so that it is impossible to establish narrow limits between these three ranges of doses. We suggest that the term *very-low-dose* may be used when the dose is low but in the range of action of natural substances on biological systems (i.e. just above the threshold dose that can be described by dose-effects plots); the term *ultra-low- dose* may be used when the dose is in the molecular range (concentrations of active principle above Avogadro's constant, that is, about 10^{-23} mol/Liter), but below the dose that is considered to be active by consensus based on most experimental systems. Evidence of the action of ultra-low doses (in the range 10^{-10} to 10^{-20} mol/liter) of substances on specific cellular and subcellular systems can be retrieved from scientific literature independently of studies on homeopathic drugs.[40]

Biological systems can achieve a high degree of sensitivity to external messages, so that they can be regulated by a few molecules. (A typical example is the response to pheromones.) The action of ultra-low-doses poses a challenge to biology because it can be seen as an "anomalous effect" to claims for the existence of amplification mechanisms of biological information. In any case, the possible action mechanism of homeopathic drugs in the potency range between first decimal (D) or centesimal (C) dilutions and 20D or 10C dilutions can be found inside the chemical-molecular paradigm. Of course, this view does not exclude the possibility that the effect of succussion during the process of homeopathic serial dilutions changes the physico-chemical structure of the medicine so that its interaction with living matter is based on further and more efficient information transfer mechanisms (for example the transfer of electric charges or protons through hydrogen bonds of water chains).[41]

As for the purported action of high-dilution/high-potency homeopathic drugs, here the problem of finding a rational and consistent explanation is much more difficult, essentially due to lack of consistent experimental data reproduced in different laboratories. There are a number of experiments showing stimulatory or inhibitory effects of highly diluted compounds[42] and showing the existence of peculiar physico-chemical states in water that are compatible with the hypothesis that structure (and information) can be stored in liquid water.[43] Moreover, these data are in agreement with quantum electrodynamic theories (QED).[44]

The basic idea of this reconsideration of QED in condensed matter, liquid and solid, is that *macroscopical* assemblies of identical *microscopic* systems, below a certain temperature (the critical temperature), and above a particular density (the critical density), behave in a way completely different from an ensemble of microscopic objects kept together by short range, electrostatic forces, as is now universally believed. The fundamental new aspect of the theory is that the interactions among the microscopical systems (atoms and molecules) are not restricted to the *nearest neighbors*, but extend over typical domains, of the size of the wavelength of the electromagnetic field that vibrates at the common frequency of the matter systems. Such *coherence domains* represent the fundamental building blocks of condensed matter, inside which matter (atoms, molecules, electrons, and nuclei) oscillates in tune (technically: *in phase*) with a macroscopic (classical) electromagnetic field, much in the same way as it happens in a familiar laser, with the fundamental difference that the coherent e.m. radiation is now trapped permanently inside the CDs, its function being to hold the system together against the wild assaults of the thermal fluctuations.[45]

In spite of these experimental and theoretical advancements, the results demonstrating the high-dilution/high-potency effect are not so consistent and reproducible as they should be for general acceptance by the scientific community.[46] The present state of knowledge does not allow definite conclusions in favor of or against the existence of specific physical states of highly diluted homeopathic remedy. Skeptics are not convinced by the available evidence. On the other hand, people with a more open-minded position are reinforced in their belief that "anomalous states" of water and "condensed matter physics" are giving to high-dilution/high potency homeopathy an increased credibility.[47] Our belief is that the phenomena described in many "high-dilution" experiments do really exist, but they are difficult to reproduce because the experiments are markedly affected by minimal technical differences and conditions, including the skill of the operator, the type of blood donors, the season and the day of the experiment, perhaps atmospheric pressure, the electromagnetic "pollution" of the laboratory, trace contaminants of the water solutions used to make the dilutions, the time left between a dilution and the subsequent, and other factors.

Homeopathy used with ultra-diluted drugs is thus a tentative approach to the bioenergetic regulation of the human body, utilizing a physical-biochemical interface due to the extreme sensitivity of biological systems to this type of regulation. The potential strength of the method consists in the fact that it attempts to achieve the maximum possible degree of *specificity* of the exogenous regulatory intervention. How can the maximum specificity of information be achieved, if we know so little about such bioenergetic systems? The answer is in the main principle of homeopathic tradition, the *law of similars*. This fundamental principle, based, as it is, essentially on the observation of *effects* (i.e. on comparison of the effects of the drug with those of the disease), is in a certain sense independent of any knowledge of the mechanism that causes the effects and thus also applies to the metamolecular level, once we have admitted the existence of the latter. Further details regarding this important point of homeopathic theory can be found in earlier sections of this book.

Homeopathy and homeostasis

The question now arises of whether the similia principle, which seems scientifically proven and which is a general law of nature, can be applied also to traditional homeopathic medicine, a method which is based essentially on *symptom similarity* as detected in human subjects.

We have not a definite answer to this point, but we would like to suggest a possible way to find the answer. Our hypothesis is based on the consideration of the complexity of physiological homeostasis.

Each living system is endowed with homeostatic systems that allow the action of a harmful agent to be counterbalanced by internal adaptation mechanisms. The concept of *homeostasis* in its essential make-up consists of a *set of anatomical, biochemical, and functional elements designed to maintain physiological variables within minimum and maximum oscillation limits.* Homeostatic systems are present at each level of biological organization: at *cell level*, (e.g. membrane transport systems, enzyme induction, heat-shock proteins, cyclic nucleotides), at *organ level* (e.g. regulation of blood flow, of numbers in cell populations, of structure and morphology), at *apparatus level* (e.g. regulation of blood pressure, thermoregulation, bowel function, sexual cycle, etc.), and at *superior function level* (e.g. mental and emotional functions, personality, character, decisions and frustrations, etc.).

All these properties may be summed up with the sophisticated *action-reaction* principle that governs homeostasis: the body (and the cell) does not simply behave passively but also actively. Reversible deviations from this norm tend to set into operation certain phenomena whose chief characteristic is reestablishment of the norm.

The concept of homeostasis, first introduced by the physiologist W.B. Cannon in 1929,[48] refers to all those activities that cooperate in the integration of all the mechanisms that allow a physiological variable to be maintained in the proper variation interval. Hundreds of years before, the principle of action and reaction was outlined by Hahnemann: "Every agent that acts upon the vitality, every medicine, deranges more or less the vital force, and causes a certain alteration in the health of the individual for a longer or a shorter period. This is termed primary action. To its action our vital force endeavors to oppose its own energy. This resistant action is a property, is indeed an automatic action of our life-preserving power, which goes by the name of secondary action or counteraction."[49]

A typical sequence of physiological mechanisms that maintain the homeostasis in the immune and endocrine system involves hypothalamic centers that are connected with higher centers and send messages to the hypophysis (corticotropin releasing hormone, CRH) and to the locus ceruleus, the main center controlling the sympathetic nervous system. The hypophysis, in turn, produces several hormones, one of which is ACTH (adrenocorticotropic hormone) that stimulates the adrenal glands to release corticosteroids. Steroid hormones have several functions. One is the suppression of production of ACTH and of CRH, thus representing a negative feedback loop with respect to its own production. Another activity of steroids is the suppression of lymphocyte proliferation and of inflammatory reactions. A similar feedback scheme is found also in the sympathetic nervous system, a system that may be activated by the hypothalamic centers and by higher centers, leading to the final production of noradrena-line, which, in turn, has inhibitory properties on white cells.

Another important pathway connects the peripheral white cells with the central nervous system, through the release of a number of specific proteins, like Interleukin-1, Interleukin-6, Tumor necrosis factor, and so on. These molecules not only serve the purpose of activating the immune system but have specific receptors at several levels of the central nervous system. They can activate the hypothalamus and thus cause various reactions including the production of CRH. This is only a small part of the neuroendocrine control of the so-called general stress response. The important thing is to focus on the multiple feedback regulatory loops that occur in these homeostatic systems.

We have said that the homeostasis is a network of molecular and nonmolecular information that is exchanged between nerve centers and endocrine glands, but one can also envisage a homeostatic network inside each tissue and each system. We have represented here a small piece of this puzzle, the piece that is being investigated regarding the relationships between the various types of inflammatory cells and immune cells.

Without entering into detail, there is a large series of both stimulatory and inhibitory cytokines that reciprocally influence the behavior of macrophages, lymphocytes, and granulocytes. It is well known that inside these cell populations there are either stimulatory (helper) cells or inhibitory (suppressor) cells. Recently, inside the helper populations, two distinct subpopulations have been described, TH1, which is involved in cellular immunity, and TH2, which is involved in humoral immunity and tends to suppress cellular immunity. These regulatory networks can be found also inside the cells, as we have discussed earlier (in connection with HSP/HSF, receptor dynamics).

Regulation of stressed homeostatic networks

Let's see what happens when a stressful stimulus is applied to such a system. To limit ourselves to the essential points, we can see that a psychosocial stress activates the neuroendocrine pathway "from above" the so-called HPA axis (hypophysis-pituitary-adrenal) and the sympathetic system, which ultimately can lead to increase of corticosteroids and decrease of inflammatory reactions. The psychosocial stress can also lead to suppression of immunity and increased susceptibility to infections. A chemical or biological stress, for example, the presence of bacterial toxins inside the tissue or inside an organ, may first activate the peripheral inflammatory reactions, and then these cells will produce cytokines, which in turn reach the central nervous system where they cause several effects, including the activation of the "response to stress" in a similar way.

In a complex system of homeostasis, using this model, it can be shown that the symptoms are produced by the increased activity of the homeostatic pathways that have been recruited by the disease process. Symptoms (headache, fever, cough, nasal discharge, skin spots, decrease of libido, anxiety, and other psychological changes) are the expression of the reaction of homeostatic systems. Even pain may be regarded as the expression of the local stimulation of sensitive nervous receptors by prostaglandins and neuropeptides, and of the complex elaboration of the signal at the central level

We have developed a model that attempts to put in more simple and general terms the structure of a typical homeostatic system and, most important, to relate it to the similia principle. This model allows prediction of the behavior of any homeostatic system. Exogenous or endogenous stressors may modify the activity of one or several systems, leading to a biphasic response.

First, there is an increased response, during which we observe that the systems that have been recruited are primed. We have represented the priming of the system as an increase of receptors that appear on the surface of the system itself. One example is a cell like a lymphocyte (that is an essential part of immune homeostasis). When a lymphocyte is stimulated by a cytokine or by a specific antigen, it is primed, or activated, and expresses on its plasma membrane an increased number of receptors for many compounds. (Of course, we are now describing a model, a general model of homeostatic systems, so we use the term "receptor" not as a precise molecular structure, but as an abstract term that means sensitivity of the system to regulation by some external signal.)

Examples of *priming* include the following:

- Cellular models (e.g. leukocytes): increase of *sensitivity* or of *response* to a second stimulus after the challenge with a first stimulus.
- Tissues (e.g. bronchial reactivity in asthmatics).
- Organs (e.g. liver induction of detoxifying enzymes after ingestion of alcohol or drugs, heart hypertrophy after repeated exercise).
- General systems (e.g. immune hypersensitivity after challenge with antigens).

The second phase of the homeostatic reaction to a stressful stimulus is represented by a decrease of response, mainly due to *desensitization*. The desensitization of a system to a specific stimulant is initially selective for that stimulant (*homologous*) while the system may remain responsive and usually is *primed* to different stimulants acting through different receptors.

The appreciation of this general biologic mechanism—confirmed in a number of experiments in our and other laboratories—is very important in order to understand the physiopathological basis of the similia principle.[50]

During the phase of desensitization the system undergoes pathologic adaptation and chronicization. As a consequence, the disease continues to be maintained due to the lack of response of one or more homeostatic systems. The important thing to note is that maintaining the disorder can continue even if the original stressor is no longer present. This may occur because the network of many interrelated homeostatic systems can be set in several different schemes of behavior (patterns), that correspond, roughly speaking, to different *dynamic attractors*. The system can be set to an attractor, "learn" and consolidate this "pathological behavior," and thus be unable to find the "right way" to change towards the healthy, primary behavior.

A typical example of loss of homeostasis is the resistance to steroids and the central resistance to cytokines that may be an important pathogenetic mechanism in conditions like AIDS,[51] allergy,[52] melancholic depression,[53] and aging.[54] AIDS patients with hypercortisolism and clinical features of peripheral resistance to glucocorticoids are characterized by abnormal glucocorticoid receptors in their lymphocytes, and resistance to glucocorticoids implies a complex change in immune-endocrine function, which may be important in the course of immunodeficiency syndrome.

Any "loss of communication" in the homeostatic systems is deleterious (meaning truly pathological) because the disorder of the homeostatic systems is maintained and can not recover spontaneously.

Possible mechanisms of the loss of communication in the homeostatic systems include the following:

- Homologous desensitization.
- Loss/inactivation of signal molecules.
- Auto-antibodies to receptors.
- Inhibitory effects of bacterial toxins.
- Chemical toxins: food, pollution, drugs, smoking.
- Endogenous toxins: free radicals, complement factors, etc. ("homotoxins").
- Connective tissue sclerosis.
- Deposition and "impregnation": cholesterol, amyloid, glycogen.
- Anomalous gene expression: oncogene activation and anti-oncogene deletion, viruses.

Coming back to our general model, the question is how to stimulate the recovery of the homeostatic communication when there is a block of normal response to the stressor and the system falls under erroneous adaptation. Here it is important to point out that desensitization of a system to a specific stimulant is initially selective (that is specific) for that stimulant (homologous), while the system may remain responsive and usually is primed to different stimulants acting through different receptors. Most biological systems (cells, tissues, organs,, and so on) have a number of different receptor sensitivities that are capable of triggering the same effector and regulating responses. The extent of expression of these sensitivities varies over time and according to the "experience" of the system itself. So it should be possible, at least in theory, to bypass homologous desensitization and utilize other sensitivities of the same system to push the homeostatic balance in the right direction.

From this perspective, the most suitable regulatory drug is the drug that is capable of directing the recovery of homeostatic equilibrium through *the stimulation of primed sensitivities* of the regulatory systems. This drug may be a specific molecule if we know precisely the level of the disorder, i.e. the specific receptor that should be stimulated (for example, a cytokine or a neurotrasmitter receptor). However, when the loss of homeostasis is due to multiple factors and to subtle causes, it is often hard to identify the specific biochemical blocks and the specific molecules to be supplied. If we deal with blood glucose concentration, we need only few hormones to keep it under control, but if we deal with complex changes and adaptation mechanisms occurring at different levels of homeostatic networks, it is very difficult to find the right stimulant or the right inhibitor for the involved systems. Moreover, the effect of a specific drug on the whole organism cannot always be predicted on the basis of the knowledge of simple models, because the same drug may sometimes have opposite effects according to the dose and the sensitivity of the patient, or may have a number of adverse effects. (These are typical problems of cytokines.)

"The more we learn, the less certain we are."[55]. In a few words: often the doctor doesn't know what to put in this syringe, doesn't know which type of cytokine could be useful to his particular patient in that particular moment of the evolution of its disease.

When the pathogenesis of the disease involves a fine balance of different regulatory systems at the neuroendocrine level, it is very difficult to apply a single or a few drugs using a molecular approach. This is the case in the most widespread diseases in Western countries. For example, it has been recently shown that the tendency to suppress emotional distress ("type-D personality") is a significant predictor of long-term mortality in patients with coronary heart disease, independently of established biomedical risk factors.[56] That means that among people with the same cholesterol levels, the same blood pressure and the same smoking habits, those with a certain personality succumb to heart disease and death much more frequently.

These types of symptoms are not reducible to a single neurobiological mechanism. We know little about the biochemical differences between the different personality profiles, but we know that these have a great impact on the health of the individuals. How can we apply a correct regulatory intervention in these conditions?

Of course, one could say that personality can be cured using psychotherapy, but though this is easy to say, it is extremely difficult to perform. Most doctors don't know how to perform psychotherapy, and most patients that would probably benefit from psychotherapy don't want to go to a psychotherapist. Therefore, the search for a medical approach is necessary, and we should try to find a medicine that helps to restore homeostasis at these levels also.

All who are familiar with homeopathy know how much importance this paradigm gives to psychological factors in the pathogenesis of the disease and in the effect of the drugs.

The logic of the simile

We now are in a position to appreciate the "logic" of the similia principle proposed by homeopathy: if we don't know the primed receptors and their stimulants, there is still the possibility of reactivating the "blocked" systems by administering the specific stimulant identified through symptom similarity. The correct drug is the drug that in a healthy (and sensitive) subject stimulates some systems of the body-mind complex, thus causing the appearance of symptoms qualitatively similar to those of natural disease. In other words: we can identify the right medicine for the right systems in the diseased body-mind complex by checking the effects caused in a healthy system. If the drug produces the same or similar symptoms that are produced by the disease, that drug is the correct one, because its specific target systems are the same systems that are involved (blocked, but still exhibiting some primed sensitivities) in the disease.

After having tried several drugs on healthy systems, and after having identified a specific drug that causes that typical pattern of that specific drug, it is time to introduce into the system information that helps to recover the correct homeostasis. If the original stressing factor is no longer present, the system will find the way to reenter the previous attractor, and thus, to become finally and definitely healthy.

The two approaches—reductionistic and holistic—are not in contrast: mainstream pharmacology uses a *structural analogy*, identified as the right molecule for the right receptor or for the right target system (if they are known). Classical homeopathy uses a *functional analogy*. We call it functional because it is identified by the function that it carries out with regard to the target system, the function being to cause the appearance of symptoms in healthy people and the reinduction of homeostasis in sick people. Functional analogy can be used also if we don't know the details of receptors and of a target system into the complex network of homeostatic systems.

Mainstream pharmacology is more precise when the exact mechanism of the disease is known, and specific remedies can be administered. Homeopathy is more effective when the complexity and subtle dynamics of disease are considered. Through the latter approach, the careful analysis of symptoms and the application of the similia principle may bypass our ignorance of the details of complex biological homeostatic networks. Symptom similarity is a possible guide at ultra-complex levels, dealing with the intimate nature of information disorders in each subject. In a few words, homeopathy may be regarded as the best exploitation of homeostasis rules in complex systems.

Moreover, the classical homeopathic approach, based on symptom analysis, has a number of advantages:

- Symptoms are the expression of the typical reaction of individual homeostatic systems.
- Symptom appearance is very sensitive and is often the earliest manifestation of a homeostatic disorder.
- Symptoms language is psychosomatic and complex by nature. It can be used also as a symbolic language of the body.
- Symptoms analysis is very cheap.

So we can say that this complexity makes working with symptoms advantageous—because it allows the understanding of the true language of complex systems—but, at the same time, is the reason for the difficulty of homeopathy to be accepted as a practical therapeutic method. It is difficult because symptom language is complex.

Hahnemann wrote: "The great, the sole therapeutic law of nature: cure by symptom similarity!" and found an empirical method of cure that was considered by many doctors and patients to be highly effective.[57] Two hundred years later, using a scientific standpoint we could say that the claim of this method as the "sole therapeutic law" is not true. As a matter of fact many years after Hahnemann, the scientific, experimental medicine discovered many effective drugs that have been employed with success to diseases according to different "therapeutic laws" (for example, antibiotics, anti-cancer drugs, insulin, anti-inflammatory agents). These new discoveries led to the erroneous belief that homeopathy was no longer necessary and without scientific bases. However, only a few decades after the discovery of these new drugs, we have found that they do not cure all diseases and have serious adverse effects. At this point the claim that symptom similarity could be a good therapeutical approach to many diseases shows its potential usefulness in a new, more rational light. From this standpoint, homeopathy may again be at the frontier of medical science.

References to Appendix 1

1. Cucherat, M, Haugh, M.C., Gooch, M, Boissel, J.P. (2000). Evidence of clinical efficacy of homeopathy: A meta-analysis of clinical trials. HMRAG. Homeopathic Medicines Research Advisory Group. *Eur. J Clin. Pharmacol.* 56: 27–33.

2. Kleijnen, J, Knipschild, P, ter Riet, G. (1991). Clinical trials of homeopathy. *BMJ* 302: 316–323.

3. Hahnemann, C.F.S. (1796). Essay on a new principle for ascertaining the curative powers of drugs, and some examinations of the previous principles. *Hufeland's Journal* 2: 391–439.

4. Guajardo G, Bellavite P, Wynn S, Searcy R, Fernandez R, Kayne S. (1999). Homeopathic terminology: A consensus quest. *Br. Homeopath. J.* 88: 135–141.

5. Bellavite, P, Andrioli, G, Lussignoli, S, Signorini, A, Ortolani, R, Conforti, A. (1997). Scientific reappraisal of the "Principle of Similarity." *Med. Hypoth.* 49: 203–212.

6. Schulz, H. (1877). Uber die Theorie der Arzneimittelwirkung. *Virchow's Archiv.* 108: 423–434; Schulz, H. (1888). Uber Hefegifte. *Arch. Fuer Physiol.* 42: 517–541.

7. Martius, F. (1923). Das Arndt-Schulz Grundgesetz. *Muench. Med. Wschr.* 70: 1005–1006.

8. Boyd, L.J. (1936). *A Study of the Simile in Medicine.* Philadelphia: Boericke and Tafel; Oberbaum, M, Cambar, J. (1994). Hormesis: dose-dependent reverse effects of low and very low doses. In: *Ultra High Dilution* (P.C. Endler and J. Schulte, eds.). Kluwer Acad. Publ., Dordrecht, pp. 5–18.

9. Calabrese, E.J. (1999). Evidence that hormesis represents an "overcompensation" response to a disruption in homeostasis. *Ecotoxicol. Environ. Saf.* 42: 135–137 ; Olivieri, G. (1999). Adaptive response and its relationship to hormesis and low dose cancer risk estimation. *Hum. Exp. Toxicol.* 18: 440–442; Calabrese, E.J., Baldwin, L.A. (1998). Hormesis as a biological hypothesis. *Environ. Health Perspect.* 106 Suppl. 1: 357–362 ; Renn, O. (1998). Implications of the hormesis hypothesis for risk perception and communication. *Hum. Exp. Toxicol.* 17: 431–438; Stebbing, A.R.D. (1998). A theory for growth hormesis. *Mutat. Res.* 403: 249–258; Luckey, T.D. (1997). Radiation hormesis. In: *Signals and Images* (M Bastide, ed.). Kluwer, Dordrecht, pp. 31–39; Calabrese, E.J., Baldwin, L,A. (1993). Possible examples of chemical hormesis in a previously published study. *J. Appl. Toxicol.* 13: 169–172; Von Zglinicki, T., Edwall, C., Ostlund, E., Lind, B., Nordberg, M., Ringertz, N.R., Wroblewski, J. (1992). Very low cadmium concentrations stimulate DNA synthesis cell growth. *J. Cell Sci.* 103: 1073–1081; Macklis, R.M., Beresford, B. (1991). Radiation hormesis. *J Nucl. Med.* 32: 350–359; Sagan, L.A. (1989). On radiation, paradigms and hormesis. *Science* 245: 574; Stebbing, A.R.D. (1982). Hormesis: the stimulation of growth by low levels of inhibitors. *The Science of Total Environment* 22: 213–234.

10. Townsend, J.F., Luckey, T.D. (1960). Hormoligosis in pharmacology. *J. Am. Med. Ass.* 173: 44–48.

11. Luckey, T.D. (1999). Nurture with ionizing radiation: a provocative hypothesis. *Nutr. Cancer* 34: 1–11.

12. Johnson, T.E., Brunsgaard, H. (1998). Implications of hormesis for biomedical aging research. *Hum.Exp.Toxicol.* 17: 263–265.

13. Calabrese, E.J., Baldwin, L.A. (2000). The marginalization of hormesis. *Hum. Exp. Toxicol.* 19: 32–40.

14. Linde, K., Jonas, W.B., Melchart, D., Worku, F., Wagner, H., Eitel, F. (1994). Critical review and meta-analysis of serial agitated dilutions in experimental toxicology. *Hum. Exp. Toxicol.* 13: 481–492; Bastide, M. (1994). Immunological examples on ultra high dilution research. In: *Ultra High Dilution* (P.C. Endler and J. Schulte, eds.). Kluwer Acad. Publ., Dordrecht, pp. 27–33; Bellavite, P., Lussignoli, S., Semizzi, M.L., Ortolani, R., Signorini, A. (1997). The similia principle: From cellular models to regulation of homeostasis. *Brit. Hom. J.* 86: 73–85; Eskinazi, D. (1999). Homeopathy re-revisited:

Is homeopathy compatible with biomedical observations? *Arch. Intern. Med.* 159: 1981–1987.

15. Davenas, E., Poitevin, B., Benveniste, J. (1987). Effect on mouse peritoneal macrophages of orally administered very high dilutions of silica. *Eur. J. Pharmacol.* 135: 313–319 ; Davenas, E., Beauvais, F., Amara, J., Robinson, M., Miadonna, A., Tedeschi, A., Pomeranz, B., Fortner, P., Belon, P., Sainte-Laudy, J., Poitevin, B., Benveniste, J. (1988). Human basophil degranulation triggered by very dilute antiserum against IgE. *Nature* 333: 816–818; Poitevin, B., Aubin, M., Benveniste, J. (1985). Effect d'Apis Mellifica sur la degranulation des basophiles humains in vitro. *Homéopathie Franc.* 73: 193–198 ; Belon, P., Cumps, J., Ennis, M., Mannaioni, P.F., Sainte-Laudy, J., Roberfroid, M., Wiegant, F.A.C. (1999). Inhibition of human basophil degranulation by successive histamine dilutions: Results of a European multi-centre trial. *Inflamm. Res.* 48: S17–S18; Sainte-Laudy, J., Belon, P. (1993). Inhibition of human basophil activation by high dilutions of histamine. *Inflamm. Res.* 38: C245–C247; Sainte-Laudy, J., Belon, P. (1997). Application of flow cytometry to the analysis of the immunosuppressive effect of histamine dilutions on human basophil activation: Effect of cimetidine. *Inflamm. Res.* 46: S27–S28.

16. Chirumbolo, S., Signorini, A., Bianchi, I., Lippi, G., Bellavite, P. (1993). Effects of homeopathic preparations of organic acids and of minerals on the oxidative metabolism of human neutrophils: A controlled trial. *Br. Hom. J.* 82: 227–244.

17. Bellavite, P., Chirumbolo, S., Lippi, G., Guzzo, P., Santonastaso, C. (1993). Homologous priming in chemotactic peptide-stimulated neutrophils. *Cell Biochem. Funct.* 11: 93–100.

18. Bellavite, P., Chirumbolo, S., Lippi, G., Andrioli, G., Bonazzi, L., Ferro, I. (1993). Dual effects of formylpeptides on the adhesion of endotoxin-primed human neutrophils. *Cell Biochem. Funct.* 11: 231–239.

19. Bellavite, P., Carletto, A., Biasi, D., Caramaschi, P., Poli, F., Suttora, F., Bambara, L.M. (1994). Studies of skin-window exudate human neutrophils: complex patterns of adherence to serum-coated surfaces in dependence on FMLP doses. *Inflammation* 18: 575–587.

20. Bellavite, P., Chirumbolo, S., Santonastaso, C., Biasi, D., Lussignoli, S., Andrioli, G. (1997). Dose-dependence of the various functional responses of neutrophils to formylpeptides: Activation, regulation, and inverse effects according to the agonist dose and cell condition. In: *Signals and Images* (M. Bastide, ed.). Kluwer Acad. Publ., Dordrecht, pp. 111–119.

21. Chirumbolo, S., Conforti, A., Lussignoli, S., Metelmann, H., Bellavite, P. (1997). Effects of Podophyllum peltatum compounds in various preparation's dilutions on human neutrophil functions in vitro. *Brit. Hom. J.* 86: 16–26.

22. See note 5.

23. Andrioli, G., Lussignoli, S., Gaino, S., Benoni, G., Bellavite, P. (1997). Study on paradoxical effects of NSAIDs on platelet activation. *Inflammation* 21: 519–30.

24. Weiner, H.L., Friedman, H., Miller, A., Khoury, S.J., Al Sabbagh, A., Santos, L., Sayegh, M., Nussemblatt, R.B., Trentham, D.E., Hafler, D.A. (1994). Oral tolerance: Immunologic mechanisms and treatment of animal and human organ-specific autoimmune diseases by oral administration of autoantigens. *Annu. Rev. Immunol.* 12: 809–837; Weiner, H.L. (1997). Oral tolerance: Immune mechanisms and treatment of autoimmune diseases. *Immunol. Today* 7: 336–343.

25. Conforti, A., Signorini, A., Bellavite, P. (1993). Effects of high dilutions of histamin and other natural compounds on acute inflammation in rats. In: *Omeomed92* (C. Bornoroni, ed.). Editrice Compositori, Bologna, pp. 163–169.

26. Conforti, A., Lussignoli, S., Bertani, S., Verlato, G., Ortolani, R., Bellavite, P., Andrighetto, G. (1997). Specific and long-lasting suppression of rat adjuvant arthritis by low-dose Mycobacterium butyricum. *Eur. J. Pharmacol.* 324: 241–247; Conforti, A., Bertani, S., Lussignoli, S., Bellavite, P. (1998). Pharmakodynamik und komplexe Systeme. In: *Biologische Mediczin in der Orthopedie/Traumatologie, Rheumatologie* (H. Hess,

ed.). Baden Baden: Aurelia Verlag, Baden Baden, pp. 39–52; Conforti, A., Lussignoli, S., Bertani, S., Ortolani, T., Brendolan, A., Cestari, T., Andrighetto, G., Bellavite, P. (1998). Suppression of adjuvant arthritis in rats by intraperitoneal Mycobacterium butyricum. *J. Chemother.* 10: 169–172.

27. Conforti, A., Lussignoli, S., Bertani, S., Ortolani, R., Cuzzolin, L., Benoni, G., Bellavite, P. (2001). Cytokine and nitric oxide levels in a rat model of immunologic protection from adjuvant-induced arthritis. *Int. J. Immunopathel. Pharmacol.* 14:153.

28. See Note 5.

29. See Note 24, Weiner.

30. Heine, H., Schmolz, M. (2000). Immunoregulation via "bystander suppression" needs minute amounts of substances-a basis for homeopathic therapy? *Med. Hypotheses* 54: 392–393.

31. Scadding, G.K., Brostoff, J. (1986). Low dose sublingual therapy in patients with allergic rhinitis due to house dust mite. *Clin. Allergy* 16: 483–491; MacDonald, T.T. (1994). Eating your way towards immunosuppression. *Curr. Biol.* 4: 178–181; Trentham, D.E., Dynesius-Trentham, R.A., Orav, E.J., Combitechi, D., Lorenzo, C., Sewell, K.L., Hafler, D.A., Weiner, H.L. (1993). Effects of oral administration of type II collagen on rheumatoid arthritis. *Science* 261: 1727–1730; Taylor, M.A., Reilly, D., Llewellyn-Jones, R.H., McSharry, C., Aitchison, T.C. (2000). Randomised controlled trial of homoeopathy versus placebo in perennial allergic rhinitis with overview of four trial series. *BMJ* 321: 471–476.

32. Bertani, S., Lussignoli, S., Andrioli, G., Bellavite, P., Conforti, A. (1999). Dual effects of a homeopathic mineral complex on carrageenan-induced oedema in rats. *Br. Homeopath. J.* 88: 101–105.

33. Iyengar, R. (1996). Gating by cyclic AMP: Expanded role for an old signaling pathway. *Science* 271: 461–463.

34. Van Wijk, R., Wiegant, F.A.C. (1995). Stimulation of self-recovery by similia principle. Mode of testing in fundamental research. *Br. Homeopath. J.* 84: 131–139; Van Wijk, R., Wiegant, F.A. (1997). The similia principle as a therapeutic strategy: A research program on stimulation of self-defense in disordered mammalian cells. *Altern. Ther. Health Med.* 3: 33–38; Van Wijk, R., Wiegant, F.A.C., Souren, J.E.M., Ovelgonne, J.H., van Aken, J.M., Bol, A.W.J.M. (1997). A molecular basis for understanding the benefits from subharmful doses of toxicants. *Biomed. Ther.* 15: 4–13; Wiegant, F.A.C., Van Wijk, R. (1996). Self-recovery and the similia principle: An experimental model. *Complem. Ther. Med.* 4: 90–97.

35. Ibid.

36. Delbancut, A., Dorfman, P., Cambar, J. (1993). Protective effect of very low concentrations of heavy metals cadmium and cisplatin against cytotoxic doses of these metals on renal tubular cell cultures. *Br. Homeopath. J.* 82: 123–124.

37. Betti, L., Brizzi, M., Nani, D., Peruzzi, M. (1997). Effect of high dilutions of Arsenicum album on wheat seedlings from seed poisoned with the same substance. *Br. Homeopath. J.* 86: 86–89.

38. Bildet, J., Guere, J.M., Saurel, J., Aubin, M., Demerque, D., Quilichini, R. (1975). E'tude de l'action de differentes diluitions de Phosphorus sur l'hepatite toxique du rat. *Ann Homeop. Fr.* 4: 425–432; Palmerini, C.A., Codini, M., Floridi, A., Mattoli, P., Buffetti, S., Di Leginio, E. (1993). The use of Phosphorus 30 CH in the experimental treatment of hepatic fibrosis in rats. In: *Omeomed92* (C. Bornoroni, ed.) Editrice Compositori, Bologna, pp. 219–226; Kundu, S.N., Mitra, K., Bukhsh, A.R. (2000). Efficacy of a potentized homoeopathic drug (Arsenicum-album-30) in reducing cytotoxic effects produced by arsenic trioxide in mice: III. Enzymatic changes and recovery of tissue damage in liver. *Complement Ther. Med.* 8: 76–81; Datta, S., Mallick, P., Bukhsh, A.R. (1999). Efficacy of a potentized homoeopathic drug (Arsenicum Album-30) in reducing genotoxic effects produced by arsenic trioxide in mice: Comparative studies of pre-, post-, and combined pre- and post-oral administration and comparative efficacy of two microdoses. *Complement Ther. Med.* 7: 62–75; Mitra, K., Kundu, S.N., Khuda Bukhsh,

A.R. (1999). Efficacy of a potentized homoeopathic drug (Arsenicum Album-30) in reducing toxic effects produced by arsenic trioxide in mice: II. On alterations in body weight, tissue weight and total protein. *Complement Ther. Med.* 7: 24–34; Lapp, C., Wurmser, L., Ney, J. (1955). Mobilization de l'arsenic fixé chez le cobaye sous l'influence des doses infinitésimales d'arseniate. *Thérapie* 10: 625–638 ; Cazin, J.C., Cazin, M., Gaborit, J.L., Chaoui, A., Boiron, J., Belon, P., Cherruault, Y., Papapanayotou, C. (1987). A study of the effect of decimal and centesimal dilutions of Arsenic on the retention and mobilisation of Arsenic in the rat. *Human Toxicology* 6: 315–320; Cazin, J.C., Cazin, M., Chaoui, A., Belon, P. (1991). Influence of several physical factors on the activity of ultra low doses. In: *Ultra Low Doses* (C. Doutremepuich, ed.). Taylor and Francis, London, pp. 69–80.

39. Fisher, P., House, I., Belon, P., Turner, P. (1987). The influence of the homoeopathic remedy plumbum metallicum on the excretion kinetics of lead in rats. *Hum. Toxicol.* 6: 321–324.

40. See Note 30, and Note 14 (Eskinazi).

41. Woutersen, S., Bakker, H.J. (1999). Resonant intermolecular transfer of vibrational energy in liquid water. *Nature* 402: 507–509; Weiss, P. (1999). Vibrations flit along water's fast lane. *Science News* 156: 358.

42. Cristea, A., Nicula, S., Dare, V. (1997). Pharmacodynamic effects of very high dilutions of Belladonna on the isolated rat duodenum. In: *Signals Images* (M. Bastide, ed.). Kluwer, Dordrecht, pp. 161–170; Sainte-Laudy, J., Belon, P., Sainte-Laudy, J., Belon, P. (1996). Analysis of immunosuppressive activity of serial dilutions of histamine on human basophil activation by flow cytometry. Application of flow cytometry to the analysis of the immunosuppressive effect of histamine dilutions on human basophil activation: Effect of cimetidine. *Inflamm. Res.* 45 (S1): 33–34; Youbicier-Simo, B.J., Boudard, F., Mekaouche, M., Bayle, J.D., Bastide, M. (1996). Specific abolition reversal of pituitary-adrenal activity and control of the humoral immunity in bursectomized chickens through highly dilute bursin. *Int. J. Immunopathol. Pharmacol.* 9: 43–51; Schiff, M. (1995). *The Memory of Water: Homeopathy and the Battle of Ideas in the New Science.* London: Thorsons; Bastide, M. (1994). Immunological examples on ultra high dilution research. In: *Ultra High Dilution* (P.C. Endler and J. Schulte, eds.). Kluwer Acad. Publ., Dordrecht, pp. 27–33; Davenas, E., Poitevin, B., Benveniste, J. (1987). Effect on mouse peritoneal macrophages of orally administered very high dilutions of silica. *Eur. J. Pharmacol.* 135: 313–319 ; Davenas, E., Beauvais, F., Amara, J., Robinson, M., Miadonna, A., Tedeschi, A., Pomeranz, B., Fortner, P., Belon, P., Sainte-Laudy, J., Poitevin, B., Benveniste, J. (1988). Human basophil degranulation triggered by very dilute antiserum against IgE. *Nature* 333: 816–818; Betti, L., Brizzi, M., Nani, D., Peruzzi, M. (1997). Effect of high dilutions of Arsenicum album on wheat seedlings from seed poisoned with the same substance. *Br. Homeopath. J.* 86: 86–89; Kundu, S.N., Mitra, K., Bukhsh, A.R. (2000). Efficacy of a potentized homoeopathic drug (Arsenicum-album-30) in reducing cytotoxic effects produced by arsenic trioxide in mice: III. Enzymatic changes and recovery of tissue damage in liver. *Complement Ther. Med.* 8: 76–81.

43. Litime, M.H., Aissa, J., Benveniste, J. (1993). Antigen signaling at high dilution. *FASEB J.* 7: A602; Elia, V., Niccoli, M. (1999). Thermodynamics of extremely diluted aqueous solutions. *Ann. N. Y. Acad. Sci.* 879: 241–248; Schulte, J. (1999). Effects of potentization in aqueous solutions. *Brit. Hom. J.* 88: 155–160; Benveniste, J. (1994). Further biological effects induced by ultra high dilutions: Inhibition by a magnetic field. In: *Ultra High Dilution* (P.C. Endler and J. Schulte, eds.). Kluwer Acad. Publ., Dordrecht, pp. 35–38; Schulte, J. (1994). Conservation of structure in aqueous ultra high dilutions. In *Ultra High Dilutions* (P.C. Endler and J. Schulte, eds.). Kluwer Acad. Publ., Dordrecht, pp. 105–115; Demangeat, J.L., Demangeat, C., Gries, P., Poitevin, B., Constantinesco, A. (1992). Modifications des temps de relaxation RMN a 4 MHz des protons du solvant dans les trés hautes dilutions salines de Silice/Lactose. *J. Med. Nucl. Biophy.* 16 (2): 135–145; Weingartner, O. (1992). *Homoopatische Potenzen.* Berlin-Heidelberg: Springer Verlag; Sachs A.D. (1983). Nuclear magnetic resonance spectroscopy of homoeopathic remedies. *J. Holistic Med.* 5: 172–177; Smith, R.B., Boericke, G,W. (1968). Changes caused by succussion on NMR patterns bioassay of bradykinin triacetate succussions

dilutions. *J. Amer. Inst. Hom.* 61: 197–212; Gregory, J.K., Clary, D.C., Liu, K., Brown, M.G., Saykally, R.J. (1997). The water dipole moment in water clusters. *Science* 275: 814–817; Fesenko, E.E., Gluvstein, A.Y. (1995). Changes in the state of water, induced by radiofrequency electromagnetic fields. *FEBS Lett.* 367: 53–55; Fesenko, E.E., Geletyuk, V.I., Kazachenko, V.N., Chemeris, N.K. (1995). Preliminary microwave irradiation of water solutions changes their channel-modifying activity. *FEBS Lett.* 366: 49–52; Liu, K., Brown, M.G., Carter, C., Saykally, R.J., Gregory, J.K., Clary, D.C. (1996). Characterization of a cage form of the water hexamer. *Nature* 381: 501–503; Widakowich, J. (1997). Microdose therapy: dilution versus potentiation? *Medical Hypotheses* 49: 437–441.

44. Arani, R., Bono, I., Del Giudice, E., Preparata, G. (1995). QED coherence and the thermodynamics of water. *Int. J. Mod. Phys.* B9: 1813–1841; Del Giudice, E., Preparata, G., Vitiello, G. (1988). Water as a free electric dipole laser. *Phys. Rev. Lett.* 61: 1085–1088; Preparata, G. (1995). *Quantum electrodynamic coherence in matter*. Singapore: World Scientific.

45. Preparata G. 1997. Regimi coerenti in Fisica e Biologia. Il problema della forma. Biology Forum. Rivista di Biologia / Biology Forum 90: 434–436; Del Giudice, E., Preparata, G., Vitiello, G. (1988). Water as a free electric dipole laser. *Phys. Rev. Lett.* 61: 1085–1088.

46. Walach, H., van Asseldonk, T., Bourkas, P., Delinick, A., Ives, G., Karragiannopoulos, C., Van Wassenhoven, M., Witt, C. (1999). Electric measurement of ultra-high dilutions: A blinded controlled experiment. *Brit. Hom. J.* 87: 3–12; Hirst, S.J., Hayes, N.A., Burridge, J., Pearce, F.L., Foreman, J.C. (1993). Human basophil degranulation is not triggered by very dilute antiserum against human IgE. *Nature* 366: 525–527; Maddox, J., Randi, J., Stewart, W.W. (1988). "High-dilution" experiments a delusion. *Nature* 334: 287–290; Walach, H. (2000). Magic of signs: a non-local interpretation of homeopathy. *Br. Homeopath. J* 89: 127–140.

47. Vallance, A.K. (1998). Can biological activity be maintained at ultra-high dilution? An overview of homeopathy, evidence, and Bayesian philosophy. *J. Altern. Complement Med.* 4: 49–76.

48. Cannon, W. (1935). Stresses and strains of homeostasis. *Am. J. Med. Sci.* 189: 1–14.

49. Hahnemann, C.F.S. (1994). Organon of Medicine. With Explanations by Joseph Reves, edited from the 5th and 6th edition. Homeopress Ltd., Haifa, para. 63.

50. Bellavite, P, Andrioli, G, Lussignoli, S, Signorini, A, Ortolani, R, Conforti, A. (1997). Scientific reappraisal of the "Principle of Similarity." *Med. Hypoth.* 49: 203–212; Bellavite, P., Lussignoli, S., Semizzi, M.L., Ortolani, R., Signorini, A. (1997). The similia principle: From cellular models to regulation of homeostasis. *Brit. Hom. J.* 86: 73–85; Eskinazi, D. (1999). Homeopathy re-revisited: Is homeopathy compatible with biomedical observations? *Arch. Intern. Med.* 159: 1981–1987; Bellavite, P., Chirumbolo, S., Lippi, G., Guzzo, P., Santonastaso, C. (1993). Homologous priming in chemotactic peptide-stimulated neutrophils. *Cell Biochem. Funct.* 11: 93–100; Heine, H., Schmolz, M. (2000). Immunoregulation via "bystander suppression" needs minute amounts of substances-a basis for homeopathic therapy? *Med. Hypotheses* 54: 392–393.

51. Norbiato, G., Bevilacqua, M., Vago, T., Baldi, G., Chebat, E., Bertora, P., Moroni, M., Galli, M., Oldenburg, N. (1992). Cortisol resistance in acquired immunodeficiency syndrome. *J. Clin. Endocrinol. Metab.* 74: 608–613.

52. Buske-Kirschbaum, A., Jobst, S., Psych, D., Wustmans, A., Kirschbaum, C., Rauh, W., Hellhammer, D. (1997). Attenuated free cortisol response to psychosocial stress in children with atopic dermatitis. *Psychosom.Med.* 59: 419–426.

53. Gold, P.W., Licinio, J., Wong, M., Chrousos, G.P. (1995). Corticotropin releasing hormone in the pathophysiology of melancholic and atypical depression and in the mechanism of action of antidepressand drugs. *Ann N.Y.Acad.Sci.* 771: 716–729.

54. Seeman, T.E., Robbins, R.S. (1994). Aging and hypothalamic-pituitary-adrenal response to challenge in humans. *Endocrine Rev.* 15: 233–266.

55. Cohen, J. (1993). AIDS research: The mood is uncertain. Science 260: 1254–1261.

56. Denollet, J., Sys, S.U., Stroobant, N., Rombouts, H., Gillebert, T.C., Brutsaert, D.L. (1996). Personality as independent predictor of long-term mortality in patients with coronary heart disease. *Lancet* 347: 417–421.

57. Hahnemann, C.F.S. (1994). Organon of Medicine. With Explanations by Joseph Reves, edited from the 5th and 6th edition. Homeopress Ltd., Haifa, para. 50.

Science and Homeopathy: From "Life Force" to Biodynamics and Biophysics

Introduction

Homeopathy raises a number of puzzles for the scientific investigator. Both clinical and basic research investigate homeopathic phenomena (effects of ultra-low-doses or high dilutions and phenomena related to the *similia principle*).

We have seen that in last ten years a number of studies have been done on cells and on animals, with findings that suggest that homeopathic drugs have specific biologic effects in different experimental models. Homeopathic principles and notably the *principle of similars* can be reevaluated in the light of modern biological, biophysical, and immunological knowledge. However, a complete theory of how homeopathic drugs may function in the body is still lacking. As a matter of fact, accumulating evidence of the consistent effects of homeopathic medicines on cells and on animals and humans is not sufficient to explain how this therapy works.

The reason for this gap in knowledge about the action mechanism of homeopathic medicines may be that the ultra-low-dose phenomena and the similia law cannot be fully understood by utilizing the reductionistic approach that is utilized for conventional, high-dose drugs. Experiments carried out on specific and small-scale models can explain and demonstrate the validity only of specific and small-scale hypotheses.

A rational approach to explaining the action mechanism of homeopathy should take into consideration three major aspects:
- the similia principle;
- the problem of dilution and dynamization of drugs;
- the homeopathic theory of health and healing.

These three aspects can be considered separately—especially from an experimental scientific standpoint—but they are strictly interrelated. A realistic interpretation of homeopathy reconciles the *integrated* view, which considers the complexity of the human being in all his or her components, with the *reductionist* view, which considers the single organ, cell, or molecular mechanism. In fact, there cannot be a contrast between the whole and the fragment that this whole contains, and therefore various medical approaches should be utilized according to which level of integration and which physiopathological mechanism(s) is the object of treatment.

Since homeopathy is a holistic approach, taking into consideration all the levels of organization of the body, in order to fully understand its possible action mechanism we need a shift of paradigm from reductionistic to complex approaches. This is not a denial of the importance of reductionism and of exact, Galileian science, but is a step further, enabling us place simple evidence into a wider, more global context. This vision of biology (and consequently of pathology) emerging from the front lines of modern science, will help apparently paradoxical phenomena claimed by homeopathy to be seen in a new light.

The "vital force"

Healing is a fact of everyday life: we heal from a wound, from influenza, from abscesses, from a common cold. Thanks to sophisticated biological systems, after most injuries, the state of health is restored spontaneously or with little medical help. This singular healing power of living beings led ancient medical investigators to conceive the existence in the body of something like a mysterious *vital force* that is ultimately responsible for subtle and unknowable biological mechanisms that regulate all the internal processes of the body and its reactions to external stresses.

According to Chinese tradition, the proper and dynamic balance of the vital force (referred to as *ch'i*) is responsible for the maintenance of health; the loss or derangement of the same force is associated with most diseases (*yin-yang* imbalance). One of the fathers of the Western medicine, Hippocrates (460–377 B.C.), called this healing principle *vis medicalis naturae* (healing force of nature) and advised doctors to take great care not to disturb it with inappropriate treatments. In fact, he used to recommend *primum non nocere* (most important, do no harm).

Hahnemann, the founder of homeopathy, adopted a markedly vitalistic standpoint: that the fundamental factor in a human being's state of health is the vital force and any disturbance of this dynamic inner principle is responsible for onset of disease, just as, conversely, the "restitutio ad integrum of the vital force necessarily presupposes the return to health of the entire organism."[1]

Paragraphs 29–31 of the *Organon* clearly define what Hahnemann meant by disease, i.e. "every disease (not entirely surgical) consists only in a special, morbid, dynamic alteration of our vital energy," whereas the pathogens are only trigger factors. "The inimical forces, partly psychical, partly physical, to which our terrestrial existence is exposed, which are termed morbific noxious agents, do not possess the power of morbidly deranging the health of man unconditionally; but we are made ill by them only when our organism is sufficiently disposed and susceptible to the attack of the morbific cause that may be present, and to be altered in its health, deranged and made to undergo abnormal sensations and functions—hence they do not produce disease in every one nor at all times."[2] We are amazed at how concepts that have only recently been espoused by the modern sciences of pathology and immunology could be so clearly perceived and expressed over 150 years ago.

Today, after the scientific developments of last century, we have accumulated an overwhelming amount of knowledge regarding the components and the mechanisms of living organisms, from single cells to higher multicellular organisms. The concept of vital force seems obsolete and unnecessary for the description of biological phenomena, including healing. Even if the term "vital force" has not completely been erased from the scientific dictionary, being still used as a synonym for *bioenergetics*,[3] the vitalistic approach has been definitely overcome and the scientifically-oriented doctor now considers the body's natural healing power as a manifestation of the evolutionary development of homeostatic and adaptive functions of cells, tissues, and humoral biochemical systems.

However, in spite of enormous scientific development, our understanding of the healing process is still primitive and unsatisfying, particularly with respect to complex, multifactorial, diseases. Unfortunately, the positive restoration of normal homeostasis after a perturbation is not always the outcome. A number of external or internal pathogenic factors—biological, chemical or physical harmful agents, or errors of diet or lifestyle—can modify permanently or semi-permanently the health state of a person, particularly when these factors interact with genetic predispositions. Moreover, internal factors (i.e. HLA molecules, blood coagulation, oxygen radical formation, amyloid deposit, platelet aggregation and so on), are linked to the defense mechanisms that may amplify to counteract the external harmful agents and become self-damaging and aggressive factors. In these conditions, the "natural" healing power shows its limits, so that chronic or even progressive diseases may develop. The inadequacy of modern medicine in the management of a number of common diseases, and the increasing problem of drug-induced diseases dramatically demonstrates that medically-assisted healing is still far from completely effective. The ultimate reason for this weakness of mainstream science is that well-being and disease are complex phenomena, and as a consequence, knowledge of single parts is not enough for regulation of the whole.

We call *biodynamic* the study of the vital force, that is, of the behavior of complex systems whose interaction and organization are responsible for the healing power of the body.[4]

A complex system presents properties which amount to more than simply the sum of its component parts. This is the main property of complex systems, and not necessarily due to the existence of a number of different components. A complex system can be composed of only a few elements, but the interaction of components on one scale can lead to complex global behavior on a larger scale that in general cannot be deduced from knowledge of the individual components.

Clearly, an entire book would not be sufficient for a thorough analysis of the mechanisms involved in healing processes, whose investigation is the field of modern biomedical sciences like genetics, biochemistry, cell biology, immunology, neurology, molecular pharmacology, and so on. Table 1 is a summary of the main systems that are responsible for the natural healing power of the body.

TABLE 1 Some mechanisms involved in the healing process at different levels of biological organization

---

Molecular mechanisms

DNA repair after mutation
Inactivation of toxins by antibodies
Free radicals scavenging
Self-assembly of collagen
Detoxification by cytochrome-P450
Buffering capacity of fluids
Action of "defensins" and lysozyme
Fibrin formation
Heat-shock proteins (chaperonins)

Cellular mechanisms

Cell adhesion and movement
Membrane exportation of toxins
Free calcium homeostasis
Virus nucleic acid degradation
Nerve fiber regeneration
Phagocytosis of foreign particles
Bacterial killing
Tumor cell destruction
Bone resorption and deposition

Systemic mechanisms

Inflammation

Immune response

Organ regeneration and remodeling

Haemostasis

Neuroendocrine response to stress

Cytokine networks

Sympathic/parasympathic balance

Rest and relaxation

Healthy diet

Psycho-social factors

Changes in lifestyle

Exercise

Solidarity

Love

Prayer

Efficiency of healthcare systems

Patient-doctor relationship

Sharing of cultural knowledge

The last part of Table 1 includes some examples of events and phenomena that are not applicable to the organic sphere, assembled under the heading "Psychosocial factors." In fact, human biology (etymologically, the "knowledge of life") can not be reduced to chemical or mechanical factors, because the human being is an *open system*, whose health state—and therefore whose healing power—is dependent not only on internal mechanisms but also on interaction with its environment. In a holistic medical perspective, the *essential rules* of homeostasis and of healing are similar at the different levels of organization that one may take into consideration.

A synthetic view of healing mechanisms

The homeopathic remedies are said to stimulate the self-healing power of the organism. Therefore any theory of homeopathy requires the definition of the healing mechanisms that are involved in the purported therapeutic effects.

The phenomena and the mechanisms involved in healing processes can be described according to two fundamental standpoints. The first one, that we may call *analytical*, considers all the single phenomena occurring in cells, tissues, and blood during the healing from damage. For example, we may investigate the molecular changes by which the integrity of the bone tissue is restored in the place where trauma broke a bone in two pieces; we may describe how an infarct heals with formation of a small connective tissue scar; how white cells, attracted by bacterial products, leave the bloodstream and migrate into the tissues where they phagocytose and kill invader microbes; or how liver cells regenerate after severe intoxication or viral infection. In these and many other healing processes, a number of molecular transformations, cell growth cycles, and metabolic modifications are activated in a specific and restricted way.

The second perspective, which we may call *synthetic*, is to try to design working models by which the *fundamental principles* and the *logic* of a complex phenomenon such as the healing process can be studied and understood. For example, we may observe that healing from trauma or from infection is due not only to local factors, like coagulation, cell chemotaxis, and angiogenesis, but also to the participation of general factors, like activation of the hypothalamus-hypophysis-adrenal axis, production of cytokines that reach all the body through the bloodstream, changes of liver protein metabolism, and so on. It is a crucial aspect of the healing process that billions of cells act in concert and in a finalized manner in order to destroy foreign invaders or tumor cells and to reestablish the healthy morphological and functional state. To achieve this coordination, soluble hormones, nervous system, cell-cell interactions and possibly long-range signals such as electromagnetic signals provide a link between general, systemic, factors and local factors.[5] The reciprocal influence of systemic and local factors is so important that a psychological stress can be associated with immune suppression and infection, while, conversely, an infectious process under a tooth can cause profound psychological depression.

A further point that is connected with the synthetic approach is the *topological* problem. This term designates the study of the position that living matter takes in space. Analysis can provide information on the *composition*, but says little about the mechanisms of development and of restitution of the *form* in a tissue. These latter, in fact, depend on a number of factors, the most important being the *self-organizing* capacity of an assembly of several different types of cells, which undertake a number of reciprocal interactions.

Both types of knowledge of the healing process, the analytical and the synthetic, are important in order to describe and, possibly, to positively influence the healing process, but here we will give a greater emphasis to the second one essentially for two reasons: first, that a thorough analysis of the biological events involved in a single healing process (for example, wound healing, bacterial killing, immune defense development, and so on) is impossible in the available space for this review; second, and more important, while the analytical approach has been intensively pursued by molecular biology in the last three decades and represents the main body of teaching in medical schools, the synthetic perspective has been and is almost completely overlooked by modern, high-tech, medicine.

Systemic thinking or *integrative thinking* is profoundly rooted in the history of physics and of mathematics in the twentieth century, representing a kind of reaction to the mechanism of the nineteenth century. The changes occurring in these sciences, in turn, prompted the development of cybernetics, informatics, ecology, and also of biology.[6] In the history of medicine, a global approach to human health and disease has received much more attention by so-called complementary medicines, which are characterized by a holistic standpoint and developed before the modern western scientific (often reductionistic) paradigms and in some case independently of them. Therefore, a rethinking of the general principles of the healing processes may serve both as a stimulus to new scientific research in the conventional, mainstream, field and as a key to understanding in a deeper and more rational way the basis of other medical traditions.

For over twenty years we have investigated the biochemical mechanisms of microbial killing and, in general, of the inflammatory process, which undoubtedly represents the first and the main biological mechanism of healing. The need for further progress in this field, combined with the admission of the overwhelming complexity of the problem itself, are the main reasons that led our research group to think about the mechanisms involved in the healing process from a holistic perspective. Our goal is integrating the current analytical approach with the possible contribution of the "science of complexity," of chaos theory, and of traditional medicines.[7] The study of homeopathy was of great inspiration and help in this integrative work. (Further discussion on the problems of pluralism in therapeutical methods, of different medical paradigms, and on the prospects for their integration, particularly as concerned with homeopathy, can be found earlier in this book.)

Biodynamic properties of living systems

Healing and life are two faces of the same coin. We can not properly understand the former without a definition of the latter. Therefore, here we will examine some essential features of living systems and of their pathological aspects. Understanding the pathogenesis of disease is a fundamental requirement for the comprehension of how disease can be reversed, either spontaneously or with medical help, and a person's health be brought back to a normal state.

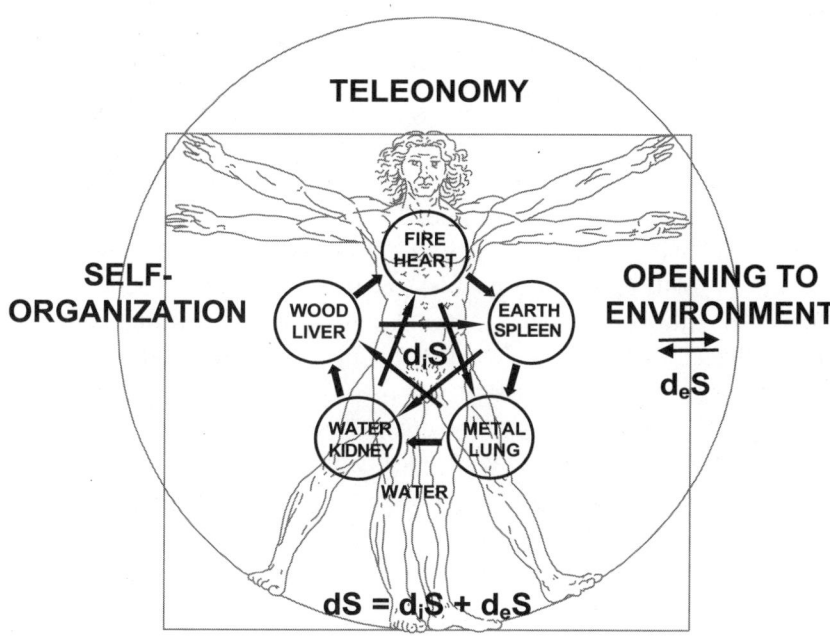

FIGURE 1 General Properties of Living Systems

The essential features that allow the birth, growth and development of life, and that include the healing capacity, are essentially two: *self-organization* and *openness* to external regulation (Figure 1). Moreover, these two features have a scope (teleonomy), that is the life of the individual, the best adaptation to the changing conditions, the survival, the healing, the reproduction, the development of human consciousness. Here is the *biodynamics* in modern terms.

Self-organization is based on the existence of multiple elements (ions, molecules, molecular aggregates, cells, organs), that are linked by multiple and reciprocal interrelations by which continuous quantitative and qualitative changes occur. A multiplicity of elements connected by physical forces, in suitable conditions and when they are subjected to a flux of energy (heat, light, mechanical agitation, etc.), tends *spontaneously* to organize as a *system*.[8] (We mean by the word *system* any organized whole of many elements.) *Organization* means the existence of a "structure" (either spatial like a *form,* or temporal, like a series of events occurring with a given *frequency*). The structure, therefore, is the existence of a state of organization (order), a state that is different from pure chance (disorder).

Many systems have been described as being capable of generating some kind of organized structure starting from a more disordered assembly of many constituents: the order may be spatial (waves, spatial structures such as rings or spirals) or temporal (oscillations, cycles, rhythms, pulsations). Often these ordered and dynamic structures can be found in biological phenomena but also in experimental chemical or physical systems. There are even chemical reactions that are capable of self-organization in nonequilibrium states in the course of time. The prototype of these reactions is the one described by Belusov-Zabotinskij: in this reaction, the reagents (we will ignore the details) generate a colored product which, however, is not always constant, nor always on the increase, but continues to oscillate in the course of time, thus giving rise to talk of a *chemical clock*.[9] Another typical example is represented by the formation of convection Bénard cells in water exposed to a flux of heat.[10]

One of the main outcomes of self-organization is the formation and maintenance of *structure*. In cells, structures have absolutely indispensable functions: we need only mention the cell membranes, which divide the cells into compartments and separate the cell itself from the surrounding environment. Through the membranes a marked *disequilibrium* of substances and electrical charges is maintained, which is necessary for a whole series of functions, such as the production of energy (mitochondria), the production and transmission of signals (neurons), and the activation of movement (muscles).

If orderly systems are formed in space (e.g. circles, target-type structures, spirals) this means that each element is affected in its position and speed by the others in the system: it takes its "orders" or information from the adjoining element and behaves accordingly. This results in phenomena of cooperation and coherence, so that the elements arrange themselves in orderly structures. If orderly structures are formed in time this means that the state of the system in any given instant *depends* on the previous one and *conditions* the next one in the series. In brief, it has been claimed that it is the very appearance of *space-time organization*, due to *broad-ranging* interactions among the elements of a system, that constitutes the most typical feature of *complexity*.[11] In other words, complexity contains not only a quantitative factor related to the number of elements involved, but also a qualitative factor associated with the appearance of *structure*, or *form*.

As a first and broad generalization, we may say that differentiation and development coincide with the expression and maintenance of a structure and with efficient storage and handling of the energy flux, while disease and death coincide with the loss of structure and dissipation of information. In order to efficiently handle the energy flux, living systems require *information*. (The word *information* refers to the special kind of energy that is required to maintain the order.) This information is present *inside* the organism from the beginning in the embryo, both as genetic (DNA) and epigenetic (other space-temporal structures that influence the DNA expression of specific genes) and penetrates from the environment as a number of signals that are perceived by specific receptor structures.

In the behavior of complex systems the *quality* of the information is far more important than the quantity, or the energy consumed to provide it. The biological system, in particular, has developed and has integrated within itself the systems of production and use of energy, utilizing various well-coordinated metabolic pathways and the rapid availability of phosphorylated intermediates. The functional reserve of these systems is considerable (except in highly pathological cases of cell damage or anoxia), so that normally the functional oscillations and the behavior patterns of cellular or organic biological systems do not depend on addition or subtraction of energy, but on control mechanisms at the *information* level. The more complex and "flexible" a system is, the scantier may be the amounts of energy capable of altering its behavior. We need only mention, for instance, the brain, which is in all probability the most complex system existing in nature. It can be mobilized—and, as a result, so can the entire body—by nonmolecular stimulations, which in a certain sense may be devoid of energy or matter. Another example is provided by molecular biology: DNA, where highly significant biological information is stored, may be changed even in a single base of the billion base-pairs of which it is composed, and this minimal change can cause a fatal disease.

The latter point brings us to consider the flux of information to which a living system is constantly exposed. Besides being endowed with self-regulating properties, it can be seen also as an *open* system, i.e. a system that is dependent from the beginning on the environment. Thus, self-organization does not mean that such an admirable capacity of increasing and maintaining complex forms and functions can occur independently of external help. On the contrary, the thermodynamic stability of a system is guaranteed by the continuous exchange with the environment. As a mater of fact, life itself, and healing in particular, can occur only because living systems are open systems (also called *dissipative structures*).

The second law of thermodynamics can be formulated briefly as follows: every *isolated* system, where any kind of transformation takes place, is subject to a series of processes tending to move from a very improbable state (that it is in) to a very probable state associated with the ensemble, where each transformation is associated with increase of *entropy* (disorder). To prevent this drift toward equilibrium, to move the system and each sub-system back toward the improbable state, work has to be constantly performed. All the vital activities of living beings that underlie differentiation, development, growth, reproduction, and healing are processes that occur far from equilibrium, a condition that can be maintained by a continuous stream of energy, matter, and information. "Any creature cut of from contact with the stream dies by asphyxiation or starvation. Structures and complex molecules come unglued, motion ceases, gradients dissipate, order decays; equilibrium is death."[12] Life implies holding out against equilibrium, converting energy into organization, and these things are possible only at the price of continuous work and continuous expenditure of energy.

The laws of physics and chemistry constitute boundary conditions that living systems must obey, but they do not usually determine which choice is performed in order to maintain and restore organization (survival and healing). Therefore, biology cannot be reduced to chemistry or physics, and to understand life other distinguishing properties have to be considered. One of these properties is the *teleonomy*, which designates the purposeful character of living things. The machinery of life *uses* the laws of chemistry and physics and the available energy (in first and fundamental instance, the sunlight) *in order to* (i.e. with the purpose to) maintain the complex organization of life itself. This purpose is evident in the evolutionary design and in the developmental behavior of each living being from zygote to adult organism.

The teleonomic character of the machinery of life is indisputable, and is documented also by the precision with which the organism tends to reintegrate its original structure after an injury. Each living system is endowed, right from the outset, with a *project* and most of its activity is used to assimilate energy and matter from the outside to match this project, notwithstanding all the perturbing factors. However, development is not *unconditioned* and the project is not pursued without problems, because the structure and function of the living organism are flexible and may *adapt* to the environment. In the proper balance of conservation of structure, adaptation is the key to healthful life.

The teleonomy of the vital force was suggested also by Hahnemann himself: "In the healthy condition of man, the spiritual Vital Force (autocracy), the dynamic that animates the material body (organism), rules with unbounded sway, and retains all the parts of the organism in admirable, harmonious, vital operation, as regards both sensations and functions, so that our indwelling, reason-gifted mind can freely employ this living, healthy instrument for the higher purpose of our existence."[13]

Time-dependent organization (rhythms)

We have seen that an organism is nothing if not *organized heterogeneity*, with nested dynamic structures over all space-time scales. Organized heterogeneity can be envisaged both on spatial and temporal scales. Spatial differentiation of the body into organs, tissues and cells is a familiar concept. The cell is partitioned into subcellular *organelles* and *compartments* separated by membranes. Molecular and electrical signals are unceasingly and rhythmically exchanged between these compartments. Within each compartment, local circuits of macromolecular *complexes* or of single enzyme proteins can be identified as responsible for cycling energy transformations or for storing biological information. Moreover, inside each sufficiently complex molecule (e.g. a protein), several *domains* can be described, whose function is to catalyze chemical reactions or to allow interaction with other molecular or electrical signals. Conformational changes of these flexible molecular structures enable proteins to absorb energy from the site where it is released, store it, and deliver it to other structures. Therefore, spatial differentiation and signal communication in living systems spans at least ten orders of magnitude, from 10^{-10} m for intramolecular interactions to meters for nerve conduction and blood perfusion in the whole organism.

Temporal organization of biological phenomena is evident in the rhythmic functional modifications of cells, tissues, and organs. These oscillating mechanical, chemical and electrical events range from 10^{-14} s for resonant energy transfer between molecules to 10^7 s for circannual rhythms and to even longer periods if one considers population dynamics. Physiological variables such as enzyme reactions, neuronal activity, heart rate, respiration, cell division, ovarian cycle, corticosteroid circadian variations, cell calcium oscillations, membrane polarization/depolarization, sleep/waking, oxidative metabolism, actin polymerization, cyclic nucleotide concentration, all undergo time-dependent oscillations. Periodical variation of molecular concentrations can be used, by living systems, as means for coding and transmitting information.[14] In other words, signals can be transmitted and perceived not only as variations in the *amplitude* of the intensity of a given phenomenon, but also in the *frequency* by which they occur. The most familiar example of *frequency-modulated* signal transmission is the action potential in the nervous system, but recently other molecular oscillations such as calcium waves and hormonal changes, have been inter-preted in this new light.[15]

Oscillations of the control parameters of the various physiological sys-tems are the norm in biology and medicine. If, however, the coordination is lost, i.e. the *connectivity* of the system as a whole and in relation to the rest of the body, certain subcomponents may oscillate in an excessive, un-predictable, and pointless manner, thus generating localized disorders which may, however, be amplified (the amplification of fluctuations is a typical behavior of chaotic systems). Oscillation thus becomes disorder and takes on the aspect of disease, in that it causes the emergence of substantial symp-toms and damage. In a complex system, loss of communication means pa-thology.

A complex system is regulated by communication modes suited to the degree of complexity. For example, communication between two molecules (fairly simple system) consists of electrostatic attraction or repulsion; com-munication between several groups of molecules (complex system) con-sists of undulatory dynamics and spatiotemporal variations (oscillations of particular signal molecules); communication between organs and systems is entrusted to further complex systems which use both chemical (hor-mones, cytokines) and physical (action potentials and probably acupunc-ture meridians) methods of communication. Communication between different individuals is achieved by other methods such as words, writing, looks, and broadcasting by cable or over the air. This means that if we want to "enter the communications network"—with a view to understand-ing and eventually influencing it—we have to use the same method or meth-ods of communication as the system we are interested in. If a system is regulated by modes of communication consisting of synergism between several molecules acting at low doses, to enter this network in an effective way theoretically we would need to use the same method: low-dose modu-lators exploiting synergism and antagonisms. If, on the other hand, we use modulators of only one molecular type and at high doses, we obtain ef-fects, admittedly, and even effects in the desired direction, but not effects in complete harmony with the system itself, resulting in a high incidence of unwanted side effects.

Analogy

In order to deal with puzzling issues like those of self-organization and regulation of biological healing, one may take advantage of cybernetic models that utilize the language of mathematics. On the basis of these models, *analogies* can be drawn with physiological phenomena, trying to understand how these mathematical concepts can be applied to living systems. What is meant by *analogy* is similarity between two distinct systems one of them to be better understood on the basis of knowledge already gained about the other. Analogy can therefore be used to construct more advanced models compared to those in current use and to make forecasts about unknown systems starting from known systems (usually physicochemical or mathematical) which act as archetypes, i.e. as *reference systems*.

The analysis proceeds in two steps. Firstly, certain analogies are traced between the observations and the behavior of physicochemical reference systems. This defines the type of model that is likely to be the most appropriate representation of the system concerned. Then an attempt is made to go beyond the stage of plain analogy, to pinpoint, within the framework of the model adopted, the specificity of each problem and to incorporate it in the description. Lastly, the predictions of the analysis are compared against experience with past behavior, and, assuming an agreement is reached on quality, these predictions are used to foresee future tendencies.

Of course, drawing an analogy does not provide the final proof of the quantitative correspondence between the model and the natural object, but analogic reasoning is a potent instrument that proves very useful in understanding complex objects and situations. Analogy is useful in order to construct hypotheses regarding complex phenomena on the basis of the knowledge of similar, more simple, phenomena that are better known. Therefore, analogic reasoning, when coupled with testable hypotheses, is integral part of the scientific proceeding when it comes to describing and understanding complex systems.

We know how important analogy is for homeopathic methodology.

Models of dynamic systems

The contribution made by the physico-mathematical approach to the problem of complexity is much greater than might be imagined: while it is true to say that a living system with its thousands of subcomponents will never resemble a chemical system with two or only a very few components, and can never be described by a mathematical formula, on the other hand, it is also true that the study of the complexity of "simple" systems may enable us to discover *basic rules* of behavior which are repeated in substantially identical forms in systems with a different evolutionary status. It has been suggested that a complex, nonlinear feedback system is something like *a universal formula for life*,[16] because it summarizes, admittedly in a very general way, most of the processes of life.

The mathematical formulation of feedback essentially describes the dynamics of a mechanism operating in living beings. As we have seen, living systems, in fact, are regulated by reaction and counteraction cycles that constitute so-called *homeostasis*. These cycles are nothing more or less than the repetition of the same operation (by analogy with mathematical iteration) in which the result of the previous cycle serves as the basis of the next one. For example, at the end of the systole-diastole cycle the heart reverts to the end-diastolic condition; at the end of a mitotic cycle the condition of the two daughter cells becomes in turn the starting condition for a new mitosis; thus, every rhythmic modification of the organism hinges upon the previous state and occurs according to fixed rules. (In the analogy we have adopted, the rule is the mathematical formula.)

The state of a dynamic system at a certain time can be seen as a point in the *space of phases*, i.e. in the space delineated by the variables of the system itself. For example, the localization of a point in a three-dimensional space is described by the value of the three (x,y,z) orthogonal axes. The dimension of the space of phases can be less or more than three, according to the number of variables of a given system. When the dynamic of the system is also considered, i.e. taking into consideration the variable of time, the evolution of a dynamic system in space-time can be also seen as series of points (a line) that follows a *trajectory*. Starting from different initial positions in the space of phases (different initial conditions), the same system may describe different trajectories that converge to a single point (so-called *point-attractor*), or trajectories that "visit" the same points (also called *orbits*, or *periodic attractors*), or finally trajectories that explore the space of phases in a way by which they never repeat the same path. The latter situation, where no regular periodicity can be seen in the system behavior, is also referred to as a *strange*, or *chaotic*, *attractor*.

Biological complexity and chaos

In recent years, considerable attention has been given to the fact that in healthy living systems all the physiological variables oscillate according to rhythms that are neither completely periodic nor totally random. These dynamic oscillations respond to complex and coordinated control systems that comply with the "laws" of deterministic chaos.[17] Introduction of chaos theory into the biological domain has a number of implications of both theoretical and practical value.

First of all, it should be pointed out that deterministic chaos is not randomness but *pseudorandom noise* or *low-dimensional aperiodic signal*.[18] While the classical phenomenological definition of chaos means absence of order (state of maximum entropy), the modern definition is based on nonlinear mathematics, whose principles were anticipated during the late nineteenth century by Poincaré and rediscovered by Lorenz in 1963, discussed in a paper with the title "Deterministic nonperiodic flow."[19] With the use of modern electronics, the mathematical analysis of chaos has developed to a point where it is beginning to have an important impact on a wide variety of fields including biology and physiology.

An important characteristic of a chaotic system is referred to as *sensitive dependence on initial conditions and to perturbations*. Sensitivity in this case refers to the situation in which two similar systems are started initially with variables having very close values but following this, their dynamic states diverge from each other quickly. Small differences in initial conditions or small perturbations produce very great differences in the final phenomena, suggesting the impossibility of long-term predictions.

Another way by which this phenomenon is exemplified is the so-called *butterfly effect*, the principle conveyed by the dictum that the flapping of a butterfly's wings in Brazil may trigger off, or stop in its tracks, a tornado in Texas.[20]

On the other hand, this also means that small applied perturbations can control chaos,[21] provided that these perturbations are specific and delivered at the right time-intervals. As stated by Elbert, "in the future it may even be possible to devise therapies for disease by manipulating control parameters back into the normal range."[22] The subtle communications between oscillators, which generate synchronism and cooperativity, are of paramount importance in many physiological functions. Regulation of these physiological and biochemical events could be possible through exploitation of the "rules of chaos," and this may have importance for the interpretation of the effects of low-energy or low-dose medical manipulations. Even signals which are extremely small, but which are endowed with highly specific information and are capable of resounding in unison with the recipient system, could act as regulators, if it is admitted that the deregulated system or systems are in a state of precarious equilibrium, near to the *bifurcation point*, where the choice whether to move in one direction or the other is related to minimal fluctuations on the border between order and chaos.

Another important example is provided by the cytokine network, which exhibits nonlinear behavior.[23] Such nonlinear cytokine interactions have important implications because they may give rise to unexpected or counterintuitive effects, that are not always recognized or taken into account in therapy. In inflammatory diseases (such as rheumathoid arthritis, multiple sclerosis and so on), inadequate immunosuppression may make things worse by inducing high-level of pro-inflammatory cytokines. So, in the context of cytokine networks, the goal of a therapeutic strategy would be not to change the concentration of one or few cytokines, but to move the whole network from one state-attractor to another (say from an inflammatory response to a noninflammatory one). Thanks to the *rules* governing chaotic systems, this could be done by using small carefully controlled interventions, rather than high doses of chemical drugs. Of course, in order to have any hope of doing this, one needs to understand the dynamics of the whole network far better than we do today.

The new concepts emerging from chaos studies tell us that at this "border" minimal variations in the conditions of the system (such as those induced even by a very small oscillatory resonance) may play a decisive role in the subsequent evolution of the system itself. In a variety of systems, the "butterfly effect" may be used to control chaos, on condition that the parameters to be controlled and changed are well known.[24]

The phenomenon of resonance is well known in physics, where it occurs in many fields: acoustics, mechanics, and electromagnetism, as well as nuclear physics. By virtue of this phenomenon, a system that is characterized by its own oscillation frequency can enter into vibration if stimulated (subjected to sound waves, electromagnetic waves, or mechanical vibrations according to the nature of the system) by frequencies close to those peculiar to the system itself. If the system is already oscillating, the resonance may greatly increase the amplitude of the oscillation, whenever the waves overlap, while the opposite may also occur, namely an arrest of oscillation, if the interaction is between two waves of the same frequency but opposite in phase.

Resonance, then, is a means whereby information is transmitted between two *similar* systems (as regards vibrational or harmonic frequencies) without the passage of matter. These linkage phenomena between oscillators, which generate synchronism and cooperativity, are of paramount importance in many physiological functions, particularly in the nervous system, but also in the cells regulating cardiac rhythm, in the cells secreting insulin in the pancreas, in the ciliated epithelia, and in the involuntary contractions of smooth muscle. Interestingly, it has been suggested that resonance may transduce information between an oscillating, low-level, electromagnetic field and molecular sub-domains of cell enzymes.[25] This type of interaction should lower the activation barrier of the rate-limiting step of enzymic reactions, thus increasing the overall catalytic activity.

Order and variability

The physiological variables controlled by the homeostatic systems oscillate continually between a maximum and minimum allowed value, but this variability may be more or less regular or rhythmic, depending upon multiple conditioning factors performing the various control functions. On changing the rate by which these transformations take place, abrupt changes between periodic and chaotic behaviors (and visa versa) are possible.

Thanks to the development of deterministic chaos theory, some processes formerly perceived as erratic, are now viewed in terms of pattern and lawful relationship. Chaotic phenomena underlie the idea of structure and the potential for describing complex systems, rhythms, shapes, and behaviors with the aid of relatively simple formulations. If an apparently random phenomenon reveals, by this mathematical analysis, the features of a chaotic phenomenon, its behavior can be better predicted and manipulated. The rate of enzymatic activities oscillates when two enzymes compete for the same substrates, and small changes in concentrations can lead to changes in the frequencies and amplitudes of oscillations, causing them to become chaotic if previously harmonic or to become harmonic if previously chaotic.[26] Analysis of temporal variations in hormone levels in healthy subjects has revealed chaotic situations in this area, too.[27] Other applications of the theory of chaos have been described in cardiology. For example, it has been reported that the heart rate of a healthy individual varies over time with an intrinsically chaotic periodicity.[28] Obviously, these are not arrhythmia, but oscillations in normal rhythm. The electroencephalogram also shows similar chaotic patterns as normal aspects of its functioning.[29]

Many, if not most, of the physiological rhythmic phenomena in healthy individuals show chaotic dynamics, and nature uses chaos in order to increase variability, flexibility and adaptation. In complex systems like heart and brain, a decrease of chaos means disease and predicts serious pathology like cardiac arrest or epilepsy.[30] In the immune system, too, chaos may play a very important role, especially because this system continually needs to generate new forms of receptors to cope with all the possible antigens that the outside world and the inside of the body may present. *Fantasy*, then, is a fundamental property of the immune system, without which the body would lack the necessary adaptability to a world in a constant state of change and the ability to defend itself against potential aggressors.[31]

Systems with mixed feedback (both positive and negative feedback) and multiple feedback with different time constants are sources of deterministic chaos. This is the case of the whole organism and of the whole cell, which can be described as dynamic systems where the *equilibrium* is a special case of attractor, the integration of a number of attractors. As a consequence, healthy and pathological states become interpretable as different types of attractors, which may be converted from each other by bifurcations or critical perturbations.[32] Rapid state changes and bifurcation are characteristic of networks that are sensitive to very weak initial conditions that lead to widespread changes in the whole system.

Networks

A peculiar property of complex systems is the ability to evolve over the course of time. This is observed both in the biological development of any organism (ontogenesis) and in the development of living species in general throughout history (evolution). In the classic Darwinian theory of evolution, the emergence of increasingly complex species is the fruit of *random variability* and *selection*, which operate to the advantage of those species which, by virtue of characteristics acquired by chance mutations, better succeed in adapting to increasingly difficult environmental conditions and in surviving the competitive struggle for vital space and food. This well-known concept of natural selection and the survival of the fittest in evolution has also been applied on a molecular and cellular scale as well as in embryology. The classic view of the origin of order and diversification of biological species—based on natural selection—has recently been contested on the basis of mathematical studies and computer models showing that, alongside natural selection, other mechanisms are involved, which have been grouped together under the term *self-organization*.[33]

As a result of the laws of chaos, nonlinear dynamic systems can easily present transition from order to disorder and vice versa, following even only minimal perturbations in control parameters or in the energy flow across such systems. Nevertheless, in these cases, we are invariably in the presence of changes somehow induced from the outside. There may, however, also be a phenomenon whereby the complex, disorderly system spontaneously "crystallizes" in an orderly state. From disorder to order thanks to *an intrinsic original property* of the system itself and with no input of outside energy; quite rightly, this phenomenon has been termed *antichaos*.

The mathematical models of self-organization were initially developed with the aim of explaining how the cell genome is organized. The genome can be viewed as a complex computer in which there is a data memory (information stored in the DNA for approximately 100,000 different proteins), but also the parallel processing of some of this information (a few hundred or a few thousand data units simultaneously). What is more, many of these protein data units influence the genome itself in its activity, in multiple control sites. In this way, many genes are coupled with the functioning of others, influencing one another reciprocally, and constituting a *network*.

Networks are complex structures because the state and the changes of each element depend, directly or indirectly, on the state and the changes of all the other elements. Therefore, a network behaves as a *coherent* system, whose health state is governed and restored depending on the connectedness of internal and external processes, that is by the value of original information, the capacity of signaling the harmful modifications, and the efficiency by which energy is channeled towards the purpose of reconstructing the original conformation.

The coordinated and sequential behavior of this network is the basic factor responsible for the functioning and differentiation of the cell, with the result that a liver cell is different from a heart muscle cell and performs different functions, despite containing the same genetic information, being composed of the same elementary materials (amino acids, sugars, lipids, carbohydrates), and obeying the same "general functioning rules" (biochemical reactions).

The concept of network is useful for describing a general organization model of complex systems:

- society: network of individuals;
- body: network of organs;
- brain: network of nerve centers;
- immune system: network of cells;
- cells: network of molecules;
- molecules: network of atoms;
- atoms: networks of elementary particles.

According to the external and internal conditions (number of components and of communication pathways, temperature, chemical concentrations, rate of changes and so on), a network system may assume different states, or *attractors*. An attractor is the state or the series of states (pattern) to which the behavior of a system is attracted. It therefore possesses an important property—stability. In a system subject to perturbations, movement tends to be towards the attractor. The theory of dynamic system shows that the attractor may be a single point, as for example in the trajectory of a pendulum when it reaches the stationary state, or a finite number of points reflecting a periodic-type behavior (orbit), or an infinite system of points generating a figure in the form of an orbit which never repeats itself identically, as may happen in chaotic systems ("strange attractors").

The choice between one state (or attractor) and another possible state (or attractor) often depends on the "experience" to which the system is exposed. The modifications that the system has undergone, are "stored" in the space-time as specific permanent and semi-permanent structures, whose existence influences further development and subsequent responses of the system itself. Unlike what happens in a system in a state of reversible equilibrium on changing the external or internal parameters, in a complex system a situation can be reached in which there is a *symmetry breaking*, or an irreversible change. While it is true that random fluctuations and perturbations can usually be damped, beyond certain threshold values, or in the presence of appropriate environmental conditions, these effects are not annulled, but with the system acting as an amplifier, a reaction is triggered which removes the system from the reference state.

Changes of attractor represent a potential problem for the healing process because by this means a certain specific behavior or structural modification can become "fixed" to a pathological attractor due to a specific perturbation, losing the possibility of fully reversible modifications. This kind of pathological modification of a dynamic system can be considered an *erroneous adaptation*, where the system finds a fixed point or a periodically oscillating behavior outside the normal, original, range of variation. In a particular sub-set of the space-time, i.e. locally or for a short period, this new attractor may appear as the most convenient in terms of energy expenditure, but for the system as a whole and for the future prospects of development of the system itself, an erroneous adaptation can be highly deleterious. Something like this process can be envisaged in the transformation of an acute inflammation into a chronic reaction, or in the heart and blood vessel hypertrophy in chronic hypertension, or in the receptor adaptation that justifies the hyperglycemia in hyperinsulinemic type II diabetic patient. Also the tissue protein or lipid deposits that can be found in amyloidal diseases (including Alzheimer disease) and in arteriosclerosis may be seen as an adaptation of tissue homeostasis to a chronic load of pathologic precursors of these deposit moieties.

We have previously shown how the concept of *change of attractor* has implications also for the understanding of the action of low doses or high dilutions of drugs selected according to the principle of similarity, traditionally proposed by homeopathic medicine.[34]

Plausibility of homeopathic high-dilutions/high potencies of drugs

The new concepts emerging from complexity theory have profound implications on the ways in which patients and diseases are investigated and treated. Since we have done a number of experimental and theoretical studies on the putative mechanism(s) of action of homeopathy, we shall attempt here to summarize a few points regarding this particular field of complementary medicine. Of course, the following points should be underlined: a) hypotheses are essential to the evolution of knowledge, but one has to guard against presenting them as certainties; b) the following discussion is based on the assumption that highly diluted remedies prepared according to the homeopathic methods are endowed with specific information of biophysical nature (superradiance, water clusters, isotopic lattices, and so on), a highly controversial issue that is discussed in other sections of this book; c) here we restrict our consideration to the possible mechanism of interaction between high-dilution homeopathic remedies and the organism, that is only one of the various questions raised by the homeopathic approach; and d) a biophysical perspective does not exclude that many effects of low- and ultra-low doses of drugs are due to "conventional" molecular interactions. The hypotheses set forth here also refer to theories proposed by other authors.[35]

A new vision of matter and life is emerging at the frontiers of science, particularly from the fields of quantum physics and mathematical theories and research that have yet to be systematized. Organisms are seen as highly regulated, complex, dynamic systems that display a characteristic metastability around certain homeostatic levels. This metastability is the net result of continual oscillations, rhythms, networks, amplifications and feedback cycles. Living systems are "suspended" between order and chaos; they partake of these two fundamental characteristics of matter and exploit them in a manner designed to promote survival. We cannot see how these new perspectives can fail to have an impact on the new orientations and trends in medicine. Medical theory, methodology, and technology have always proceeded hand in hand with the general scientific theory and socioeconomic situations of the times.

On this basis, a hypothetical model of the possible action mechanism of homeopathic drugs can be advanced. The following hypothesis is formulated starting from the assumption that some type of structural or dynamical information storage actually occurs in water. This assumption is based on the preliminary evidence provided by biological and biophysical studies reviewed throughout this book and in Appendix 1.

From a biophysical standpoint, disease may be regarded not only as a functional or molecular-structural abnormality, as in the classic view, but also (and not by way of contrast) as a disturbance of an entire network of electromagnetic communications based on long-range interactions between elements (molecules, nerve centers, organs, to mention but a few) which oscillate at frequencies which are coherent and specific and thus capable of resonance. This would be a *disturbance of internal oscillators and their communications*. Our knowledge is still too scanty to say whether or not these oscillators can be identified with certain nerve centers in particular (the ability to oscillate at characteristic frequencies is typical, though not exclusively so, of nerve centers) or with the collective behavior of nerve centers and/or other tissues or cells. With regard to cell-to-cell and intracellular communication, biophoton research suggests the existence of extensive coherent fields of interaction in the visible range.[36]

If the disease process involves a disturbance of oscillation frequencies— and of the communications associated with them—it should be brought back to a state of equilibrium by means of *syntonization or tuning, i.e. by means of a change in frequency imposed by interaction with another oscillator.* According to this notion, the homeopathic remedy might act in the patient as an external guide frequency.

A potentized homeopathic drug might be regarded as a small amount of matter containing elements oscillating in phase (coherently), capable of transmitting these oscillatory frequencies, via a process of resonance, to biological fluids (in turn mostly made up of water), but also to complex "metastable" structures, subject to nonlinear behavior patterns and capable in turn of oscillating (macromolecules, a-helixes, membranes, filamentous structures, receptors). There would thus be the possibility of a link between drug frequencies and oscillators present in the living organism perturbed by the disease.

It is very likely that in the near future studies on fractals and on deterministic chaos will be applied to physiology and pathology to an increasing extent. In fact, if chaotic dynamics is a *normal* aspect of physiological processes, investigating this may furnish more complete predictive information for characterizing the therapeutic effects of various types of periodical stimuli (including physiological stress, acupuncture, electric pacing, psychotherapy, and so on), of pharmacological compounds[37] and of highly diluted homeopathic remedies.[38]

The pathogenesis of many diseases, at least in their initial phases, is characterized by communication defects arising in the complex networks of integrated systems (control of cell proliferation, immune system, equilibrium between pro- and anti-inflammatory factors, coagulation and fibrinolysis, and so on), for which models can be created like the Boolean networks. In a network in which many homeostatic systems (molecular, cellular, systemic) are interconnected, the information of the entire system "passes through" cycles (attractors) which have variable, fluctuating spatiotemporal forms, but which can always be traced back, in states of normality, to a harmonic pattern where the whole is viewed in its entirety, aimed at the survival of the organism with the least possible consumption of energy. If one or more elements in these networks is delayed, or loses its information connections (i.e. something snaps in the homeostatic system itself, or some erroneous adaptation process follows an external perturbation) a pathological process occurs precisely because disorder is generated, or rather the system goes over to another attractor. According to these models, the new attractor, regarded as "pathological" in the case in question, may be preserved even if the initial perturbation is only temporary. Under these conditions, one could speak of a *tendency towards chronicity*.

As a consequence, if pathology is loss of communication, healing is increase of communication, establishment of connections between different systems, integration of responses. Sometimes, healing requires external perturbations that remove pathological adaptations. The "science" and the "art" of the doctor are to help the natural, but often erroneous healing power by providing the right information for the extremely complex, unique, and open system that is a human being affected by some disturbance of its homeostasis. Since biological communication is frequency-modulated and all the transformation processes in the body are networked and correlated, the organism can be seen not as an ensemble of mechanisms, but, instead, as a playing orchestra. Different parts (instruments) are harmoniously linked because they follow a series of guiding-frequencies. All the parts of an orchestra resonate and communicate, thus contributing to the overall performance. If an important part (an instrument) breaks down or goes out of the rhythm, that constitutes a threat for the functioning of all the orchestra. In analogous manner, a correlation in the rhythms of functioning organs and of the frequencies of oscillating cellular processes is established and maintained in the body. Every change in these rhythms affects, more or less profoundly, the correlated functions and spreads to other structures triggering a homeostatic reaction whose main purpose is to save the whole harmony of the organism.

Extrapolating these concepts to homeopathy, it is possible to envisage that major changes in the homeostatic systems and eventually the healing of the entire body could be obtained through light but carefully selected stress such as inserting a needle into an acupoint, administering a low-dose remedy, or even providing the right psychological advice. Signals which are endowed with highly specific information and are capable of specific interactions with the recipient system, could act as regulators, if it is admitted that the deregulated system or systems are in a state of meta-stability, or precarious equilibrium, where different behaviors (attractors) can be followed and where the choice whether to move in one direction or the other is related to minimal fluctuations. Homeopathic drugs are thus thought to act as substitutes for an endogenous regulatory signal that, for various reasons, may be inadequate or ineffective because the system is no longer sensitive to it, being "blocked" in a pathological attractor by the disease itself. The traditional similia law presupposes that the intrinsic tendency to self-recovery can be supplemented and actively assisted by the employment of suitable stimuli to a system when it is in a specific sensitive state.

Despite all the limitations related to difficulties in rendering the homeopathic approach objective, it is clear that it entails an attempt to explore the patient's medical history at the level of the neuroendocrine system and thus to calibrate some form of therapeutic intervention at this level, too. Homeopathy regards inflammation as a *symptom* (i.e. as a signal or message) and not as a *disease*, and regards this symptom as the expression of an alteration of the relationship between subject and environment and/or between systems in the same subject.

The "secret" of homeopathy lies in the meticulous gathering of information both in the proving phase and in the homeopathic history-taking phase. This information can come from the hidden depths of the homeostatic regulatory system under investigation, but is still information. In the homeopathic method it is used directly in the therapeutic intervention, trusting in the fact that the body will know how to receive, decode, and utilize this informational input for the purposes of restoring the lost equilibrium. Another "secret" of homeopathy is that it deals with the human being as a whole, devoting the maximum attention to symptoms of a psychological type and those peculiar to each individual subject (individualization). In this way, it achieves a very substantial measure of specificity, inasmuch as it is now well known that the response to drugs can vary on the basis of the characteristics of the individual user.

Further insights into the analysis of symptoms

We integrated our experimental results and the resulting model with clinical homeopathic experience. This yielded a theoretical model of the similia principle based on observations of cellular and systemic homeostasis. The operating model used for reference is that of cellular and tissue stress with its phenomena of a) regulation and integration of the response to the stimulus, and b) of physico-chemical adaptations. These have several similarities with the so-called primary and secondary drug actions cited by Hahnemann.

Ultimately a careful analysis of symptomatology with an attempt to connect biological changes and the evolution of symptoms must be included in a discussion of the rule of similars. Our point of departure is the conviction that every symptom has its own significance and origin, which is almost invariably connected to biological changes (biophysical and/or biochemical), to the function and/or structure of protein molecules, cells, tissues, nervous center, and body systems.

One aspect of this definition ought to be considered: in explaining the law of similars Hahnemann uses the relatively original concept of the artificial disease produced by the medicine which should be capable of reducing the natural disease. Both Hahnemann's explanation of the law of similars and practitioners' clinical observations may be explained by our biological model and are curiously connected by it. Our model of the law of similars is based on the concept of homeostasis and biological communication. In this model homeopathy constitutes a reactivation of biological communication.

These hypotheses have the benefit of connecting our experimental observations with those of clinical homeopathy, for example, homeopathic aggravation, the return of old symptoms, the origin of symptom modalities, artificial drug-induced disease, the similarity and difference between pathogenesis and treatment.

The model we are using to better study the law of similars is basically that of classical feedback, where the points of regulation derive from the regulatory system ("RS") and from a variable "A" which oscillates between the two conditions "A/A'" in a reversible equilibrium. The model is presented in Figure 8 in this book and its implications for homeopathic similia rule are discussed in Chapter 6.

In light of the above, we need to consider how symptoms change in the acute phase (of alarm), and in the chronic phase (of adaptation). We have already mentioned that as a result of the decreased sensitivity of the RS and its deficient response, disorder may continue in the absence of the pathogenic agent. At this point the system remains blocked in pathological behavior and is incapable of finding the original attractor associated with health.

The production of regulatory signal r is no longer integrated with the physiological circuit connected to variable "A/A'," but will depend on other signals connected to heterologous receptors. After adaptation and down-regulation, the level of factor r will follow other governing factors that translate into different and more characteristic symptoms.

Perhaps these events of priming and down-regulation occur dozens of times before the reserves of the organism are exhausted and constitute a true mechanism of pathology, i.e. appearance of chronic disease. When the dysfunction of the regulatory system impinges upon areas of marginal importance, other compensatory regulatory systems come to the rescue. However, if the dysfunction strikes in a region of central importance in the regulation, the alterations in these functions become functionally irreversible (pathologic adaptation). Here the homeopathic "simile" could help to recover the teleonomical functions of the RS.

As long as the organism has supplementary regulatory systems that can regulate the advancing disorder, probably only the mildest and most nebulous of symptoms will manifest. While these are of no great significance to conventional medicine, they carry weight in homeopathy. Examples include premenstrual headaches, acidic sweat, or sun intolerance. When finally many regulatory systems are in disequilibrium, true diseases will manifest in various tissues or organs.

Developing our hypothesis further we may place symptoms in various groups: a) direct or strong symptoms, which are related to the increase or decrease of a molecular signal, and are probably those which are more evident, immediate and perceptible and which transform a crisis into a disease (e.g. fever, pain, vomiting, hemorrhage, etc.), and b) complex or weak symptoms connected to changes in sensitivity and reactivity of the networks of regulatory systems.

In the latter group they are more complex, and while not being determined by a specific abnormal molecular concentration, are only of minor intensity and accordingly less felt by the subject. As they are governed by a large series of variables determined by the homeostatic network, they may only manifest under certain circumstances. But it is precisely for this reason that they are the richest in information because they provide a more complete idea of the current disequilibrium.

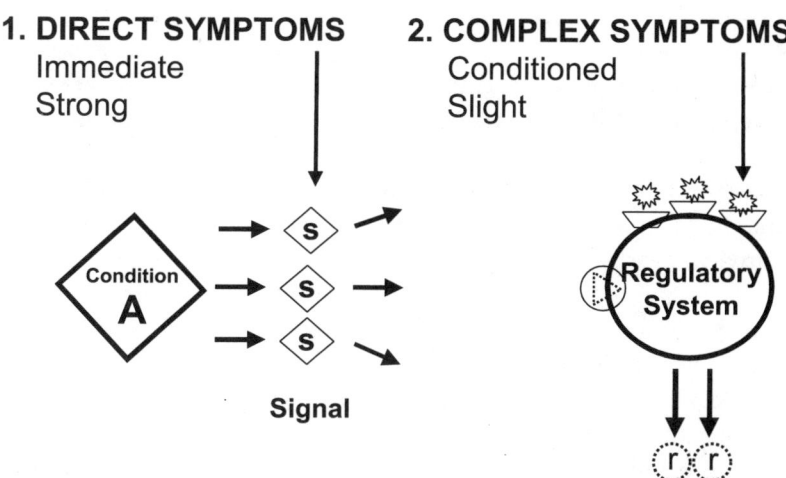

1. DIRECT SYMPTOMS
Immediate
Strong

Signal

2. COMPLEX SYMPTOMS
Conditioned
Slight

FIGURE 2 Two types of symptoms observed during the pathological phases. Symptoms due to increased quantity of molecules (i.e. fever) and symptoms due to change of system sensitivity. If our *in vitro* observations are correct, we should anticipate that in diseases where the endogenous signal is excessively stimulated, sooner or later a loss of sensitivity should occur, for example in diseases with an excess of inflammatory stimulation.

If our *in vitro* observations are correct, we should anticipate that in diseases where the endogenous signal is excessively stimulated, sooner or later a loss of sensitivity in one or more regulatory systems should occur, for example in diseases with an excess of inflammatory stimulation.

We have seen that symptoms almost always originate in biological (physico-chemical) changes in the structure and or function of enzymes, receptors, cells, tissues, etc., so the totality of symptoms of the body, of necessity, comprises all the functional and organic changes (tissues, cells, enzymes, or receptors) present within the organism.

Moreover, if we knew the correct hierarchy of symptoms and how to group them correctly, and if we knew "specific" medications for each of these possible groupings, then of necessity the appropriate utilization of such medications would address or modulate the microscopic disequilibrium connected to the symptomatology in question.

The specificity of which we speak could be viewed either homeopathically (law of similars) or as antidoting (law of opposites). It must be noted that the specificity of the drug in relation to the symptoms in question could be close only if the drug is capable of producing similar symptoms; otherwise the similarity would be significantly limited to a tissue or a cellular function.

This is due to the mechanism of divergence of signals and homeostatic networks that are regulated in a complex fashion and by agonist/antagonist couplings that differ from one tissue to another, as with subtypes of receptors to adrenaline, histamine, serotonin, and many other mediators.

If it is true, as follows from our hypothesis, that homeopathic modalities of symptoms are more connected to receptor sensitivity and homeostatic networks than to the action of high-dose molecular signals, the use and hierarchy of such symptoms would correspond to an indirect study of such sensitivity. And the difference between studying network sensitivity or molecular actions on the cell is quite different, because the latter is very similar to the action of an external drug, while the former is of necessity dependent on the body as a whole.

Consequently, a drug intended to regulate these types of symptoms (modalities) should address (in a more or less gentle fashion) such receptor sensitivities and their homeostatic networks. The hypothesis we propose is that the action of the drug on key-points of altered regulatory systems would force the cell or the system to recover the functional sensitivity which had been lost, including recovery of superficial receptors. This last idea is a fascinating hypothesis, as yet unconfirmed, to interpret the biological mechanism of the law of similars.

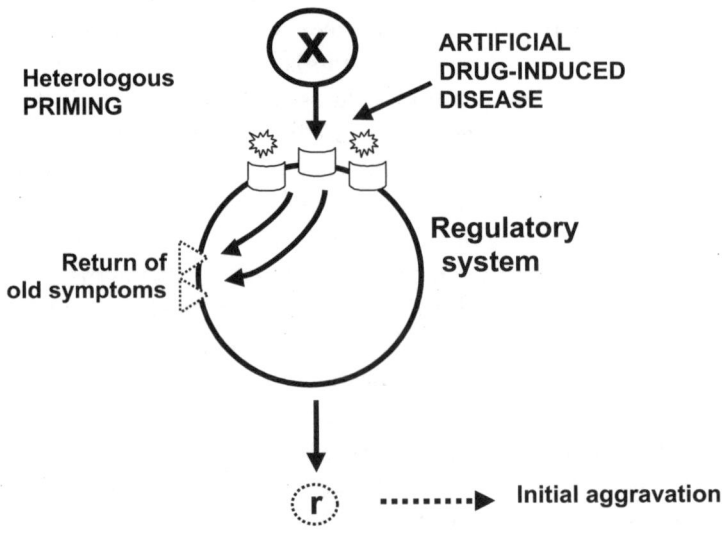

HYPOTHETICAL ACTION OF HOMEOPATHIC MEDICINE

FIGURE 3 Some phenomena of the peculiar homeopathic healing response.

Could this idea be the corresponding phenomenon to Hahnemann's hypothesis in explaining the similia principle with the "artificial drug-induced disease"? If the true illness of a homeostatic system is the loss of communication, then true healing will be the recovery of this communication.

Thus, if our remedy acts on the stimulated receptors, the first effect to be expected is an increase in symptoms (initial aggravation) until this leads to a definitive change in regulatory receptors. Moreover, the possibility that the disabled receptor recovers its function would explain the repeated observation under homeopathic treatment of the return of old symptoms after an absence of years. In fact, given that the input signal has remained overactivated for a long time (years), the reactivation of receptors must lead to a reappearance of symptoms that disappeared when their function was lost.

Let us see where the rule of similars is situated according to this model.

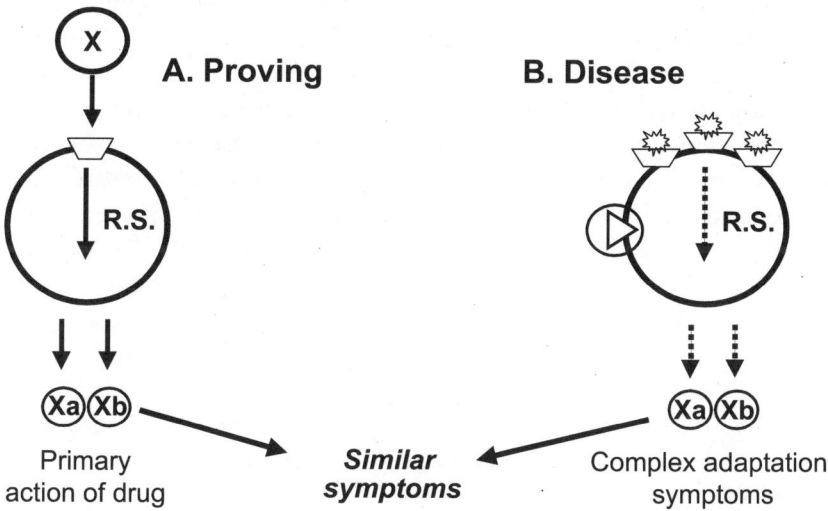

FIGURE 4 Biological hypothesis of the rule of similars.

As we see in A (proving), as a result of excessive molecular signalling, certain symptoms develop. In disease (B), desensitisation (down-regulation) occurs accompanied by heterologous hyperactivity. This determines a certain functional disequilibrium, accompanied by heterologous hyperactivity whose expression is other symptoms. Thus, we will observe two kinds of symptoms—direct symptoms (probably due to excessive quantity of molecules), and adaptation symptoms (probably due to cell hypersensitivity connected with network disequilibrium). The latter are the more interesting because they express the level at which the system is acting. These two types of symptoms are quite different because they correspond to quite different pathways of biological communication. Moreover, direct symptoms, owing to their force, are poorly affected by modalities, those due to adaptation, and precisely because of their weakness, are more sensitive to modulation and to present themselves as a consequence of a particular modality.

If the doses used during homeopathic experimentation (proving) are quite attenuated, it is possible that the symptoms that arise may be due to an unknown physico-chemical phenomenon. This would be associated with an increase in sensitivity of the same receptors. The resulting onset of particular symptoms will derive from the modulation or integration of homeostatic networks for the action of low dosages on cellular targets. This is more than a hypothesis because the priming effect of low dosage substances is well- known, and we have seen experiments at very low dosage that confirmed it.

Coming back to pathological state (B), during a disease, symptoms similar to those caused by a particular drug could arise as a consequence of homeostatic adaptation during the chronic phase. In other words, the receptors in question should generate the same symptoms in their totality, either from hypersensitivity of the pathological state or due to hyper-modulation of homeostatic systems during experimentation. However, during experimentation symptoms are directly caused by the primary action of the drug. In pathology, the symptoms arise from the relative hypersensitivity of the same receptors as a complex result of homeostatic adaptation.

In simple terms the rule of similars in our model would exist between

a) *direct* symptoms (primary action) of experimentation; and

b) *complex* adaptation symptoms of the disease.

There are at least two advantages with this model: firstly, its biological bases are quite solid (priming and down-regulation); secondly, it leads to a sensible interpretation of several homeopathic phenomena such as initial aggravation and the return of old symptoms.

However, a limitation of our model could be the fact that we do not know if it holds true for all symptom groupings or is limited to those of the excitatory remedies, as it is more probable in our observations. Two more consistent objections to our model may consist in the lack of experimental proofs regarding the possibility that a) homeopathic dilution interacts with membrane receptors and that b) this action may invert the microscopic dynamic disequilibrium of homeostatic systems.

In proposing our tentative hypotheses we take heart from Claude Bernard's statement, that only by daring to make, and hopefully to verify scientific hypotheses, may human knowledge progress.

Summary

Our working hypothesis on the pharmacological action of homeopathic drugs could be summarized as indicated in the following points:

1. The *therapeutic similarity* of drug action may be fundamentally based on the widespread phenomenon of *inversion of biological effects* dependent on the *dose* and/or on the *physiological state* of the receiver.
2. Medicine that has been chosen according to the similia principle may be perceived by *specific* regulatory systems—that have a crucial role in the dynamic of the disease–as a *heterologous "similar" signal.*
3. Specificity of information may be based on the *sensitization* (priming) of the receiver due to biological stress, on the use of *ultra-low- doses/ high- dilutions* of medicines and on the *complexity* of the remedy actions at various levels.
4. The specific signal may trigger a homeodynamic reaction that shifts the global dysequilibrium of the ill person toward a *new dynamical attractor*, proximal to the healthy state.
5. In acute diseases, homeopathic regulation may be regarded as homeodynamic regulatory feedback, in chronic disease as *unblocking* of pathologic adaptation and orientation towards correct responses.
6. The clinical application of the similia principle (*symptom analysis in the complex field of the whole person*) may allow the identification of specific remedies even with the lack of detailed knowledge about the single molecular mechanisms of disease and of drug action.
7. The information of homeopathic medicines may have either *chemical* nature (ultra-low-dose) or *physical* nature (high-dilution/dynamization), or both.

References to Appendix 2

1. Hahnemann, C.F.S. (1994). *Organon of Medicine*. With explanations by Joseph Reves, edited from the 5th and 6th edition. Homeopress Ltd., Haifa, para.12.

2. Ibid., para 29–31.

3. Harold, F.M. (1986). *The Vital Force: A Study of Bioenergetics*. New York: Freeman and Company.

4. Bellavite, P. (1998). *Biodinamica: Basi fisiopatologiche e tracce di metodo per una medicina integrata*. Milano: Tecniche Nuove.

5. Endler, P.C., Pongratz, W., Smith, C.W., Schulte, J. (1995). Non-molecular information transfer from thyroxine to frogs with regard to homeopathic toxicology. *Vet. Hum. Toxicol.* 37: 259–260; Fesenko, E.E., Gluvstein, A.Y. (1995). Changes in the state of water, induced by radiofrequency electromagnetic fields. *FEBS Lett.* 367: 53–55; Goodman, E.M., Greenbaum, B., Marron, M.T. (1995). Effects of electromagnetic fields on molecules and cells. *Int. Rev. Cytol.* 158:279–338; Ho, M.W., Popp, F.A., Warnke, U. (1994). *Bioelectrodynamics and Biocommunication* Singapore: World Scientific; Adey, W.R. (1993). Whispering between cells: Electromagnetic fields and regulatory mechanisms in tissue. *Frontier Perspect.* 3: 21–25; Smith, C.W. (1989). Coherent electromagnetic fields bio-communication. In: *Electromagnetic Bio-Information* (F.A. Popp, U. Warnke, H.L Konig, and W. Peschka, eds.). Urban Swarzenberg, Munchen, pp. 1–17; Tsong, T.Y. (1989). Deciphering the language of cells. *Trends Biochem. Sci.* 14: 89–92.

6. Capra, F. (1996). *The Web of Life*. New York: Doubleday-Anchor Book.

7. Bellavite, P., Signorini, A. (1996). Pathologie, komplexe systeme, und resonanz. In: *Homoopathie und Bioresonanztherapie: Physiologische und physikalische Voraussetzungen Grundlagenforschung* (P.C. Endler, J. Schulte, eds.). Medizinverlag Maudrich, Wein, pp. 65–76; Bellavite, P. (1997). Disease as information disorder. *Advances—Journal of Body-Mind Health* 13: 4–7; Bellavite, P., Signorini, A. (1998). Pathology, complex systems and resonance. In: *Fundamental Research in Ultra-High Dilution and Homoeopathy* (J. Schulte and P.C. Endler, eds.). Kluwer Acad. Publ., Dordrecht, pp. 105–116; Conforti, A., Bertani, S., Lussignoli, S., Bellavite, P. (1998). Pharmakodynamik und komplexe Systeme. In: *Biologische Mediczin in der Orthopedie/Traumatologie, Rheumatologie* (H. Hess, ed.). Aurelia Verlag, Baden Baden, pp. 39–52; Bellavite, P., Semizzi, M.L., Lussignoli, S., Andrioli, G., Bartocci, U. (1998). A computer model of the five elements theory of traditional chinese medicine. *Complem.Ther.Med.* 6: 133–140.

8. Nicolis, G., Prigogine, Y. (1991). *La complessità. Esplorazioni nei Nuovi Campi della Scienza* Torino: Einaudi; Coffey, D.S. (1998). Self-organization, complexity and chaos: The new biology for medicine. *Nature Medicine* 4: 882–885; Kauffman, S.A. (1993). *Origins of Order: Self-Organization and Selection in Evolution*. Oxford: Oxford University Press; Kauffman, S.A. (1995). *At Home in the Universe: The Search for Laws of Self-Organization and Complexity*. Oxford: Oxford University Press.

9. Petrov, V., Ga'spa'r, V., Masere, J., Showalter, K. (1993). Controlling chaos in the Belusov-Zhabotinsky reaction. *Nature* 361: 240–243.

10. Nicolis, G. (1995). *Introduction to Nonlinear Science*. Cambridge: Cambridge University Press.

11. Goldberger, A.L. (1996). Non-linear dynamics for clinicians: Chaos theory, fractals, and complexity at the bedside. *Lancet* 347: 1312–1314; Nicolis, G., Prigogine, Y. (1991). *La complessità. Esplorazioni nei Nuovi Campi della Scienza* Torino: Einaudi; Coffey, D.S. (1998). Self-organization, complexity and chaos: The new biology for medicine. *Nature Medicine* 4: 882–885

12. Harold, F.M. (1986). *The Vital Force: A Study of Bioenergetics*. New York: Freeman and Company.

13. Hahnemann, C.F.S. (1994). *Organon of Medicine*. With explanations by Joseph Reves, edited from the 5th and 6th edition. Homeopress Ltd., Haifa, para. 9.

14. Breithaupt, H. (1989). Biological rhytms and communication. In: *Electromagnetic Bio-Information* (F.A. Popp, ed.). Urban & Schwarzenberg, Munchen, pp. 18–41; Matthews, D.R. (1991). Physiological implications of pulsatile hormone secretion. *Ann. N. Y. Acad. Sci.* 618: 28–37.

15. Berridge, M.J., Morewton, R.B. (1991). Calcium waves and spirals. *Curr. Biol.* 1: 296–297; Strogatz, S.H., Stewart, I. (1994). Oscillatori accoppiati e sincronizzazione biologica. *Le Scienze* 306: 62–68.

16. Cramer, F. (1993). *Chaos and Order: The Complex Structure of Living Systems* Weinheim:.VCH Verlagsgesellschaft.

17. Holland, J.H. (2000). *Emergence: From Chaos to Order Reading.* MA: Addison-Wesley; Solomon, G.F. (1997). Stress, hormones, immunity, the complexity of interwined systems, and the simplicity of humanism. *J. Intensive Care Med.* 12: 219–222; Mainzer, K. (1994). *Thinking in Complexity: The Complex Dynamics of Matter, Mind, and Mankind.* Berlin-Heidelberg: Springer-Verlag; Bellavite, P. (1997). Disease as information disorder. *Advances—Journal of Body-Mind Health* 13: 4–7; Coffey, D.S. (1998). Self-organization, complexity and chaos: The new biology for medicine. *Nature Medicine* 4: 882–885; Kauffman, S.A. (1995). *At Home in the Universe: The Search for Laws of Self-Organization and Complexity.* Oxford: Oxford University Press.

18. Elbert, T., Ray, W.J., Kowalik, Z.J., Skinner, J.E., Graf, K.E., Birbaumer, N. (1994). Chaos and physiology: Deterministic chaos in excitable cell assemblies. *Physiol. Rev.* 74: 1–47.

19. Lorenz, E.N. (1963). Deterministic nonperiodic flow. *J. Atmos. Sci.* 20: 130–141.

20. Lorenz, E.N. (1979). Predictability: Does the flap of a butterfly's wings in Brazil set off a tornado in Texas? Address at the Annual Meeting of the American Association for the Advancement of Science Washington, DC.

21. Shinbrot, T., Grebogi, C., Ott, E., Yorke, J.A. (1993). Using small perturbations to control chaos. *Nature* 363: 411–417; Garfinkel, A., Spano, M.L., Ditto, W.L., Weiss, J.N. (1992). Controlling cardiac chaos. *Science* 257: 1230–1235; Weiss, J.N., Garfinkel, A., Spano, M.L., Ditto, W.L. (1994). Chaos and chaos control in biology. *J.Clin.Invest.* 93: 1355–1360.

22. See Note 18.

23. Callard, R., George, J.T., Stark, J.S. (1999). Cytokines, chaos, and complexity. *Immunity* 11: 507–513.

24. Cotton, P. (1991). Chaos, other nonlinear dynamics research may have answers, applications for clinical medicine. *J. Am. Med. Assoc.* 266: 12–18; West, B.J., Zhang, W., Mackey, H.J. (1994). Chaos, noise and biological data. In: *Fractals in Biology and Medicine (T.F. Nonnemacher, G.A. Losa, and E.R. Weibel, eds.).* Birkhauser Verlag, Basel, pp. 38–54; Bellavite, P., Semizzi, M.L., Lussignoli, S., Andrioli, G., Bartocci, U. (1998). A computer model of the five elements theory of traditional chinese medicine. Complem.Ther.Med. 6: 133–140.

25. Tsong, T.Y., Gross, C.J. (1994). The language of cells: Molecular processing of electric signals by cell membrane. In: *Bioelectrodynamics and Biocommunication* (M.W. Ho, ed.). World Scientific, Singapore, pp. 131–158.

26. Cramer, F. (1993). *Chaos and Order: The Complex Structure of Living Systems* Weinheim:.VCH Verlagsgesellschaft.

27. Nugent, A.M., Onuoha, G.N., McEneaney, D.J., Steele, I.C., Hunter, S.J., Prasanna, K., Campbell, N.P.S., Shaw, C., Buchanan, K.D., Nicholls, D.P. (1994). Variable patterns of atrial natriuretic peptide secretion in man. *Eur. J. Clin. Invest.* 24: 267–274.

28. Goldberger, A.L. (1996). Non-linear dynamics for clinicians: Chaos theory, fractals, and complexity at the bedside. *Lancet* 347: 1312–1314.

29. Freeman, W.J. (1991). The physiology of perception. *Sci. Am.* 264: 34–41.

30. Babloyantz, A., Destexhe, A. (1986). Low dimensional chaos in an instance of epilepsy. *Proc. Natl. Acad. Sci. USA* 83: 3513–3517; Kleiger, R.E., Miller, J.P., Bigger, T., Moss, A.J. (1987). Multicenter post-infarction rg.: Decreased heart rate variability and its

association with increased mortality after acute myocardial infarction. *Am. J. Cardiol.* 59: 256–262.

31. Varela, F.J., Coutinho, A. (1991). Second generation immune networks. *Immunol. Today* 12: 159–166.

32. Bellavite, P. (1997). Disease as information disorder. *Advances—Journal of Body-Mind Health* 13: 4–7; Bellavite, P., Semizzi, M.L., Lussignoli, S., Andrioli, G., Bartocci, U. (1998). A computer model of the five elements theory of traditional chinese medicine. *Complem.Ther.Med.* 6: 133–140; Elbert, T., Ray, W.J., Kowalik, Z.J., Skinner, J.E., Graf, K.E., Birbaumer, N. (1994). Chaos and physiology: Deterministic chaos in excitable cell assemblies. *Physiol. Rev.* 74: 1–47.

33. Kauffman, S.A. (1993). *Origins of Order: Self-Organization and Selection in Evolution.* Oxford: Oxford University Press.

34. Bellavite, P., Semizzi, M.L., Lussignoli, S., Andrioli, G., Bartocci, U. (1998). A computer model of the five elements theory of traditional chinese medicine. *Complem.Ther.Med.* 6: 133–140.

35. Vithoulkas, G. (1980). *The Science of Homeopathy.* New York: Grove Press Inc.; Rubik, B. (1995). Energy medicine and the unifying concept of information. *Altern. Ther. Health Med.* 1: 34–39; Popp, F.A. (1990). Some elements of homoeopathy. *Br. Homeopath. J.* 79: 161–166; Endler, P.C., Schulte, J. (1994). *Ultra High Dilution: Physiology and Physics* Dordrecht: Kluwer Academic Publishers; Poitevin, B. (1993). Les grandes directions de la recherche en homéopathie. In: *Encycl. Med. Nat. Editions Techniques*, Paris: Editions Techniques; Del Giudice, N., Del Giudice, E. (1999). *Omeopatia e Bioenergetica.* Verona.: Cortina International; Eskinazi, D. (1999). Homeopathy re-revisited: Is homeopathy compatible with biomedical observations? *Arch. Intern. Med.* 159: 1981–1987; Schulte, J. (1999). Effects of potentization in aqueous solutions. *Brit. Hom. J.* 88: 155–160; Endler, P.C., Schulte, J. (1997). *Homoopathie und Bioresonanztherapie: Physiologiche und Physikalische Voraussetzungen Grundlagenforchung.* Wien.: Medizinverlag Maudrich.

36. Ho, M.W., Popp, F.A. (1993). Biological organization, coherence, and light emission from living organisms. In: *Thinking About Biology* (W.D. Stein and F.J. Varela, eds.). Addison-Wesley Publ. Co., Reading, pp. 183–213.

37. van Rossum, J.M., de Bie, J.E.G.M. (1991). Chaos and illusion. *Trends Pharmacol. Sci.* 12: 379–383.

38. Garner, C., Hock, N. (1991). Chaos theory and homoeopathy. *Berlin J. Res. Hom.* 1: 236–242; Shepperd, J. (1994). Chaos theory: Implications for homeopathy. *J. Am. Inst. Homeopathy* 87: 22–29; Ruiz, G., Torres, J.L., Michel, O., Navarro, R. (1999). Homeopathic effect on heart rate variability. *Br. Homeopath. J.* 88: 106–111; Torres, J.L., Ruiz, G. (1996). Stochastic resonance and the homoeopathic effect. 85: 134–140; Schwartz, G.E., Russek, L.G., Bell, I.R., Riley, D. (2000). Plausibility of homeopathy and conventional chemical therapy: The systemic memory resonance hypothesis. *Med. Hypotheses* 54: 634–637.

Index

About the Authors

PAOLO BELLAVITE is a medical doctor specializing in hematology who has been an Associate Professor of General Pathology at Verona University Medical School in Italy since 1984. He completed a post-doctoral degree in biotechnology at the Cranfield Institute of Technology in Bedford, U.K., is a member of the European Society of Clinical Investigation, and is a founder of the Observatory for Complementary Medicine at Verona University. Dr. Bellavite has published more than 150 papers in medical and scientific journals on inflammation, free radicals, leukocyte biology, and cellular pharmacology. He is currently involved in the investigation of the scientific basis of homeopathy and the integration of leading alternative therapies into mainstream medicine.

ANDREA SIGNORINI holds a medical degree with specialization in Clinical Biology from the University of Verona. He completed studies at the Verona Homeopathic School and has worked as a practitioner in the field since 1986. He currently teaches homeopathy at the Homeopathic Medical School of Verona and is director of the Scientific Department in the Italian Federation of the Homeopathic Medical Association. Since 1998 Dr. Signorini has worked towards proving homeopathic methodology. He has recently published accounts of the proven efficacy of remedies, including *Hypericum* (St. John's Wort) and *Piper methysticum* (mint).

THE EMERGING SCIENCE OF
HOMEOPATHY

THE EMERGING SCIENCE OF

HOMEOPATHY

*Complexity, Biodynamics,
and Nanopharmacology*

Paolo Bellavite, M.D.
and Andrea Signorini, M.D.

Translated by Anthony Steele

North Atlantic Books
Berkeley, California

Published by
North Atlantic Books
P.O. Box 12327
Berkeley, CA 94712

Printed in the United States of America

Cover design by Jan Camp
Book design by Ayelet Maida
Photos and illustrations courtesy the authors
Illustrations produced by Catherine Campaigne and Jan Camp
Cover photo ©1980 Sondra Barrett, Ph.D.
    The cover photograph is of pure sodium chloride taken through an Olympus polarizing light microscope (magnification 31X). The salt was dissolved in sterile distilled water and allowed to recrystallize at room temperature.

The Emerging Science of Homeopathy is sponsored by the Society for the Study of Native Arts and Sciences, a nonprofit educational organization whose goals are to develop an ecological and crosscultural perspective linking various scientific, social, and artistic fields; to nurture a holistic view of arts, sciences, humanities, and healing; and to publish and distribute literature on the relationship of mind, body, and nature.

North Atlantic Books' publications are available through most bookstores. For further information, call 800-337-2665 or visit our website at www.northatlanticbooks.com. Substantial discounts on bulk quantities are available to corporations, professional associations, and other organizations. For details and discount information, contact our special sales department.

Library of Congress Cataloging-in-Publication Data
Bellavite, Paolo
    [Homeopathy, A Frontier in Medical Science]
    The Emerging Science of Homeopathy: Complexity, Biodynamics, and Nanopharmacology / by Paolo Bellavite and Andrea Signorini ; translated by Anthony Steele
        p. cm.
    Includes bibliographical references and index.
    ISBN 1-55643-384-0 (pbk.)
    1. Homeopathy. I. Signorini, Andrea. II. Title.

RX71 .B45 2002
615.5'32—dc21   2001055853
                                                                        CIP

1 2 3 4 5 6 7 8 9 / 07 06 05 04 03 02

Contents

Contents